DERMATOLOGY - LABORATORY AND CLINICAL RESEARCH

SUPERFICIAL MYCOSES – AN OVERVIEW

Dermatology - Laboratory and Clinical Research

Additional books in this series can be found on Nova's website
under the Series tab.

Additional e-books in this series can be found on Nova's website
under the e-book tab.

DERMATOLOGY - LABORATORY AND CLINICAL RESEARCH

SUPERFICIAL MYCOSES – AN OVERVIEW

AVNER SHEMER

WITH

NICOLE SAKKA

AND

SHARON BAUM

NOVA BIOMEDICAL

New York

Library of Congress Cataloging-in-Publication Data

ISBN: 978-1-63482-406-4
Library of Congress Control Number: 2015932296

Published by Nova Science Publishers, Inc. † New York

Contents

Preface		**vii**
Chapter 1	Introduction	**1**
Chapter 2	Epidemiology	**5**
Chapter 3	Human Immunity and Fungal Infections	**9**
Chapter 4	Diagnostic Techniques of Fungal Infections	**15**
Chapter 5	Cytochromes P450	**21**
Chapter 6	Treatment and Drug Interactions	**27**
Chapter 7	Antifungal Drugs in Pregnancy	**33**
Chapter 8	Tinea Capitis	**37**
Chapter 9	Tinea Faciale	**61**
Chapter 10	Tinea Barbae	**77**
Chapter 11	Tinea Corporis	**83**
Chapter 12	Tinea Cruris	**99**
Chapter 13	Tinea Pedis	**113**
Chapter 14	Tinea Manuum	**133**
Chapter 15	Onychomycosis	**141**
Chapter 16	Pityriasis Versicolor	**179**
Chapter 17	Tinea Nigra Palmaris	**193**
Chapter 18	White Piedra and Black Piedra	**195**
Chapter 19	Cutaneous Candidiasis	**199**
Chapter 20	Erythrasma	**211**
Chapter 21	Conclusion	**215**

Appendix: Drug Interactions 217

References 231

Authors' Contact Information 245

Index 247

Preface

The superficial mycoses are those that include the pathogenic, keratinizing fungi.

Contamination by different fungi may induce an inflammatory response whose intensity depends upon the particular fungus and the sensitivity of the host to the fungus.

As a group, the superficial mycoses account for up to 50% of all skin diseases. This book will not discuss subcutaneous mycoses or deep systemic mycoses.

The superficial mycotic infections include tinea corporis, tinea capitis, tinea faciale, tinea barbae, tinea cruris (jock itch), tinea pedis, tinea manuum, onychomycosis, pityriasis versicolor, black and white piedra, tinea nigra palmaris, and several superficial candidiases.

This book introduces the clinical presentations of superficial mycoses, explains how to establish diagnosis, and provides treatment methods and ways to prevent over-treatment. This book differs from other books especially from the point of view of differential diagnosis. While other books provide a list of differential diagnoses of each superficial mycosis disease, this book takes each variant of a specific disease (e.g., different clinical representations of tinea capitis), and for each of those variants, provides the relevant differential diagnosis and broadly discusses how to differentiate and correctly diagnose other diseases resembling the mycotic disease. The differential diagnosis focuses on important clinical presentation details such as size and location of the lesion/s, the borders of the lesion/s, the lesion/s' lack or presentation of well-circumscribed borders, the level of elevation of the well-circumscribed borders compared to the rest of the lesion, the uniformity of lesion color (i.e., is the color uniform on the entire lesion or is there a dark or light shade in the border area compared to the center?). This book focuses on questions such as: Does the lesion/s have central healing or almost central healing compared to the circumference of the lesion? Is the lesion/s covered by thin/thick/rough scales? Are the scales located all over the lesion/s or only around the lesion or only in the center area of the lesion/s? Are the scales silver/white/yellowish in color? Do the scales stick strongly to the lesion or peel off easily by gentle scratching? Is there any bleeding (pinpoint/oozing) from the lesion/s itself after gentle scratching?

As some saprophyte fungi may exist alongside certain skin diseases or even at a normal skin level, a mycological sample may reveal a saprophyte fungus, which can wrongfully lead to over-diagnosis.

It is not rare for a mycological analysis to be taken (by mistake) from a non-mycotic lesion, revealing non-pathogenic fungi that are irrelevant to the basic disease, causing it to be wrongfully interpreted as a fungal disease and therefore disrupt proper treatment.

This book focuses broadly on the interpretation of mycological analysis results and clarifies the difference between the pathogenic and non-pathogenic fungi. Due to the fact that there is a broad group of fungi that is generally considered non-pathogenic – the non-dermatophyte molds – it is possible in certain circumstances for the non-dermatophyte molds to be pathogenic and thus should be treated properly. This book discusses the differences between the pathogenic and non-pathogenic fungi from two points of view: the mycological analysis results and the relevant clinical presentation. This differentiation is very important from the aspect of unjustified topical and systemic treatment.

This book is accompanied with clinical images that help the reader to visualize the different skin conditions while focusing on the relevant clinical differences between different diagnoses.

In addition, this book contains a unique table specifying interactions between common drugs and different systemic antifungal drugs, showing which other medications the patient may be taking may be disruptive to the antimycotic treatment and prevent cure. The drugs are presented clearly in groups in order to enable quick and easy access to the relevant interactions.

The drug interactions between the antimycotic drugs and many other drugs occur because many of the antimycotic drugs and other drugs metabolize in the same cytochrome enzyme system – mainly CYP450. There are several possible results – the action of the antimycotic drug will decrease, remain the same, or increase combined with decrease/increase/no change of the other drug/s. Not only is the change itself mentioned but also the level of change, varying between mild, moderate, and major changes in the blood level of the antimycotic/other drug/s. In common practice, many adults use several or many drugs, and the combination of drugs should be taken into consideration when deciding on treatment.

This book is suitable for dermatologists, general physicians, PhDs with a specialization in mycology, and medical students.

Professor Avner Shemer, MD
Associate Clinical Professor of Dermatology
Specialist in Skin and Venereal Diseases

Chapter 1

Introduction

Fungi are a large group of organisms. They are very common and found worldwide. They are eukaryotic, but they vary from plants and animals in several major respects [1]:

1. The fungal cells are coated with a firm cell wall, composed of polysaccharides, chitin, and glycoproteins. The sterol present in their cell membranes is principally ergosterol.
2. The fungi are heterotrophic, meaning that they require organic carbon compounds for their nutrition. Fungi secrete enzymes that digest proteins and absorb nutrients via pinocytosis through their cell wall. They are essentially aerobic with limited anaerobic capabilities.
3. The basic structure of the fungus is a chain-like tubular filament (hyphae) or a round single cell (yeast) with no clustering of cells into organs or tissues. Many fungal pathogens can alter their form while changing environments from natural to contaminated tissues. When there is a mass of hyphae, it is termed a mycelium. Under certain conditions, a chain of elongated budding cells, termed pseudohyphae, is formed. The fungi can reproduce asexually but often hold sexual reproduction ability. Sexual reproduction is often difficult to demonstrate in the laboratory. This is important for their classification as many species have two labels: one terming their asexual state (termed anamorph) and the other the sexual state (termed teleomorph).

The Fungal Kingdom

The fungal kingdom is one of the six kingdoms of existence, containing a wide range of organisms. The criteria for classification depend mainly on the morphology of macroscopic forms and filamentous or yeast-like microscopic structures, as well as on the specialized cell wall that produces them [2]. It is important to choose a specific culture medium for different types of fungi since each may favor a different kind of culture medium [3, 4].

The fungal kingdom is divided into seven phyla, which include the **Ascomycota** and **Basidiomycota**.

Classification of fungi has historically been based on the method of sexual spore production. However, the asexual stage (anamorph) has been used successfully with some fungi as a means of rapid dispersal to new habitats, diminishing the effectiveness of classification according to the sexual stage (teleomorph). The shape of the [asexual] spores along with the arrangement of their spore-bearing structures have been of major importance in the classification and identification of fungi.

Sexual reproduction – For practical purposes, in clinical laboratories one should be aware that most filamentous fungi do not spontaneously produce their sexually productive configurations. Sexual reproduction is limited to few species, namely: *Aspergillus*, *Chaetomium*, and *Pseudallescheria*. Only these organisms form fruiting bodies called "ascomata" that are observed as spherical or carafe-shaped structures containing free ascospores that scatter by extruding through an opening or split to release their content under pressure.

Asexual reproduction – The majority of filamentous fungi are identified by the morphology of their asexual structures. For example, the Hyphomycetes are categorized by their conidia – blastic conidia – and act by budding to form a new wall to separate the new cell from the mother cell at the time of maturation; by contrast, thallic conidia are the product of hyphal segments that are already surrounded by a septum and differentiate as specialized conidia.

To simplify the characterization of conidia, they are classified into seven types:

Blastoconidia – These are formed by budding and may be solitary or a branched chain.

Phialoconidia – These are bottle-shaped cells that produce conidia collected in a mucoid mass or attached in dry chains. Their growth terminates with the production of the initial conidium.

Annelloconidia – These produce conidia collected in a mucoid mass or attached in dry chains, but unlike phialoconidia, they continue growing during conidiation, and they have a series of annular rings at the apex.

Poroconidia – These conidia are formed through pores in the cell wall of the conidiophore. They are often melanized and multiseptate and have a geniculate shape.

Arthroconidia – These conidia arise from the transformation of cells along the hyphae. They may be contiguous or intercalated, and at maturity the former separate by forming double walls and splitting, while the latter separate after detachment of the cells.

Chlamydospores – These are formed from preexisting cells within a hypha. They are inflated round cells with thick walls. Unlike other spores and conidia, they lack a dehiscence mechanism at maturity.

Aleurioconidia – These conidia are formed by the lysis of the cells that support them. They have a truncate base bearing small annular additions that are the remnants of the broken walls. This type is characteristic of dermatophytes.

How to Recognize the Different Groups of Fungi

Advances in DNA sequencing have led to fungal species today being defined as groups of organisms with sequence homologies at multiple loci, in contrast to organisms sharing common morphological characteristics or those that succesfully mate with one another. It has also allowed assignment of asexual, anamorphic, or mitosporic fungi to genera within the phyla Ascomycota or Basidiomycota even in the absence of the sexual stage.

Colony forms – The texture and color of colonies remain typical of species although they can be influenced by the culture medium and the age of the isolate. Some colonies are glabrous and others are wooly or powdery. The color can be pale while others can be brightly colored. Some fungi possess pigment that can be concentrated in the conidia so that the colony is dark on the surface and pale on the bottom; those that elaborate melanin to the hyphal wall possess darkened colonies of both surface and the bottom.

Growth rate – Under the controlled conditions of culture medium, temperature, and amount of inoculum used, the colony growth rate remains constant. This is also an important fact in the process of identification. Certain dermatophytes grow slowly – 0.5 cm in diameter in a week of incubation – in comparison to mucorales that grow very fast and cover the entire surface of a petri dish in two to three days.

Hyphae – Three categories of hyphae can help to identify certain groups of fungi (Fig. 1.2): 1) large aseptate hyphae are characteristic of the **Mucoromycotina,** 2) vegetative hyphae with clamp connections indicate the **Basidiomycota,** and 3) narrow septate hyphae are characteristic of most medically important filamentous fungi.

Scientific Names

The scientific names of fungi are based on the International Botanical Code of Nomenclature. In practice, this means that the earliest published name following this code is adopted as the correct name for any given species, and subsequent names are considered mere synonyms. Nevertheless, to avoid confusion, the Code of Nomenclature permits exceptions. For instance, the existence of an earlier generic name that has been largely overlooked or a later name that has achieved general use, while reversion to the earlier name would be problematic. Transfer of a species of fungus from one genus to another on the basis of new findings, e.g., that establish it as a new genus, constitute an acceptable reason for renaming a fungus.. Indeed, many fungi bear two names, one based on its sexual phase and another its asexual phase.It is accepted practice, therefore, to refer to a fungus with regard to its asexual phase if this is typically found in cultures. Names of fungal diseases, unlike the names of fungi, are not subject to firm international regulations. They are usually related to the generic names of the causative agent, e.g., cryptococcosis or aspergillosis.

Since the development of mycological science and medicine, there has been an enormous change in our understanding of, diagnosis of, and treatment options for fungal infections.

Chapter 2

Epidemiology

Fungal Infections

At least 100,000 species of fungi have been named. Fewer than 500 of these, however, are associated with disease in humans, while less than 100 are capable of producing infection in immunocompetent individuals. The remaining species are capable of producing disease only in hosts that are immunocompromised in some manner. Some are important as pathogens of animals and plants. Most fungal infections in humans are caused by those growing in the environment as saprophytes, and are acquired through direct contact, autoinoculation, ingestion, inhalation, or via traumatic implantation. Yeasts, which may exist symbiotically with humans, nevertheless cause endogenous infections in the context of imbalance in the host.

Fungal diseases share a wide distribution, though some are restricted to specific geographical regions, usually because the etiological agents are saprophytes, themselves restricted in their distribution by environmental conditions.

The incidence of fungal infections globally is changing today due to a variety of factors including the percentage of immunosuppressed patients in the population (e.g., HIV, organ transplanted patients, malignancies) and geographical mobility (i.e., immigration from endemic to non-endemic locations). Urban development and changes in land use in the endemic regions have also contributed to this trend, as has the seasonal migration of unexposed populations from one region to another. An increase in the overall number of people traveling internationally has also contributed to the rise in the reported outbreaks and sporadic cases of fungal diseases such as histoplasmosis and coccidioidomycosis. This is most striking with regard to individuals normally residing far from the regions where these diseases are endemic; for example, US residents treated for travel-related mycoses acquired while visiting an endemic region within the Americas, Africa, or Asia. Such infections have also been seen in foreign travelers, primarily those returning to Europe, Australia, or Japan. With tourism from Asia to the US constantly increasing, migration-related infections are now reported from specific regions, e.g., the Indian sub-continent. It has been estimated that nearly a million cases of cryptococcal meningitis occur worldwide in HIV positive individuals each year. Sub-saharan Africa heads the list where with 720,000 cases it is among the leading locations of fungus-related mortality with about 500,000 deaths/year. Southwest and

Southeast Asia are tied for second place with 120,000 cases each. It may be useful to point out that cryptococcosis is estimated to cause more deaths in this region than diseases such as tuberculosis, despite being less common in the population. The increasing use of invasive monitoring and aggressive therapeutic interdictions has, it should be said, resulted in improved survival rates for this and many other life-threatening illnesses. Yet this fact has also contributed to a rise in the number of people at risk for fungal infections.

Other developments in clinical practice that have impacted the incidence of invasive fungal diseases in various at-risk populations include the now-common use of triazole antifungal agents for both treatment and chemoprophylaxis, and of amphotericin B in suspected fungal infection. It is nevertheless true that opportunistic infections by well-recognized organisms including *Aspergillus fumigatus*, *Candida albicans*, and *Pneumocystis jirovecii*, represent an ever-increasing threat. Previously regarded as harmless saprophytes, these are today widely pointed to as the cause of serious and even lethal infections in immunocompromised individuals. Thus, the *Fusarium* species, long recognized for its role in nail and corneal infections, are now considered to be the cause of invasive and frequently fatal infections in neutropenic patients.

The identification of these organisms as significant pathogens in human disease has important implications for diagnosis and management. This is so not only because the clinical presentation can mimic a more common disorder, e.g., aspergillosis, but also because they are typically resistant to the most commonly prescribed drug for empirical treatment of suspected fungal infections in febrile neutropenic patients—Amphotericin B.

Superficial fungal infections are generally divided into a number of broad groups with regard to the initial site of infection. This approach emphasizes the degree to which the different groups of fungi adapt, as well as the manner in which the affected site is related to the route by which the fungus enters the host.

Superficial mycoses – These fungi, the most common type, infect the outermost, keratinized layers of skin, the nails, hair, and mucous membranes. The principal pathogens in this group are the dermatophytoses NDM (non-dermatophyte molds) and superficial forms of candidiasis. These diseases, affecting millions worldwide, include markedly distinct subtypes. They are often easily diagnosed and usually respond well to treatment. Most are unable to survive in competition with other keratinophilic organisms as free-living saprophytes in the environment and are thus dependent for their survival on passage from host to host. These obligate pathogens appear to have evolved from unspecialized saprophytics. The result is that the majority of dermatophytoses are no longer capable of sexual reproduction, with some even incapable of asexual reproduction. In general, however, these organisms have become well adapted to humans, inducing little or no inflammatory reaction from the host. Only dermatophyte infections are truly contagious.

The etiological agents of candidiasis, including the dermatophytes, are largely dependent on their host for their survival. They differ, however, in the manner by which this is achieved. Such organisms, among which *Candida albicans* is the most important and the most common pathogen of candidiasis, are normal commensal inhabitants of the human digestive tract and skin. Acquisition of such organisms from another host seldom results in overt disease and also results in the setting-up of a symbiotic relationship with the new host. These organisms do not produce disease unless some change in the host environment lowers natural defences. In which case, infection from the host's own reservoir of the organisms may evoke mucosal, cutaneous, or even systemic infection.

Other common superficial infections, e.g., pityriasis versicolor, a mild, often recurrent infection of the stratum corneum, are caused by lipophilic yeasts of the genus *Malassezia*. These fungi are skin commensals. Disease is likely related to host and environmental factors. Pityriasis versicolor is most common in tropical climates.

The subcutaneous mycoses – These are infections of the dermis, subcutaneous tissues, and underlying bones that generally spread slowly in a restricted manner and usually result from traumatic insertion of saprophytic fungi from soil or vegetation. More widespread, ematogenic or lymphatic dissemination, while uncommon, can occur in immunocompromised individuals. The subcutaneous mycoses include mycetoma, sporotrichosis, phaeohyphomycosis, and chromoblastomycosis. The infections they produce are most frequently encountered among the rural populations in tropical and sub-tropical regions where individuals go barefoot and wear minimal clothing.

The systemic mycoses – Fungi residing within the body produce infections that most frequently originate in the lungs, and may spread to other organs. These infections are most commonly acquired as a result of inhaling spores of fungi growing as saprophytes or as pathogens from plants.The organisms that cause systemic fungal infection can be divided into true pathogens and what are termed opportunists. True pathogens comprise a handful of organisms, mostly dimorphic fungi that invade and develop in the tissues of a healthy host, typically with no recognizable predisposition. The principal diseases they cause are blastomycosis, coccidioidomycosis, histoplasmosis, and paracoccidioidomycosis.

The opportunists are less virulent and less well-adapted organisms that are capable of invading only immunocompromised hosts. While new species of fungi are regularly identified as disease-causing agents in immunocompromised patients, five diseases still account for the majority of reported infections: aspergillosis, candidosis, cryptococcosis, mucormycosis, and pneumocystosis. Infections with true pathogenic fungi are frequently asymptomatic or mild and of short duration. They generally occur in geographical regions where the etiological organisms are native and gain entry to the host who inhales the spores. Recovery from these infections may leave a marked and longstanding resistance to reinfection, although chronic or residual infection may sometimes occur, resulting in a less stable, more dangerous situation.

True pathogenic fungi have emerged as important players in diseases in immunocompromised individuals. For example, histoplasmosis and coccidioidomycosis are today recognized as AIDS-defining diseases. Both are frequently seen in HIV-positive patients throughout North and South America. In such cases infections with true pathogenic fungi are often life-threatening and unresponsive to antifungal drugs, or relapse following discontinuation of treatment.

Opportunistic fungi typically infect immunosuppressed individuals, and often result in significant disease. Resolution of the infection does not confer protection, and reinfection or reactivation may follow if compromised resistance in the host recurs. In contrast to the generally restricted geographical distribution of the true pathogenic fungi, opportunistic fungi tend to be ubiquitous, residing in soil, in the air, or on decomposing organic matter. These infections are associated with high fatality rates, although estimates of their occurance are thought to be conservative compared to their actual incidence since many cases go undiagnosed or unreported.

Chapter 3

Human Immunity and Fungal Infections

For many years, it has been known that family genetic history influences a human being's susceptibility to fungal skin infections [5-7]. In other words, an individual with a family medical history of fungal skin infection and/or a genetic relative (tinea pedis, tinea corporis, onychomycosis, etc.) is at greater risk of contracting a fungal skin infection compared with the general population. Two important genetic mutations were identified: the CARD9 mutation and Dectin-1, which are associated with vaginal *Candida* infection. [8, 9]

Fungi may penetrate the human body via several possible portals. Newborns may be exposed to the yeast *C. albicans* in the vaginal canal during birth. As a result, the fungus may colonize the mouth and other parts of the upper and lower gastrointestinal tract as a life-long commensal (symbiotic) organism.

Another symbiotic fungus, *Malassezia furfur*, can routinely be found in areas of the skin densely populated with sebaceous glands, although the colonization process of this fungus is still unknown.

Both of the above mentioned fungi, *M. furfur* and *C. albicans* are unique in having achieved symbiotic relationships with humans, and are therefore considered as part of the indigenous flora. Hence, certain unusual circumstances are required for these fungi to inflict disease.

Fungi causing human diseases originate from the exterior environment, where they typically exist in the form of plant parasites or as saprobes on decaying fauna. Despite the constant exposure to infectious propagules, healthy humans with an intact immunological system, rarely contract fungal disease. It is only following the "accidental" penetration through the human body's natural barriers, the skin or the mucous membrane linings, or in the context of a compromised immune system or other debilitating condition in the host that fungal colonization can occur. For example, diagnosing the fungus *C. albicans* in a sick patient may indicate an underlying endocrine (e.g., diabetes mellitus), immunological (e.g., HIV) or other disorder that must first be controlled in order to effectively treat the fungal infection.

Fungi rarely cause disease in healthy hosts. Rather it is the result of accidental penetration of host barriers, particularly in the context of diminished immunologic capacity or other debilitating conditions. Hence, it is the underlying immunological condition of the individual that would largely determine if a fungal infection is contracted as well at its severity more so than the pathogenic potential of the specific fungi. Both the humeral and the cell-mediated immunity (CMI) components are important in combating fungal infections. The worse severity of fungal infections in patients with impaired CMI seems to indicate its greater importance over the humeral system in fighting fungal infections. Induction of specific immune responses requires that fungal infection first cross non-specific barriers .These consist of the integument, naturally occurring long-chain (unsaturated) fatty acids, competition with local bacterial flora, and the epithelial turnover rate. Additionally, the epithelial cells lining the mucous membranes are submerged in a fluid containing antifungal agents and frequently cilia that actively remove microorganisms.

Fungi are ubiquitous in nature, and exist as free-living saprobes with little known advantages derived from a parasitic infection of humans or animals. Because they are so prevalent and are readily cultured from body surfaces, it is sometimes difficult to discern whether a particular fungus obtained from a sick individual is a pathogen or alternately a transient environmental contaminant. Prior to confirming a diagnosis of a specific fungus as inflicting a disease, elements morphologically consistent with the isolate must be observed in lesion samples obtained in a series of specimens. In general, because of the nature of the relationship between fungi and their hosts, diseases resulting from fungal infection are incidental. As mentioned, some fungi have evolved from a parasitic to a commensal (symbiotic) relationship with humans, becoming part of the indigenous microbial flora (e.g., various species of *Candida*, especially *Candida albicans*, and *Malassezia furfur*). Although a plethora of data exists regarding the molecular basis of bacterial pathogenesis, the mechanisms of fungal pathogenesis are poorly understood. Infection, defined as entry into bodily tissues and subsequent reproduction of the organism, may be hidden or result in injury to cells from accumulation of toxic metabolites, or from interference or competitive metabolism, or from fungus replication, or from a variety of immune responses. Immune responses may manifest clinically as acute and transient or as chronic and prolonged. They may be cell-mediated (CMI), or humeral (producing specific antibodies to components of the infecting organism), or both. An infection may cause disease, defined as an interruption or a deviation from normal structure or function of organs or systems.

Human beings as well as animals has different meananisms which prevent different fungi spp penetrating to the skin of their hosts.

Among these protecting mechanisms there are the normal bacterial flora which affecting the level of the PH the long chain unsaturated fatty aeids, the long chain unsaturated fatty aeids , the rithrm of the turnover of the epidermis

Fungi are recognized by cells of the innate immune system (e.g., dendritic cells and macrophages), which bind components of fungal cell walls using pattern recognition receptors (PRRs) on their surface. C-type lectin receptors (CLRs, e.g., Dectin-1) are particularly important PRRs in anti-fungal immunity, although several other PRRs are also involved, including the Toll-like receptors (TLRs, e.g., TLR2) [10].

Immune responses vary with regard to the fungal species encountered. The relative importance of defense mechanisms, both specific innate and adaptive, differs with respect to the organism and the anatomical location of infection. The fungal morphotype (e.g., yeast, pseudohyphae, and hyphae) is likely an important factor in the host reaction. In contrast to yeasts and spores, which are often effectively phagocytosed, the larger size of hyphae impedes ingestion.

In addition, pathogenic fungi have developed mechanisms to avoid and disrupt host defenses. Some fungi, having evolved as intracellular parasites, can even survive within phagocytes, using them to avoid being targeted by other host defence elements.

Indeed, fungi have developed many mechanisms that enable them to colonize human hosts. One of the most important is the ability to survive and grow at 37°C. Another, the synthesis of keratinase enables dermatophytes to penetrate the body's principle barriers by digesting keratin in skin, hair, and nails. Dimorphism allows many fungi existing as molds to tranform to a yeast form within the host and thus become pathogenic. In contrast, *C. albicans* usually exists in normal flora as yeast capable of morphing into an invasive filamentous form. In yet another example, the antiphagocytic properties of the *Cryptococcus neoformans* capsule and the adherence abilities of *C. albicans* give them pathogenic potential. Dermatophytes and related fungi may spread locally on the skin or eumycotic mycetomas in subcutaneous tissue. Another subcutaneous pathogen, *Sporothrix schenckii,* spreads via local lymphatics. The fungi-producing systemic mycoses initially cause pulmonary infections. They are phagocytosed by alveolarmacrophages but not destroyed. Instead, the fungi successfully spread hematogenously. An exception to this pathologic path is *Cryptococcus neoformans*, which disseminates without being first phagocytosed. The pathogenesis of some fungi may at least be in part due to the host reaction to the specific invaded organism. An example of this is the allergic reactions provoked by some fungi.

The interdependence of several parts of the immune system and the interaction between host defenses and fungal pathogenic mechanisms are important characteristics of the human immune response. Several common defense mechanisms are effective against a range of fungi. For example, dendritic cells initiate innate and adaptive immunity in an attempt to respond to a wide variety of microorganisms. They capture and process antigens, migrate to lymphoid organs, express co-stimulatory lymphocyte molecules, and secrete cytokines to initiate immune responses. They play a key role in linking innate and adaptive responses to a range of pathogenic fungi, such as *Aspergillus fumigatus*, *Cryptococcus neoformans*, and *C. albicans*. The signals transmitted by dendritic cells, moreover, differ depending upon the particular fungus or morphotype encountered, with the outcome reflecting the nature of elicited adaptive immune responses. Whether dendritic cells employ intracellular or extracellular antifungal mechanisms depends on a number of factors, including the infecting species, morphotype, and route of exposure. Neutrophils, macrophages, and monocytes are the primary antifungal effector cells. At the time of infection, tissue phagocytes attempt to damage or kill invading fungi. Neutrophils and monocytes, and other effector cells are recruited to sites of infection by the action of cytokines, chemokines, and complement components. Fungi are killed or damaged by production and/or release of reactive oxygen intermediates and antimicrobial peptides.

The differentiation of CD4+ T cells along with a T-helper (Th) cell type 1 (Th1) or type 2 (Th2) pathway, and the generation of specific Th responses are essential determinants of the host response vulnerability or resistance to the invasive fungal infections. The development of Th1 responses is governed by the intensive activity of cytokines, such as interferon-c, interleukin-6, IL-12, tumor necrosis factor-α, , and the relative absence of Th2 cytokines, such as IL-4 and IL-10. The predominance of Th1 over Th2 type cytokines correlates with protection against various mycoses. Within this context, however, are nuances relating to temporal and quantitative aspects of cytokine production and ultimately to development of particular T-cell responses. They relate as well to the role the modulation of immunity plays in limiting autoimmune injury. Both human cells and fungi are eukaryotic. In addition to anatomic similarities, therefore, both possess a nucleus surrounded by a nuclear membrane, 80S ribosomes, and Golgi apparatus; they possess similar mechanisms for gene transcription and translation, and protein synthesis. This fact significantly limits the number of potential antifungal targets since the vast majority of such compounds are also toxic to human cells. For this reason, antifungal drugs are designed to target those features of fungal cells that differ from human cells. For example, the plasma membrane of most fungal cells contains ergosterol rather than cholesterol, the sterol in human cell membranes. Of course, the major distinguishing feature of fungal cells, the rigid cell wall containing chitin, mannans, and glucans, is a favored target of antifungal drug developers.

The cell wall provides physical protection, making it resistant to certain host defences, including complement-mediated lysis. Innate immune defenses such as β-glucan receptors, mannose receptors, and toll-like receptors (TLRs), have evolved to recognize and respond to the components of fungal cell walls. For instance, TLRs at the phagocytic cell surface that identify conserved molecular patterns are found on many microbes (including fungi). They are characterized by a distinguishing extracellular domain and a cytoplasmic domain that transmits signals to intracellular adapter proteins. One such, MyD88, initiates a signaling cascade leading to the expression of cytokines and microbicidal molecules. The proportional role of individual receptors, e.g., TLR2, TLR4, and TLR9, in MYD88 activation depends on the particular infecting fungus and the location of infection. Specific receptors differentially activate antifungal actions leading to varying responses and susceptibility to infection.

The risk for increase in mycotic infections is expected to continue for the foreseeable future. This is the result of the rapidly growing immunedeficient population as a result of the HIV pandemic, coupled with the increasing use of immune-suppressive drugs for the treatment of numerous diseases. On the positive side, these developments have led to exciting biotechnology advances into the immune response to fungi in recent years. The relative importance and interconnected responses of innate and adaptive immunity in protection, for example, are being actively investigated. At the same time, methods of immune manipulation and reconstitution have become promising research topics.

Future therapeutic strategies for managing invasive fungi may include application of agents that augment the natural antifungal activity of effector cells and alter Th balance. While clinical experience has been gained in the use of recombinant cytokines as adjuncts to antifungal drug therapy, clinical trials conducted in highly compromised hosts are lacking. Many questions remain regarding their safety, efficacy, and manner of optimal use. Another potentially efficacious approach is the manipulation of signaling cascades. The finding that innate and adaptive immunity in response to common fungal pathogens is mediated by the coordinated action of TLR family members acting through MYD88, suggests that TLR manipulation may be a useful intervention for inducing antifungal resistance. Development of antifungal vaccines represents yet another strategic direction, and requires trials in patients. Similarly, transfusion of dendritic cells exposed to fungi or fungal products and the adoptive transfer of T cells have both been successful in animal trials. It is clear that a better understanding of host–pathogen interactions is needed to achieve further efficacy of these and other novel antifungal therapies.

Dermatophyte Infections – The dermatophytes are fungi that colonize skin, nails, and hair in living hosts. They possess more extensive invasive properties than those involved in superficial infections, but are mostly limited to the keratinized tissues(such as hair and nails). In a 2005 paper, Baran, McLoone, and Hay [11], assert that unlike previous perceptions in dermatology, there is a unique form in which the dermatophyte exists below the proximal nail fold (the stratum corneum, the ventral part of the proximal nail fold). From this location it spreads distally along the nail plate, involving the fingernail and/or the toenail, while no port of entry is visible. In this case, the cuticle and the dorsal part of the nail plate look normal, and the entire pathological process (the fungus itself) is located just beneath the nail plate, so no other possibility exist for penetration other than from the internal organ [12]. The fact that several fingernails and/or toenails simultaneously have transverse bands proves that the infection travels from the blood stream towards the distal parts of the extremities, creating the white bands. Baran et al. raised the question was raised about the potential role of lymphatic or deep spread in some types of onychomycosis, in endogeneous reactivation, or auto-reinfection from a deeper part of the nail rather than another or new external reinfection.

Trauma plays an important role in infection, by facilitating entry through the uppermost layers of integument. They accomplish this with the help of keratinase, which they produce to metabolize the insoluble, tough fibrous protein. It is not known why they spread no deeper, but the possibility that cell-mediated immunity and/or the transferrin in serum inhibit deeper fungal propagation thereby preventing systemic disease. Hence, Dermatophytes produce skin alterations in humans and other animals but do not lead to systemic disease for reasons not fully understood.

Some dermatophytes are isolated from the skin in the absence of disease as an indication of evolving a commensal relationship with the host. The CMI essential role is to destroy the fungi and produce an immunoprotective response aimed at preventing re-infection. The resolution of the disease is associated with a delayed hypersensitive response. There are many effective veterinary vaccines against dermatophytoses.

Chapter 4

Diagnostic Techniques of Fungal Infections

Laboratory diagnosis should be employed prior to the initiation of treatment [13-16]. Clinical criteria provide only probable identification of fungal infection. The lesions may resemble other diseases, or they can be attenuated by previous treatments such as topical steroids or partially treated by topical antifungal cream. The laboratory- established procedure often provides the information needed for confirmation of the diagnosis – either by identifying the fungal cause of the disease or by excluding fungal infection when there are several optional diagnoses. The laboratory can help monitor the disease, select the antifungal treatment, and confirm that a mycological cure has been achieved.

The specimens should be obtained properly to ensure the accurate diagnosis and prompt appropriate treatment. Samples should include information about the patient including age, sex, part of the body in which the specimen was collected, and certain epidemiological data including prior contact, geography, and immunosuppressive treatment. The success of the laboratory diagnosis depends on the expertise of the mycologist and quality of the specimen collected.

The most common laboratory examinations to establish diagnosis are direct microscopy (smear) and culture. Direct microscopy may reveal the existence of fungal elements such as hyphea, pseudohyphea, spores, and yeast cells. The positive findings of these fungal elements do not lead to the precise type of the fungus and/or the vitality of the fungus. In other words, live fungus and dead fungus elements may appear about the same in direct microscopy.

Fungi are examined in potassium hydroxide or a fluorescent stain such as Calcofluor and can be cultured on Sabouraud's medium in which the specific identification of the fungus can be made. Skin scales, hair, and nails can be sent to a laboratory enclosed in a card (transport packs are available). Material from mucosal surfaces is best sent on a moistened swab.

Routine molecular diagnostic measures are not available commercially. This is due to the price of these methods, which are more expensive than the old traditional methods. On the other hand, yeasts and/or non-dermatophyte molds can be identified more easily by different biochemical tests. Although microscopic morphology might be sufficient in general, in many cases of these types of fungi (yeasts and non-dermatophyte molds) there is some difficulty in identifying the final species; thus more advanced techniques are needed. These techniques are based mainly on identifying the fungus DNA, but as there is great difficulty in the standardization of validating the diagnosis; in borderline cases is it impossible to determine for certain whether the fungi are pathogenic or saprophytic. Molds are identified almost exclusively by their morphology, particularly how they sporulate on agar. Fungi can often be identified in tissue, even in the absence of culture, by taking into account the clinical findings, body site, inflammatory response, and fungal appearance.

Culture diagnosis is potentially more accurate than diagnosis by histologic features, but many smaller laboratories encounter difficulties in isolating and identifying fungi. The histologic features of a biopsy specimen aid diagnosis when mycoses are caused by slow-growing fungi. Biopsy slides are mailed to consultants more readily than cultures, which may arrive nonviable or contaminated. Skin biopsy may be used also for the diagnosis of fungnal infection of the skin/nails. This kind of histopathological examination is rarely needed to confirm the fungal infection of the skin. Stains with PAS (periodic and schiff) is required for established the final diagnosis of fungal infection of the skin, scalp and nails. Furthermore, a biopsy may provide proof that the fungus is invading tissue and is not just a contaminant or saprophyte growing on debris in a lung cavity or skin ulcer. Ideally, both histologic examination and culture should be done together. As yet, detection of fungal DNA by polymerase chain reaction has not proved useful for detecting or identifying fungi in tissue. In contrast, luminescent DNA probes for hybridization to fungal RNA are commercially available and valuable for identifying colonies of *Histoplasma capsulatum*, *Coccidioides* spp., *Blastomyces dermatitidis*, and *Cryptococcus neoformans*. Identification of fungi in tissue by immunohistochemistry and molecular methods remains experimental.

Serologic Diagnosis

Despite the rich history of serologic studies on mycoses, the only mycosis for which serodiagnosis has an established role is coccidioidomycosis. Even with this infection, the lack of standardization of tests among laboratories and among methods has made it difficult for the clinician to interpret results. The situation is even worse for histoplasmosis and blastomycosis, for which the most promising test cited in the medical literature, complement fixation, has been considered too labor intensive and has been replaced in commercial laboratories by tests of unknown significance. Serodiagnosis for any mycosis should be used with great caution and with knowledge of the technique and laboratory performing the test.

Diagnosis by antigen detection has proved very useful in disseminated histoplasmosis and cryptococcosis. Severe cases of aspergillosis, coccidioidomycosis, and blastomycosis may also be amenable to diagnosis by antigen detection. Tests are commercially available for detecting β-glucan, a cell component, in patient serum. Further discussion of these tests is included in the relevant chapters.

New directions in diagnosis – Among the challenges in contending with opportunistic invasive fungal infections, none is more critical than early diagnosis. This is essential to reduce the case fatality rates observed in immune compromised individuals. In recent years some progress has been reported in diagnosing such infections, largely due to the increased use of computed tomographic scanning and other imaging procedures. It is very important to stress that the precise location of the suspected fungal infection is critical, because taking the mycological specimen from the wrong location might be interpreted as a negative result. Therefore, all samples should be taken by a skilled technician. For example, let's look at two common onychomycosis forms: DLSO (distal and lateral subungual onychomycosis) and SWO (superficial white onychomycosis). In DLSO, the fungus is located under the nail in the ventral part of the nail and the upper part of the nail bed; therefore, the deeper we penetrate the nail, the greater the probability to find fungi. If by mistake, as it often happens, the sample is taken from the dorsal part of the nail plate, a false negative is likely to appear. In SWO, the fungus is located on the dorsal part of the nail plate and not under the nail, which requires the sample to be taken from the dorsal part of the nail plate. Another example is taken from tinea corporis. In tinea corporis, the fungal source is known to be centrifugal and creates a clinical presentation of elevated red edges in comparison to the center of the lesion, while in many cases the center of the lesion itself is clean of fungi. If by mistake the sample is taken from the central part, a false negative could be returned. On the other hand, a false positive can be returned in many cases where there are saprophyte fungi that have nothing to do with the skin condition. Such conditions may be psoriasis or lichen planus, and taking allergy tests may reveal several allergens, which are clearly irrelevant for the correct diagnosis. There is a need to find the delicate balance between the lab tests on one hand and the relevance on the other, which some new techniques are trying to accommodate. It should be differentiated from the white opaque color that is obtained from long term use of nail lacqures (Figure 4.1).

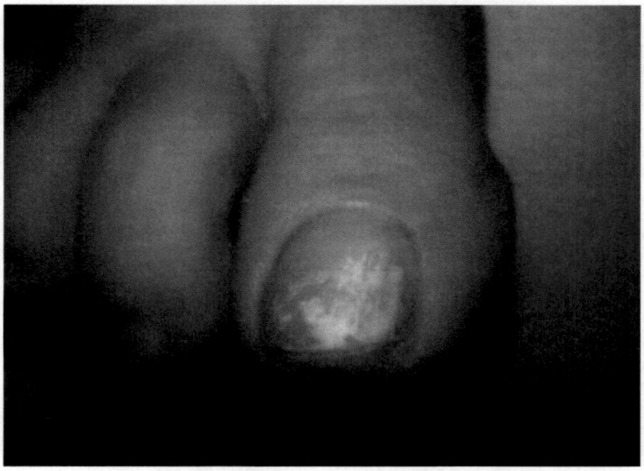

Figure 4.1. After nail lacquer.

In addition, it is important to make sure the patient hasn't recently received an antifungal medication so the result won't be affected by that previous treatment.

The following are leading factors for false negative cultures:

1. Wrong sample location
2. Recent use of an antifungal agent prior to sampling
3. Insufficient material sampled
4. Obsolescence of sample
5. Sample mix up
6. Irrelevant fungal culture medium
7. The mycologist did not interpret results correctly

8. A wrong answer is sent back to the physician

These are the most common factors for false positives:

1. Non-sanitized sampling tools that may contain remains of fungi from another patient or from the same patient but at a different location
2. The fungus exists, but it is a saprophyte and not pathogenic
3. Samples mix up
4. The mycologist did not interpret results correctly
5. A wrong answer is sent back to the physician

Promising approaches to diagnosing invasive fungal infections include the detection of certain components of the cell wall or metabolites and the detection of fungal DNA in clinical specimens. Novel methods for species determination use isolated fungal DNA for fingerprinting or PCR analysis based on differential sequence elements. Polymerase chain reaction (PCR) is used to amplify desired section of DNA from any source (i.e. virus, fungi, bacteria, plant, human) generating thousands to millions of copies of a particular DNA sequence. PCR reaction is composed of the DNA sequence of interest, DNA polymerase (Taq polymerase), DNA primers (short DNA sequences) and the four different nucleotides. The method relies on repeated cycles of heating and cooling. By heating the system you break the hydrogen bonds between the two different DNA strands into single strand. By decreasing the temperature each primer anneal to the 3' prime end of complementary matches on the target DNA sequence. The next step (at a slightly higher temperature) is the binding of the DNA polymerase to the DNA sequence with the primer which adds nucleotides to extend the second strand. Once it is completed there are two strands that are identical to the first one. In the following cycles the same steps of denaturing, annealing and extending are repeated to make additional DNA copies. After 3 cycles the target sequence which is defined by the primers starts to accumulate after 30 cycles, millions of copies of the target sequence are produced from a single starting molecule. When Polymerase chain reaction based detection of fungi in specimens is performed the primers selection is according to known published DNA sequences and the PCR products of amplification from each species are sequenced and recognized. As an alternative to DNA-dependent methods, mass spectral analysis and identification of microorganisms has become increasingly recognized. In a number of studies, matrix-assisted laser desorption /ionization time-of-flight (MALDI-TOF) mass spectrometry has been employed for the rapid classification and identification of microorganisms, and is becoming more prevalent in microbiology laboratories. Because of its ability to characterize a wide arrey of microorganisms, including viruses, bacteria, and fungi, MALDI-TOF-MS is both useful and innovative. Potential applications for this technology include medical diagnostics, environmental monitoring, biodefense, and food quality control. Because it can provide high-throughput and microbial identification at low-cost,MALDI-TOF-MS is an attractive alternative to conventional biochemical and molecular identification systems.

This approach also allows detection of [highly abundant] proteins in a mass range between 2 and 20 kDa, serving as taxon-specific biomarkers.

A striking advantage of mass spectral over genetic or morphological approaches is its straight-forward sample preparation procedure and the short time required for analysis. By analyzing colonies, an accurate classification of microorganisms at the levels of species, subspecies and strain can be made within a few minutes. MALDI-TOF-MS is a revolutionary approach to the identification of living organisms that will likely modify strategies for identification over the next years. It will potentially replace many phenotypic and genetic identification methods, due to its contained cost and excellent performance. Over the past decade, MALDI-TOF-MS tools have been successfully adapted for microorganism identification including for specific identification of fungi.

A publication by Welham et al (2000) described fungal identification by utilizing the MALDI-TOF-MS. Three fungal species (*Penicillium spp.*, *Scytalidium dimidiatum,* and *Trichophyton rubrum*) were distinguished from each other by their mass profiles. Recently, many studies have focused on the application of the MALDI-TOF-MS technique to characterize more strains of diverse fungal species and groups and to create mass spectra databases for further identification. Several species of *Penicillium* were identified by Chen et al. and Hetick et al. at the species and genus levels using MALDI-TOF-MS analysis of intact fungal spores or short chemical extractions. However, intact-spore MALDI-TOF mass spectra did not correctly classify 4 closely related *Aspergillus* spp. MALDI-TOF-MS tools were then applied to identify *Aspergillus* spp. at the species level. This technique was extended to identify *Aspergillus* strains, with an accuracy rate of 95% for *Aspergillus flavus* and 100% for *Aspergillus fumigatus*. The challenge of identifying *Aspergillus niger* strains, which were classified in the *Aspergillus chevalieri* cluster, has been noted. The application of *Aspergillus* spp. identification by automated MALDI-TOF-MS in clinical laboratories requires reliable reference databases of several strains of different species of *Aspergillus* spp. (~180 species). The identification of *Fusarium* spp. by MALDI-TOF-MS was reported in many studies. Marinach-Patrice et al. [17] updated the BioTyper database by adding 13 strains of five *Fusarium* spp. and accurately identified 89.7% of 49 clinical *Fusarium* isolates at the species level compared with molecular methods. Only one *Fusarium pseudonym gamai* isolate was misidentified, and four unidentified *Fusarium* isolates had no reference in the database.

MALDI-TOF-MS has been also applied to identify the species of *Fusarium* spores. Other fungal species have also been successfully identified, with human *Microsporidia* spp., *Candida* spp., *Cryptococcus* spp., *Saccharomyces* spp., *Trichosporon* spp., *Geotrichum* spp., *Pichia* spp., *Blastoschizomyces* spp., *Trichoderma* spp., *Rhizopusoryzae*, *Trichoderma reesei*, *Phanerochaete chrysosporium,* and *Saccharomyces cerevisiae* as examples. Several recent publications demonstrated the identification of fungal species using MALDI-TOF-MS analysis of direct samples, such as positive blood culture specimens from patients with candidemia, or nail samples from patients with onychomycosis.

Identification of fungi continues to rely mostly on phenotypic traits. Obtaining mature fungi with phyalids (i.e., conidiogenous cells observed in a type of asexual reproduction leading to the production of conidia) still requires several days, however. This delay in diagnosis may carry clinical implications in light of the morbidity and mortality associated with fungal infections, especially common among neutropenic patients. Thus, like other diagnostic techniques such as PCR and sequencing, MALDI-TOF has the potential to improve diagnosis by allowing for accurate and objective identification at species level, with the added values of timely and cost contained analyses compared with PCR and sequencing. MALDI-TOF-MS has mainly been utilized for the routine identification of yeasts; further development is needed in creating libraries of databases as well as standardizing protocols for sample preparation in order to optimize this approach with other groups of fungi, such as filamentous fungi and dermatophytes. As with other microorganism such as bacteria, the no identification or misidentification of fungal species by MALDI-TOF-MS analysis is due to either absence, mistakes, or incomplete reference spectra in the database. Usually, high quality MS spectra are readily obtained with both fungal hyphae and spores, following the manufacturer's instructions or based on the recommendation of reference studies.

Chapter 5

Cytochromes P450

These enzymes belong to a large superfamily of heme-thiolate proteins responsible for the metabolism of a wide arrey of endogenous and exogenous compounds [18,19]. They were discovered in rat liver microsomes in 1955 and are characterized by an intense absorption band at 450 nm in the presence of carbon monoxide.

Cytochrome P450 (CYP) mixed function monooxygenases reside on the smooth endoplasmic reticulum of cells throughout the body, with the highest concentrations found in liver (hepatocytes) and small intestine. They are responsible for the oxidative (Phase I) metabolism of numerous compounds, including medications, e.g., the biotransform of lipophilic drugs to more polar compounds capable of being excreted by the kidneys. The metabolites are typically less active than their parent compound, although some undergo biotransformation to pharmacologically active agents. In some cases, the metabolites are toxic, carcinogenic, or teratogenic. These enzymes are critical for the metabolism of many compounds including a variety of medications. Although CYP includes more than 50 iso-enzymes, 6 of these are responsible for the metabolism of approximately 90% of drugs. The two most clinically significant are CYP2D6 andCYP3A4. Polymorphism of these enzymes may lead to altered responses to commonly prescribed drugs, including beta blockers and antidepressants. While some drugs inhibit others induce CYP enzymes activity, causing potentially clinically significant drug-drug interactions that may lead to unanticipated adverse reactions or therapeutic effect (enhanced or reduced). Indeed, interactions with antidepressants, antiepileptic drugs, warfarin, and statins frequently involve CYP enzymes. Thorough understanding of the potential for CYP enzymes metabolism to impact common drugs as well as the agents that affect these enzymes is instrumental in minimizing the possibility of adverse drug reactions. Although genotype testing can identify specific enzyme polymorphism, the correlation between the genotype tests and the possibility of adverse reactions and interactions is currently not fully predictable.

There are more than 50 CYP enzymes, but the mayrity of the drug (90%) are metabolized by just 6, namely CYP1A2, CYP2C9, CYP2C19, CYP2D6, CYP3A4, and CYP3A5. Predominantly expressed in liver, and less common in the small intestine fangs kidneys.

Synthetic versions of different essential molecules such as steroids, cholesterol, and prostacyclins are produced by the CYP enzymes. They are also required for detoxifying foreign chemicals and metabolizing drugs. Cytochrome P450 owes its name to its binding to intracellular membranes (i.e., "cyto") and to the heme pigment protein it contains (i.e., "chrome" and "P") which absorbs light at the 450 nm wavelength upon exposure to carbon monoxide.

At least 12 CYP gene families have been identified in humans, although just three of these are involved in the majority of drug biotransformations, CYP1, CYP2, and CYP3. Cytochrome P450 families are based on amino acid sequence similarities, which can be further separated into subfamilies that are designated by capital letters following the family designation (e.g., CYP3A). Individual enzymes in a subfamily are indicated by Arabic numerals (e.g., CYP3A4). A given CYP is considered as belonging to a family when its amino acid sequence possesses greater than 40% homology; enzymes with greater than 55% homology are placed in a subfamily, and discrete enzymes can have up to 97% sequence homology. A single hepatocyte can contain a variety of cytochrome P450 enzymes. An individual CYP is capable of metabolizing numerous drugs, though a given drug may be primarily metabolized by a single enzyme.

In humans, CYP3A subfamily members are the most rich cytochrome enzymes, accounting for 30% of the cytochrome enzymes in the liver and 70% in the gut. In the adult liver, CYP3A4 is the major form of CYP, and it metabolizes the highest proportion of drugs. This enzyme, along with CYP3A3, which are 97% homologous and are indistinguishable on the basis of the substrates they metabolize, are the major enzymes expressed in the small intestine. CYP3A5 is the principle isoform expressed in the stomach. Interestingly, CYP3A5 is present in < 30% of Caucasians, yet deficiency in this isoform poses no danger since the CYP3A4 enzyme is available to assume its functions.

A widespread division of P450-containing monooxygenase systems exists as two types: bacterial/mitochondrial (type I) and microsomal (type II). Mitochondrial P450 systems have three compounds: a FAD-containing flavoprotein (NADPH or NADH-dependent reductase), an iron-sulfur protein, and P450. The eukaryotic microsomal P450 system contains two components: NADPH-P450 reductase, a flavoprotein containing both FAD and FMN, and P450.

Only in their third postnatal week do infants develop a mature enzyme system. The elderly have age-related decreases in liver mass, hepatic enzyme activity, and hepatic blood flow. In addition, they exhibit a reduced overall metabolic capacity of the liver, though the considerable inter-individual variability in age- and disease-related changes encountered in organ function makes it difficult to generalize. Two of the most common causes of altered

Twenty percent (one in five) of Asian descents, poorly metabolizes CYP2C19 dependent drugs, an important isoform that is responsible for the metabolism of phenytoin (Dilantin), phenobarbital, omeprazole (Prilosec), and other drugs.

Induction – Induction refers to an increased synthesis of the enzyme associated with exposure to drugs. The induction can occur when a drug stimulates biotransformation of administered drugs, either through the same enzyme pathway or an alternative one. Inducers, however, are normally specific for a given CYP family. Occassionally a drug will induce its own biotransformation in addition to that of other agents. The effects of induction are apparent within the first two days of therapy, although it will usually take more than a week for new enzymes to be synthesized and the maximal effect to occur. The time course for induction of enzyme onset and offset is closely related to the plasma concentration of the inducer, the half-life of enzyme production, and protein degradation.

Inhibition – Competitive inhibition is the principle mechanism of inhibition, and is induced when two or more drugs compete for the same enzyme. The clinical significance of an inhibition interaction principally depends on the relative concentrations of the drugs, as well as on a array of additional patient-specific factors. Some drugs are capable of binding to, and acting as competitive inhibitors of P450 enzymes different than those responsible for the biotransformation of that particular drug. The heme-binding site of different drugs could be bound in a reversible or irreversible mechanism, depending on the drugs and the CYP450 enzyme system.

Mechanism-based inhibition occurs when active metabolites of certain drugs that bind to the enzyme result from interaction with CYP, causing irreversible loss of function. Restoration of activity requires the synthesis of new enzymes, which may take several days. More complex mechanisms of inhibition are also known. For example, some drugs undergo metabolic activation by CYP and may inhibit the production of different metabolized products. The metabolites may generate relatively stable complexes with CYP such that the cytochrome is held in an inactive state. This interaction can be of great clinical significance since it is relatively long lasting. Additionally, there is potential for toxicity when the interaction involves drugs with narrow therapeutic ranges (Table 5.1).

Unlike induction, enzyme inhibition is typically initiated with the first dose of the inhibitor. It is maximal when the inhibitor reaches steady state (i.e., four to seven half-lives); the maximum concentration of the inhibited drug is achieved when the inhibited drug reaches steady state at its new, longer half-life. Similarly, the time required for the interaction to resolve is also dependant on the half-lives of the drugs involved.

Drug Interactions – Drugs interact with CYP450 enzymes in several ways. They may be metabolized by a single enzyme (e.g., metoprolol is metabolized by CYP2D6) or by multiple enzymes (e.g., warfarin [Coumadin] by CYP1A2, CYP2D6, and CYP3A4) (Table 5.2).

As a resultof the interaction betweenany antifungal drugwith the CYP450, the drug level in the blood may increase or decrease. This interaction may result in potentiation or blockage of the CYP450. Inhibitors block themetabolizing activity of one or more CYP450 enzymes.The extent to which an inhibitor affects the metabolism of a drug depends on factors such as the dose and the ability of the inhibitor to bind to the enzyme.

In addition, a drug can be both metabolized by and inhibit the same enzyme (e.g., erythromycin). Alternately, it can be metabolized by one enzyme and inhibit another (e.g., terbinafine [Lamisil]). Drugs may intentionally be combined to take advantage of CYP450 inhibition. Ritonavir (Norvir), a protease inhibitor and potent CYP3A4 inhibitor, is given together with lopinavir (Kaletra) to boost serum levels in patients positive for HIV.

Genotype Testing – Genotyping for CYP450 polymorphism has been used in both research and in clinical drug trials. The first genotype test was recently approved by the FDA. It is designed to inform the selection of drugs metabolized by CYP450 enzymes. The Amplichip CYP450 test is a DNA microarray capable of simultaneous detection of 29 polymorphisms of CYP2D6 and two polymorphisms of CYP2C19 in a blood sample. Although there is evidence linking polymorphisms coding for reduced CYP450 activity and adverse effects, large prospective clinical trials are needed to determine whether the use of genotyping in clinical practice is cost effective and improves clinical outcomes, presumably by preventing adverse drug effects or by identifying poor responders.

Table 5.1. Significant Cytochrome P450 Enzymes and their Inhibitors, Inducers, and Substrates [18]

Enzyme	Potent inhibitors*	Potent inducers†	Substrates
CYP1A2	Amiodarone (Cordarone), cimetidine (Tagamet), ciprofloxacin (Cipro), fluvoxamine (Luvox‡)	Carbamazepine (Tegretol), phenobarbital, rifampin (Rifadin), tobacco	Caffeine, clozapine (Clozaril), theophylline
CYP2C9	Amiodarone, fluconazole (Diflucan), fluoxetine (Prozac), metronidazole (Flagyl), ritonavir (Norvir), trimethoprim/sulfamethoxazole (Bactrim, Septra)	Carbamazepine, phenobarbital, phenytoin (Dilantin), rifampin	Carvedilol (Coreg), celecoxib (Celebrex), glipizide (Glucotrol), ibuprofen (Motrin), irbesartan (Avapro), losartan (Cozaar)
CYP2C19	Fluvoxamine, isoniazid (INH), ritonavir	Carbamazepine, phenytoin, rifampin	Omeprazole (Prilosec), phenobarbital, phenytoin
CYP2D6	Amiodarone, cimetidine, diphenhydramine (Benadryl), fluoxetine, paroxetine (Paxil), quinidine, ritonavir, terbinafine (Lamisil)	No significant inducers	Amitriptyline, carvedilol, codeine, donepezil (Aricept), haloperidol (Haldol), metoprolol (Lopressor), paroxetine, risperidone (Risperdal), tramadol (Ultram)
CYP3A4 and CYP3A5	Clarithromycin (Biaxin), diltiazem (Cardizem), erythromycin, grapefruit juice, itraconazole (Sporanox), ketoconazole (Nizoral), nefazodone (Serzone‡), ritonavir, telithromycin (Ketek), verapamil (Calan)	Carbamazepine,Hypericum perforatum (St. John's wort), phenobarbital, phenytoin, rifampin	Alprazolam (Xanax), amlodipine (Norvasc), atorvastatin (Lipitor), cyclosporine (Sandimmune), diazepam (Valium), estradiol (Estrace), simvastatin (Zocor), sildenafil (Viagra), verapamil, zolpidem (Ambien)

CYP=cytochrome P.

*These will slow down substrate drug metabolism and increase drug effect.

†These will speed up substrate drug metabolism and decrease drug effect

Table 5.2. Examples of Common Drug-Drug Interactions Involving the Cytochrome P450 Enzyme System [18]

Drug(s) /product	Enzyme inhibitor or inducer	Drug(s)	Metabolizi ng enzyme	Possible clinical effect
Amiodarone (Cordarone)	CYP2C9 and CYP3A4 inhibitor	Warfarin (Coumadin)	CYP2C9	Increased risk of bleeding caused by increased warfarin level
Carbamazepine (Tegretol), phenobarbital, phenytoin (Dilantin)	CYP3A4 inducer(Bactrim, Septra)	Ethinyl estradiol containing contraceptives	CYP3A4	Unplanned pregnancy caused by reduced estradiol level
Clarithromycin (Biaxin), erythromycin, telithromycin (Ketek)	CYP3A4 inhibitor	Simvastatin (Zocor), verapamil (Calan)	CYP3A4	Myopathy or rhabdomyolysis caused by increased simvastatin level. Hypotension and QT interval prolongation caused by increased verapamil level
Diltiazem (Cardizem), verapamil	CYP3A4 inhibitor	Prednisone	CYP3A4	Immunosuppression caused by increased prednisolone serum levels
Fluoxetine (Prozac), paroxetine (Paxil),	CYP2D6 inhibitor	Risperidone (Risperdal), tramadol (Ultram)	CYP2D6	Increased risk of extrapyramidal adverse effects caused by increasedrisperidonelevel. Decrease in analgesic effect caused by low level of active metabolite
Grapefruit juice	CYP3A4 inhibitor	Buspirone (Buspar)	CYP3A4	Dizziness and serotonin syndrome caused by increased buspirone level
Metronidazole (Flagyl)	CYP2C9 inhibitor	Warfarin	CYP2C9	Increased risk of bleeding caused by increased warfarin level
Terbinafine (Lamisil)	CYP2D6 inhibitor	Amitriptyline	CYP2D6	Dry mouth, dizziness, and cardiac toxicity caused by prolonged increase in amitriptyline and nortriptyline (Pamelor) levels

CYP=cytochrome P.

Chapter 6

Treatment and Drug Interactions

Definition

Antifungal agents are drugs that selectively eliminate fungal pathogens from a host while causing minimal toxicity. Several important differences between fungi and bacteria have led to a lag in the development of antifungal agents in comparison with antibacterial agents. The differences between the prokaryotic nature of bacteria and the eukaryotic nature of human cells allow for the targeting of several structural and metabolic targets specific to bacteria. Fungi, on the other hand, are eukaryotes, causing most antifungal agents to also be toxic to the host. Fungi typically grow slowly and often times in multicellular forms, making their quantification more difficult compared to bacteria. The quantification difficulty complicates the evaluation of *in vitro* or *in vivo* efficacy of a potential antifungal agent in experiments. Despite these limitations, numerous advances have been made in developing new antifungal agents and in understanding the existing ones [20-23].

Fungal cells, like many other eukaryotic cells, have many common biochemical targets. Therefore the drugs that interact with the cells of fungi will usually not interact with the eukaryotic cells. Ketoconazole was excluded by the FDA and other regulatory authorities in other countries worldwide due to the fact that in as many as 1 in 15,000 cases severe hepatic disorder may be caused. The fungal cells and human cells have several targets that the ketoconazole could not differentiate between. Since there is a huge difference between fungal cells and bacterial cells, antibacterial antibiotics do not interfere with the fungal cells [20, 24, 25].

In general, there are four major mechanisms of action of the different antifungal drugs:

1. Inhibition of the cell wall
2. Inhibition of cell division
3. Inhibition through cell membrane disruption
4. Direct toxic effect, caused by pH distribution dysfunction of the membrane.

The inhibition of cell wall biosynthesis is accomplished by many chemicals in different steps. Clinically it is less successful *in vivo* than *in vitro* and the targeting such mechanism is through the β-glucan synthesis.

The inhibition of cell division is done by nucleoside antifungal agents directly through the microtubules in the fungal cells.

Inhibition through cell membrane disruption is done either by attaching to the ergosterol, by binding the sterol-causing direct effect on the fungal cell membrane (e.g., amphotericin B), or by inhibition of the ergosterol synthesis.

Toxic effect to the fungal cell membrane occurs by accumulation of squalene via inhibition of the squalene epoxidase (e.g., Terbinafine).

The classes of drugs and their actions are:

Polyenes – bind ergosterol
Azoles – inhibit ergosterol synthesis
Echinocandins – inhibit glucan synthase
Allylamines – inhibit squalene epoxidase and inhibit ergosterol synthesis
Nikkomycins –inhibit chitin synthesis
Sordarins – inhibit protein synthesis
N-Myristoyltransferase inhibitors
Sphingolipid synthesis inhibitors

Polyene Antifungal Drugs

The polyene agents differ by containing alternating conjugated double bonds in the macrolide ring structure. Polyene antifungal drugs are produced by different *Streptomyces* species. By interacting with sterols in the plasma membrane (ergosterol in fungi, cholesterol in humans), channels are formed that allow for the leakage of small molecules from inside the fungal cell. Polyene antifungal agents include nystatin, amphotericin B, and pimaricin. Amphotericin B, discovered in 1956, is the most widely used drug for treatment of mycoses, with the possible exception of the dermatophytoses. It has a broad spectrum of activity that spans most of the clinically important molds and yeasts, including dimorphic pathogens, e.g., *Coccidioides immitis, Histoplasma capsulatum, Blastomyces dermatitidis,* and *Paracoccidioides brasiliensis.* It is also the drug of choice for most fungi induced opportunistic mycoses caused by such as *Candida* species, *Cryptococcus neoformans, Aspergillus* species, and the Zygomycetes. Resistance to amphotericin B is rare, but not unknown. Notable examples are *Pseudallescheria boydii*, *Fusarium* spp., *Trichosporon* spp., some isolates of *Candida lusitaniae,* and *Candida guilliermondii.* Administered intravenously, the drug is unfortunately known to cause several potential side effects, ranging from phlebitis at the infusion site to occasionally severe renal toxicity. Due to the fact that the polyene antifungal drugs are widely in use there is awareness of the renal toxicity, and the understanding of the renal mechanism pathology led to major progress in preventing and decreasing side effects. The impairment caused to glomerular filtration can be addressed by administration of volume by infusing sodium chloride. Nystatin, the first effective antifungal developed, is still in general use. It is indicative of newer polyene antifungal agents developed. Unfortunately, its broad-spectrum antifungal activity is counterbalanced by the host toxicity. It is therefore limited to topical administration, where it has demonstrated to be effective against yeasts such as the *Candida* species. Pimaricin (natamycin), a polyene utilized against both yeasts and molds, is applied topically for the treatment of superficial eye mycotic infections.

Azole Antifungal Drugs

In general, the azole antifungal agents are thought to inhibit cytochrome P450-dependent enzymes (particularly C14-demethylase) which are known to be responsible for the synthesis of membrane sterols, required for the structure and function of fungal cell membranes. The azole antifungal agents have five-member organic rings containing either two or three nitrogen molecules (i.e., the imidazoles and triazoles, respectively). Clinically used imidazoles include clotrimazole, miconazole, and ketoconazole,. Clinically important triazoles include itraconazole and fluconazole. Ketoconazole introduced a better-tolerated, orally administered systemic antifungal although it can also be applied topically. Given itsrange of targets, including infections by *Histoplasma capsulatum* and *Blastomyces dermatitidis*, it is often employed in non-immunocompromised patients. In addition, it is active against mucosal candidiasis and a variety of cutaneous mycoses, including dermatophytes, pityriasis versicolor, and cutaneous candidiasis. Most recently, the FDA prohibited the systemic use of ketoconazole due to the frequency of hepatic side effects and its ineffectiveness against *Aspergillus*. The above mentioned triazoles (fluconazole, itraconazole) are now the standard, having replaced azoles such as amphotericin B, especially for treating certain forms of systemic mycoses. Fluconazole, which is routinely prescribed for the management of candidemia in non-neutropenic hosts, is now also utilized in cryptococcosis and selected forms of coccidioidomycosis. Itraconazole has been demonstrated to be effective in treating histoplasmosis, blastomycosis, sporotrichosis, coccidioidomycosis, consolidation treatment for cryptococcosis, and certain forms of aspergillosis. Fluconazole may be administered orally or intravenously. The currently approved formulation of itraconazole is for oral use, however an intravenous formulation is under development and could prove effective in addressing limitationof absorption/bioavailability seen with the oral formulation. It must be said that side effects are observed less with the azoles than with amphotericin B, although severe life-threatening hepatic toxicity is a risk with prolong use. Liver toxicity like that seen with ketoconazole has not been a concern with the triazoles, although other side effects have been reported, including nausea and vomiting. In addition, drug interactions between azoles and several other drug classes pose a potential challenge. These include cyclosporin, anticoagulants, certain antihistamines, anti-seizure drugs, oral hypoglycemics, and other medications undergoing similar metabolism in the liver.

Allylamine and Morpholine Antifungal Drugs

Allylamines (naftifine, terbinafine) inhibit ergosterol biosynthesis at the level of squalene epoxidase as well as the 14 alpha-demethylase enzyme just as with the azole drugs, thus the allylamins act as fungistatic medications. The morpholine drug amorolfine has a dual mechanism of action; it inhibits the D14 reductase and D7-D8 isomerase resulting in a decrease in the creation of ergosterole molecules as a fungistatic mode of action, and accumulation of ignosterole at the fungal cytoplasmatic cell membrane as a fungicidal mechanism of action.

Antimetabolite Drugs – 5-Fluorocytosine

Unlike antibacterial agents, only a few antimetabolite drugs are available for treatment of mycoses. One, 5-fluorocytosine, is a fluorinated analog of cytosine that inhibits both RNA and DNA synthesis via intracytoplasmic conversion of 5-fluorocytosine to 5-fluorouracil. The latter is converted to 5-fluorouridine triphosphate, which inhibits RNA processing, and 5-fluorodeoxyuridine monophosphate, which inhibits thymidylate synthetase. This, in turn, inhibits the formation of the deoxythymidine triphosphate needed for DNA synthesis. As with other antimetabolites, the emergence of drug resistance is a problem. Therefore, 5-fluorocytosine is seldom used alone. In combination with amphotericin B, 5-fluorocytosine is the treatment of choice for cryptococcal meningitis and is effective against a variety of other mycoses, including some caused by the dematiaceous fungi and perhaps even by *C. albicans*.

Other Antifungal Agents

Griseofulvin is an antifungal produced by *Penicillium griseofulvum*. It is the drug of choice for certain chronic fungal infections (e.g., those of the nails with *Trichophyton rubrum*) since it is orally administered and presumably incorporated into constitutively growing tissue. It has also shown activity against most dermatophytes *in vitro*. Griseofulvin is still considered a gold standard for tinea capitis. The drug inhibits mitosis in fungi. The treatment has to be continued up to the complete cure of the tissue.

Potassium iodide administered orally as a saturated suspension is uniquely employed to treat cutaneous and lymphocutaneous sporotrichosis. Potassium iodide has no effect against *Sporothrixs chenckii in vitro*. It appears to act by augmenting the transepidermal elimination process in an infected host.

The two allylamines (naftifine and terbinafine) inhibit ergosterol synthesis at the level of squalene epoxidase and also the 14 alpha-demethylase enzyme; one morpholene derivative (amorolfine) inhibits a subsequent step in the ergosterol pathway.

Selection of Antifungal Agents

Susceptibility testing with fungi *In vitro* is yet to become standardized, and *in vitro* test results are not always comparable with the results obtained *in vivo*. Accordingly, choosing an antifungal agent for clinical use is based primarily on the specific pathogen involved. For each given licensed antifungal agent there is a well determined spectrum of activity as determined by preclinical and clinical testing of common fungal pathogens. Adopting such an approach allows for an informed selection of drugs based on known resistant to specific agents by various species of fungi. However, it is less effective in informing the selection of antifungals for fungi species that may develop secondary (i.e., drug-induced) resistance.

Resistance to antifungal drugs is an emerging problem as a larger armamentarium of antifungal agents is being developed. . Resistance to the polyene antifungals is consistently primary rather than secondary. That is, susceptibility profiles for this species are characteristic and inherent, and rarely vary in response to the agent. Amphotericin B-resistant species, e.g., *Pseudallescheria boydii* and *Candida lusitaniae,* are well documented, and do not seem to have resulted from exposure to the antifungal. The widespread use of amphotericin B to treat *Candida albicans* infections rarely leads to the development of secondary resistance. In contrast, both primary and secondary resistance to 5-fluorocytosine occur in strains of *Candida* spp., a fact that explains the increasingly precaution of using this agent in combination with other antifungal drugs.

Questions regarding fungal resistance to the azole drugs are considerably more complex. Examples of both primary and secondary resistance are documented for the medically important yeasts as well as for selected azole antifungals. *Candida krusei* as a species is typically resistant to fluconazole. Different strains of *Candida albicans* show some resistance to fluconazole due to overtreatment with systemic fluconazole, especially in HIV patients. The issue of drug resistance is complicated by limitations in the available methodologies for susceptibility testing and in their ability to distinguish between microbiological and clinical drug resistance. The latter typically becomes relevant when an inhibitory antifungal agent reaches the limits of its activity in an immunocompromised host.

The updated formulation of the azoles, polygenes, and fluorocytosine are given now to those patients whose disease was considered in the past as mycotic (see Figures 6.1 and 6.2). However, as advances in modern medicine continue to extend lifespan, particularly through aggressive therapies in life-threatening diseases such as cancer, new and larger patient populations are at risk today for opportunistic fungal infections. These patients pose unique challenge as they are often left with a dangerously diminished immune function and must be treated by fungicidal rather than fungistatic agents. The search for fungicidal agents less toxic to the host continues. Active research is also increasingly directed towards developing immunomodulating agents that could address the perilous loss of native host immunity.

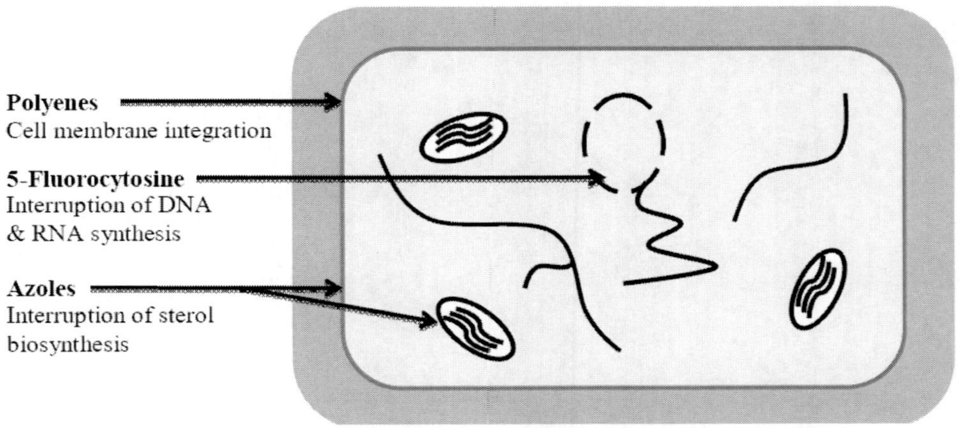

Figure 6.1. Generalized fungal cell showing the sites of action of the common antifungal agents.

Table 6.2. The Major Antifungal Agents and their Common Uses

	Clinical application				
	Opportunistic Mycoses				
Drug	Aspergillosis	Candidiasis	Cryptococcosis	Dermatophytosis	Other
Polyenes					
Amphotericin b	+	+	+	-	
Nystatin	-	mc*	-	-	
Pimaricin	-	-	-	-	mycotic keratis
Imidazoles					
Clotrimazole	-	mc	-	+	
Miconazole	-	mc	-	+	
Ketconazole	-	+**	-	+	
Triazoles					
Itraconazole	+	mc	+	+	sporotrichosis
Fluconazole	-	+	+	+	sporotrichosis
Antimetabolite					
5-Flucrocytosine	+	+	+	-	phaeohyphomycosis

* including mucocutaneous but not systemic candidiasis.

**insufficient data.

***used only in combination with amphotericin B.

Chapter 7

Antifungal Drugs in Pregnancy

Topical antifungal treatment and, of course, systemic antifungal treatment for pregnant women should be always considered as a potential risk factor to the fetus. The antifungal medication, mainly the systemic and less commonly the topical treatment – as other drugs, are to be considered for the benefit of the pregnant woman and the fetus. In 1980 the FDA published a classification of antifungal drugs and their potential risk in pregnant women (Table 7.1). This classification is graded A, B, C, D, X, and N, where category A is defined as the safest drug, and category X is defined as having the highest potential risk for the fetus.

Table 7.1. FDA classification of antifungal drugs and their potential risk in pregnant women

Category	
A	Controlled studies have not revealed a risk to the fetus in the first trimester of pregnancy. There is no evidence of risk in later trimesters.
B	Animal studies have not revealed risk to the fetus, and there are no controlled studies that prove risk to pregnant women.
C	Animal studies have shown a risk to the fetus, and there are no available controlled studies in women.
D	There is positive evidence of risk to the fetus, but there are cases in which potential benefits may be superior to the potential risks.
X	There is a definite risk to the fetus, and the risks are greater than the potential benefits.
N	FDA has yet to classify the drug.

The following section provides a broad discussion of the different antifungal drugs that may or may not be given to pregnant women topically, through vaginal therapy, and via systemic treatment.

Topical Antifungal Treatment

Topical anti-fungal medications are widely used in mild to moderate fungal infections. Tinea capitis, onychomycosis, tinea manuum, and tinea pedis require, in principal, systemic treatment, but the mild involvement of each of the mentioned fungal diseases may be treated topically. Tinea corporis of mild to moderate involvement is treated topically, while severe cases are treated systemically. Stubborn mild to moderate cases that do not react to conventional topical antifungal medication should also be treated systemically.

Several topical antifungal creams are nonprescription and others are prescription.

Different countries have different rules regarding the need for prescribed drugs, while other topical antifungal preparations are considered to be over-the-counter (OTC; nonprescription medications).

Table 7.2. Summary of the most common topical antifungal drugs with their risk category

Agent	Risk Category
Nonprescription	
Clioquinol	N
Clotrimazole	B
Miconazole	C
Naftifine	B
Nystatin	B
Tolnaftate	N
Undecylenic Acid	N
Prescription	
Amphotericin B	B
Butoconazole	C
Ciclopirox	B
Econazole	C
Haloprogin	B
Ketoconazole	C
Oxiconazole	B
Sulconazole	C
Terbinafine	B
Terconazole	C
Tioconazole	C
Triacetin	N

Vaginal Antifungal Treatment

Vaginal antifungal preparations are very widely used during pregnancy. Among the most common vaginal antifungal medications are the polyenes (amphotericin B and nystatin) and the imidazoles, such as miconazole nitrate, clotrimazole, butoconazole, tioconazole, and terconazolesliders – which are allgenerally considered as safe antifungal agents in pregnancy based on retrospective and prospective comparative clinical trials. The fact that the first trimester of pregnancy is well known to be far less safe for many drugs compared to the second and the third trimesters, has led many drug manufacturers to caution against the use of the vaginal – or even topical – antifungals in the first trimester, although many studies as well as data regarding the use of vaginal antifungal medication show these drugs to be relatively safe (Table 7.3).

Table 7.3. The common vaginal antifungal drugs

Topical	Systemic	Contraindicated in pregnancy
Imidazoles Clotrimazole Micanazole Butoconazole Tioconazole	**Imidazoles** Terconazole	-
Polyenes Nystatin	**Polyenes** Amphotericin B Amphotericin B lipid complex Amphotericin B cholesteryl sulfate Amphotericin B liposomal complex	-
-	-	**Antimetabolites** Flucytosine
-	**Echinocandins** Caspofungin	-
-	**Triazoles** Ketoconazole Itraconazole Fluconazole	**Triazoles** Voriconazole
	Squalene epoxidase inhibitors Terbinafine	
		Miscellaneous Poatassium iodide Griseofulvin

Systemic Antifungal Drugs

The systemic antifungal drugs, for unknown reasons, are traditionally considered to be dangerous drugs for healthy people, and all the more so in pregnant women. Antifungal drugs have been given to pregnant women only to fight life-threatening fungal infections; therefore, there is not enough experience regarding systemic antifungal drug use in pregnant women. In a paper published by Varsha and colleagues in the *Expert Opinion on Drug Safety* [26], there is a list of antifungal drugs and their risks in pregnant women. Tables 7.1 and 7.2 summarize the topical antifungal medications and the antifungal drugs that are contraindicated in pregnancy. Fungal infection in pregnant women is not less common than in non-pregnant women. On the contrary, vaginal candidiasis is more common in pregnant women. When using topical antifungal treatment and especially systemic antifungal treatment, the benefit of the mother versus the risk to the fetus should be carefully considered.

Several antimycotic drugs may penetrate through the placental barrier to the fetus. Giseofulvin, potassium iodide, ketoconazole, flucytosine, and voriconazole are known to potentially have serious risks regarding fetal malformations.

Chapter 8

Tinea Capitis

Synonym: ringworm of the scalp

Definition: Tinea capitis is a dermatophyte infection of the scalp and associated hair by a dermatophyte fungus.

Epidemiology

The epidemiology of tinea capitis varies within different geographical areas throughout the world. In Northern and Western Europe, it is estimated to account for 1% of all superficial fungal infections [27]. Tinea capitis is a common dermatophyte infection of the scalp most commonly encountered in children and much less frequently in adults. The exact incidence remains unknown but is most commonly found between the ages of 3 to 14 years. Children of African descent living in tropical and underdeveloped countries are more commonly infected with tinea capitis. Tinea capitis, caused by the *Trichophyton* species, affects males and females equally, and in the cases caused by *Microsporum audouinni* and *Microsporum canis*, males are more likely to be infected compared to females [28]. Infection in adults is considered uncommon, possibly because the increased triglycerides in the sebum produced following puberty increase fungistatic action. Immunocompromised patients are predisposed to developing tinea infections.

Pathogens

The etiological agents of dermatophytes can be classified in three anamorphic genera: *Trichophyton*, *Microsporum,* and *Epidermophyton*. Tinea capitis can be caused by any pathogenic dermatophyte from the genera of *Trichophyton* and *Microsporum.* Based on host preference and natural habitat, dermatophytes can be classified as anthropophilic, zoophilic, and geophilic. Anthropophilic species usually infect humans, and animals are rarely affected. Zoophilics are pathogens of animals, but transmission from animals to humans does occur. Geophilic species inhabit the soil and infect both humans and animals. The etiologic agents of tinea capitis are usually anthropophilic and zoophilic. Worldwide, the most common dermatophytes isolated causing tinea capitis are [27]: *M. canis* (*M. gypseum, M. fulvum, M. nanuum), Trichophyton mentagrophytes,* and *Trichophyton verrucosum.* On the European continent, *M. canis*, *Trichophyton tonsurans*, *Trichophyton violaceum*, *T. verrucosum,* and *Trichophyton soudanense* are the most frequently encountered etiologic agents. *M. canis*, a zoophilic dermatophyte, is the most common reported causative agent of tinea capitis in Europe. Countries reporting high incidence of *M. canis* infection are mainly in the Mediterranean area but also in Austria, Hungary, Germany, and Poland. In the UK, there has been an increase of *T. tonsurans,* especially in urban areas. In Central America, the Caribbean, and South America, *T. tonsurans* predominates. In the rest of South America, the most frequent organism is *M. canis*. In Australia and New Zealand, the most frequent organisms causing tinea capitis are *M. canis* and emerging *T. tonsurans.* In Western and Southern Asia, the most common is *T. violaceum* and in the Middle East countries *M. canis, T. mentagrophytes,* and *T. violaceum.* In Africa, the most common organisms include *T. violaceum, T. audouinii*, *T. soudanense, T. mentagrophytes,* and *M. canis*. In Israel, the most common fungi causing tinea capitis are *M. canis* and *T. violaceum* [28].

The causative pathogens more frequently involved are *T. tonsurans,* which is the most prevalent worldwide, followed by *M. canis*. Tinea capitis due to *M. audouinii* or *T. tonsurans* is more likely to occur in children. Among different geographic locations, there is a variation of the pathogens involved. This can be related to several factors such as movements of populations, changes in habits, and availability of medical supplies.

The most frequent pathogen of tinea capitis reported in adults is *T. tonsurans* [27].

Transmission is increased with poor personal hygiene, areas that are overcrowded, and low socioeconomic status. The offending pathogens are cultured from items such as combs, caps, pillowcases, toys, and theater seats. Even after shedding, hairs may harbor infectious organisms for more than a year.

The main reservoirs for *M. canis* are cats and dogs, but numerous other mammalian species may also serve as endemic reservoirs. *M. canis* causes lifelong infection in these animals and appears to be in active evolution. Without its animal reservoir, *M. canis* appears to lose virulence after about four human-to-human transmissions and infection is re-established by new contact with an animal carrier [29].

Presentation

Tinea capitis has a broad spectrum of presentation that can be influenced by many factors such as the causative organism, the host's immune resistance, and the degree of inflammatory host response.

Anthropophilic endothrix infection (within the hair shaft), for example in the case of *T. tonsurans* and *T. violaceum*, results in hair breakage at the level of the scalp and leaves a "black dot" appearance. This is the least inflammatory form of tinea capitis. Alopecia may or may not occur, but when it does, hairs break at the level of the level of the scalp leaving grouped black dots within the areas of the alopecia with poorly demarcated margins. An amount of normal hair usually remains within the patches of partial or complete alopecia. The affected hairs may have a grey appearance because they are coated with arthroconidia. Scaling is often present, and inflammation can vary but usually is minimal.

Infections caused by anthropophilic ectothrix organisms (around the hair shaft), as in for example *M. auouinii* or *M. canis*, result in dry, scaly patches of alopecia also known as "grey patch" or the seborrheic form of tinea capitis. The noninflammatory pattern of tinea capitis lesions has prominent scaling and minimal inflammation. Hairs in the affected area have a greyish appearance and break off just above the level of the scalp. Sometimes there is no noticeable hair loss. Plaques often appear as well-defined, round to oval hyperkeratotic, scaly areas of alopecia. Hairs that are present exhibit green fluorescence under Wood's lamp. The most frequent location of the lesions is the occiput.

Another significant factor affecting clinical presentation is the host's immune response. The inflammatory type of tinea capitis usually presents with zoophilic or geophilic pathogens such as *M. canis* and *M. gypseum*. The spectrum ranges from pustular folliculitis to kerion, which often presents as a purulent plaque, which is boggy and oozing with pus that may result in abscess formation and alopecia. Alopecia may affect discrete areas of the scalp or occur more extensively and cover the entire scalp with multiple plaques. The hair tends to regrow, but the longer the infection persists, the likelihood that the alopecia will be permanent increases. This often occurs when a kerion is misdiagnosed as a bacterial abscess. Commonly, patients presenting with kerion have an associated lymphadenopathy of the posterior cervical or posterior auricular lymph nodes, which can be helpful when differentiating other scalp disorders that cause alopecia. Other associated features are pain on palpation, and patients can exhibit signs of systemic illness such as fever. Additional lesions on glabrous skin can present. With infection by *T. tonsurans,* it is unusual for scarring to occur.

Clinically, tinea capitis can be divided into several groups, as follows:

a) Black dot tinea capitis
b) Grey patch tinea capitis
c) Seborrheic dermatitis-like/diffuse scale tinea capitis
d) Diffuse pustular tinea capitis
e) Kerion celsi
f) Favus

A. Black Dot Tinea Capitis

Black dot tinea capitis is one of the most common subtypes of tinea capitis and is characterized by round/oval patchy areas of broken-off hair stubs of 1-3 mm (Figure 8.1). This subtype usually occurs due to zoophillic fungi, namely *T. violaceum* and *T. tonsurans* (large spore endothrix), and therefore it does not produce fluorescence under Wood's lamp.

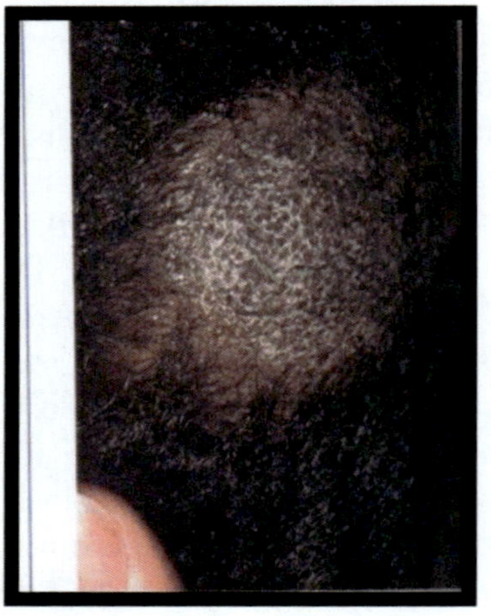

Figure 8.1. Black Dot Tinea Capitis characterized by round/oval patchy areas of broken-off hair stubs of 1-3mm

B. Grey Patch Tinea Capitis

Gray patch tinea capitis is characterized by scaling without inflammation, causing broken-off short hair (not too close to the scalp level) and with a gray/discolored appearance (Figure 8.2). This type of tinea capitis is usually caused by zoophilic fungi (*M. Canis, M. ferrigieum, M. distortum*, etc.) and therefore they produce fluorescence under Wood's lamp. The gray tinea capitis is usually seen in Africa and Asia.

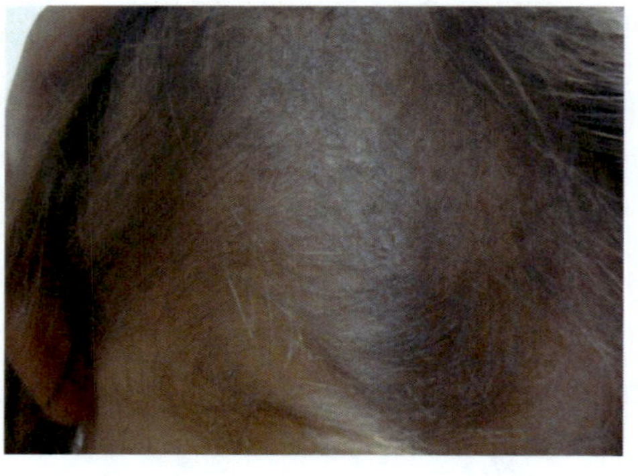

Figure 8.2. Grey Patch Tinea Capitis and with a gray/discoloured appearance.

C. Seborrheic Dermatitis-Like/Diffuse Scale Tinea Capitis

The diffuse scale type of tinea capitis should be differentiated from atopic dermatitis and psoriasis (Figure 8.3). Usually atopic dermatitis appears in locations such as cubital fossa and popliteal fossa, and a personal or familial atopic background often exists. In psoriasis patients we usually see psoriatic lesions on other parts of the body, and the scalp scales in psoriasis are thicker, more massive, and the scalp lesions' borders are better circumscribed. In seborrheic dermatitis or seborrhea, which rarely occur in young children, the well-known *Pityrosporum ovale/P. orbiculare* or other *Malassezia* spp. should not be interpreted as the cause of tinea capitis, which is caused by dermatophytes and not by yeast cells.

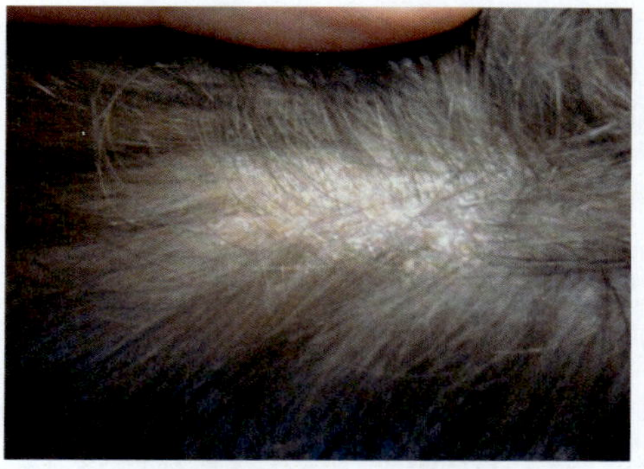

Figure 8.3. Seborrheic Dermatitis-Like diffuse scale Tinea Capitis differentiated from atopic dermatisis and psoriasis.

D. Diffuse Pustular Tinea Capitis

The diffuse pustular type of tinea capitis (Figure 8.4) should be differentiated from folliculitis abscedens et suffodiens, scalp impetigo, folliculitis decalvanse, id reaction, impetigo, and pustular psoriasis.

Perifolliculitis capitis abscedens et suffodiens is also known as perifolliculitis capitis or dissecting cellulitis. Perifolliculitis capitis abscedens et suffodiens is a type of chronic folliculitis that usually attacks young adults and adults and rarely affects children. It is more common in dark-skinned people (male > female). This disorder is associated with severe acne. On the scalp are red papules, pustules, and furuncle/carbuncle-like abscesses that are accompanied by cicatricial/scaring alopecia.

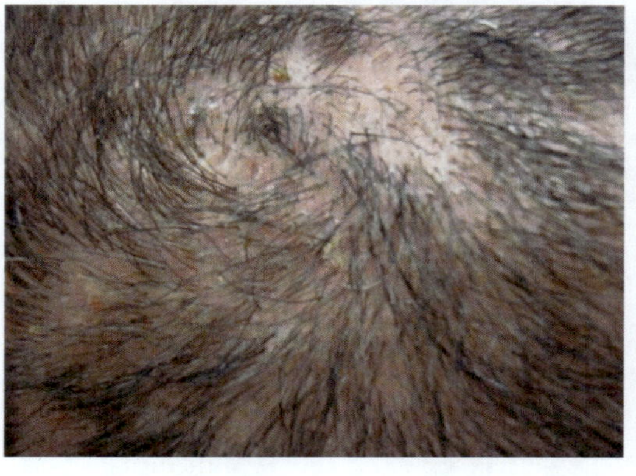

Figure 8.4. Diffuse Pustular Tinea Capitis.

E. Kerion Celsi

Kerion celsi is one of the most inflammatory types of tinea capitis, which is a type of abscess – a combination of the immune system and the fungus itself. It usually appears on the scalp but can appear on the face and beard area. Clinically, kerion celsi is presented as a boggy, pus-filled lump, with size varying from one to several cm (Figure 8.5). Usually the kerion celsi contains elements of fungi and bacteria that cause the body to react with severe inflammation. The most common fungi that cause kerion are *M. canis, T. tonsurans, T. verrucosum,* and *T. mentagrophytes*. Diagnosis can be done by Wood's lamp, which may result in yellow-green fluorescence. However, if it is negative, it may be due to the fungus being obscured by the inflammation. In such a case, bacterial analysis should be done and relevant systemic antibiotics should be given, and afterwards mycological analysis from the superficial and deep areas should be conducted.

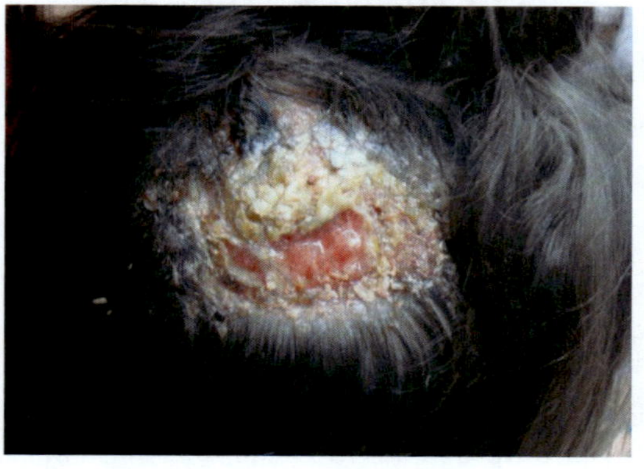

Figure 8.5. Kerion Celsi with size varying from one to several cm.

F. Favus/Tinea Favosa

Favus is a fungal infection caused by *Trichophyton schoenleinii* (Figure 8.6). It is rarely caused by *Trichophyton violaceum, Trichophyton mentagrophytes* var. *quinckeanum,* or *Microsporum gypseum*. Favus may attack children and adults, and both females and males are affected equally. Favus is considered a severe inflammatory type of tinea capitis but can also attack the beard area or skin. Unlike typical subtypes of tinea capitis, there is no effect on hair growth. Microscopically, air spaces separating hyphae elements can be seen. Favus is rare in the US and is more prevalent in third world countries.

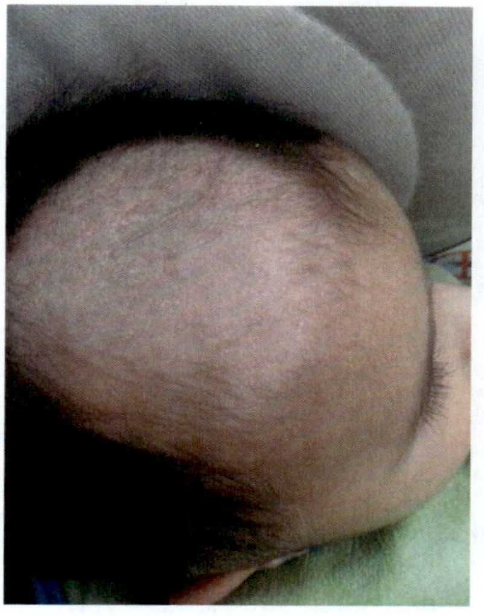

Figure 8.6. Favus/Tinea favosa caused by Trichophyton schoenleinii.

Carrier Stage

Carrier stage, also known as occult disease, refers to the cases of tinea capitis that elicit absent or minor clinical symptoms yet have a positive fungal culture (Figure 8.7). This is seen more frequently in adults who have had close encounters with infected children.

Household contacts are at increased risk from infection as there exists the opportunity for close and prolonged contact. In addition to the household setting, the spread of conidia may also occur in residential schools, day-care centers, and hospital wards. Data suggest that viable fungal conidia are present in the environment surrounding patients with tinea capitis and in a variety of inanimate objects such as combs, hair brushes, caps, backs of theater seats, pillows, blankets, curtains, bed sheets, and instruments used by barbers and can remain viable for up to two years. The prolonged survival can also explain the transmission of infection in the absence of a clearly defined host. Infection is more frequent in males than in females. The carrier stage is considered contagious, and some physicians recommend treating occult disease with either oral or topical antimycotic treatment modalities. Asymptomatic carriers are common and are a significant reservoir for the disease, spreading spores, making tinea capitis difficult to eradicate [29]. Hay et al. demonstrated that individuals whose culture plates exhibited fewer than 10 colonies were regarded as being carriers, whereas those with positive cultures yielding growth from 50% to 100% of the inoculum points were considered to be infected [31].

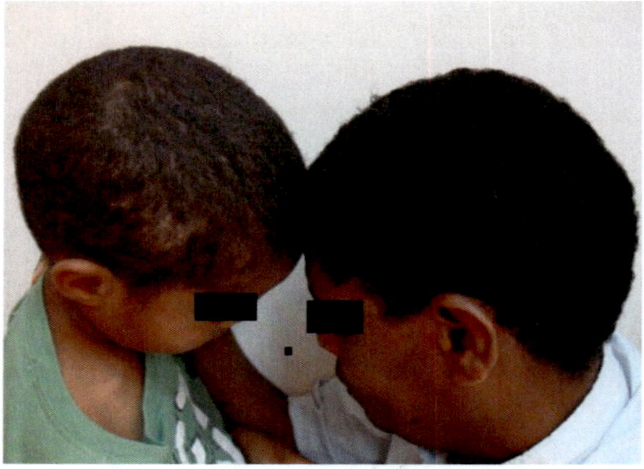

Figure 8.7. Carrier Stage –A father and his son have a positive fungal culture.

Anthropophilic rather than zoophilic species can present more frequently with asymptomatic carriage. The asymptomatic state may persist between 6 weeks and 6 months in 10–25% of untreated individuals [32].

Differential Diagnosis

There are many scalp disorders that can cause scalp alopecia. Scarring and non-scarring scalp causes of alopecia should be considered in the differential diagnosis as tinea capitis can present in both ways. Fungal infection should always be excluded in the case of scalp alopecia but usually not in scarring alopecia unless kerion celsi occurs – the more the severe the kerion celsi, the more scars that remain. Hence, the majority of the cases of tinea capitis do not leave scars. The following differential diagnoses are related to the non-scarring alopecia areata, except the unique subtype kerion celsi, which may leave scars and which will be discussed later in this chapter.

Differential Diagnosis of Black Dot Tinea Capitis

A. Alopecia Areata

Alopecia areata is a type of noncicatricial alopecia that causes loss of hair on various hair-bearing areas of the body, mainly on the scalp. Alopecia areata usually starts with the appearance of one (Figure 8.8) or more (Figure 8.9) round or elliptic bare patches, usually with a diameter between 1 and 5 cm, sometimes larger; short hairs, which are narrower at the base, may appear inside or around the patch, due to their appearance they are named "exclamation point" hairs.

Alopceia areata may involve fingernails and toenails and cause nail pitting.

Alopecia areata presents in children, young adults, and adults, while alopecia areata usually presents in young children and rarely in adults. Regarding the morphological presentation, in untreated tinea capitis, broken hairs may be seen 1–3 mm above the scalp level, the broken hairs pull out very easily, and there is no an exclamation point (!) as may be seen in alopecia areata.

In tinea capitis (at the bald areas) mild erythematous lesions covered by fine scales with or without (mild to severe) secondary infection (kerion celsi) can be seen, while in alopecia areata no erythematous inflammatory reaction is seen (although histologically mild inflammation may appear).

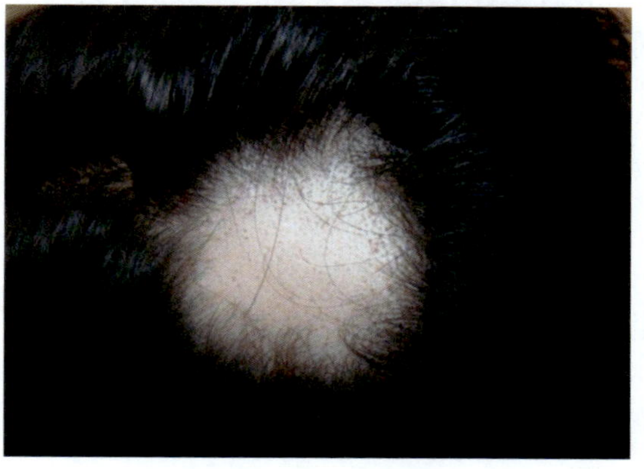

Figure 8.8. Alopecia Areata.

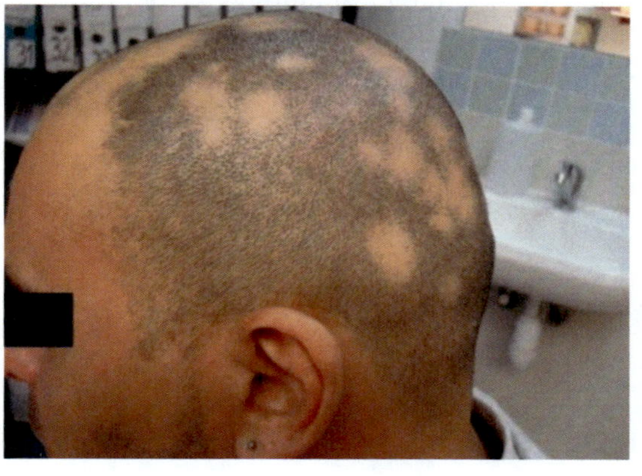

Figure 8.9. Multiple lesions of alopecia areata.

With tinea capitis, it is very important to take the mycological analysis properly; otherwise false negative results may occur. The hair shaft, which is located just beneath and within the superficial skin of the scalp, should be included, together with a sample of the deeper part of the scalp. This is achieved by holding the hairs gently with two fingers and then quickly pulling them out. For painless procedures, very few hairs from the bald area or the peripheral area should be collected together and use of a very rapid pulling action may prevent pain for the patient.

B. Trichotillomania

Trichotillomania is a type of neurological disorder that involves a compulsive urge to pull hair, leading to hair loss mainly on the scalp (Figure 8.10), eyebrows, eyelashes, and face. This disorder can range between small patches of baldness to complete hair loss.

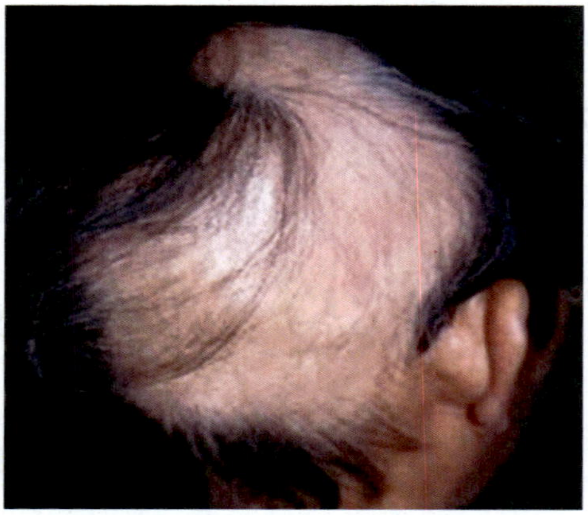

Figure 8.10. Trichotillomania.

This phenomenon sometimes appears with other neurological disorders such as nail biting and/or lichenification (lichen simplex chronicus) or neurotic excoriations that may appear on different parts of the body – usually on the dorsal part of the hands. There are no clinical signs of scalp inflammation, namely erythema, edema, or desquamation. Focusing on the clinical appearance at the hair shaft, different lengths of hair may be seen, and the exclamation point should not be seen. The hairs are not pulled out easily, and no broken hairs should be noted as is seen in tinea capitis.

C. Scalp Psoriasis

Psoriasis is an inflammatory disease that usually involves areas such as the knees, elbows, scalp, lumbosacral areas, intergluteal clefts, and glans penis, but any location can be involved.

The psoriatic rash is characterized by the appearance of reddish papules and/or plaques that are covered by fine scaling or white/silver thick scaling. Following moderate to severe scratching, bleeding spots may appear on the lesions (Auspitz's sign).

Scalp psoriasis may resemble different types of tinea capitis such as black dot tinea capitis, diffuse scale tinea capitis, and in unique circumstances favus.

Psoriatic lesions located on the scalp usually do not cause hair loss and/or broken hairs as can be seen in tinea capitis (Figure 8.11).

It is very important to distinguish between the two disorders. Another point by which to distinguish between scalp psoriasis and tinea capitis is that the scales that cover the psoriatic plaques are usually thick and tightly adherent to the psoriatic plaques. In tinea capitis the scales are much more delicate and can be peeled off very easily.

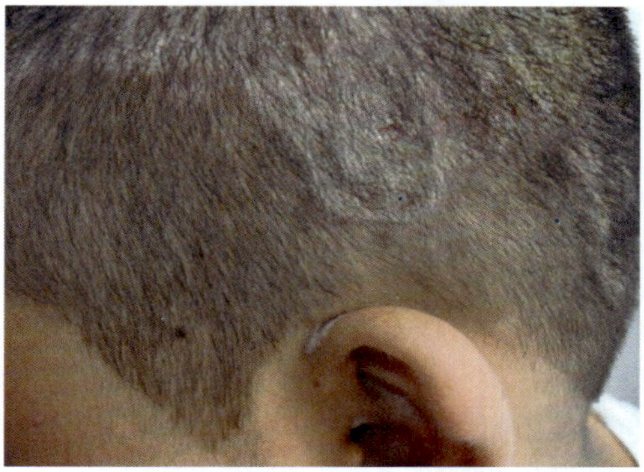

Figure 8.11. Scalp Psoriasis.

Similar to tinea capitis, scalp psoriasis may appear as a single lesion or as multiple lesions.

D. Seborrheic Dermatitis

Seborrheic dermatitis is a chronic inflammatory disorder that mainly involves areas rich with sebaceous glands and is usually located on the scalp (Figure 8.12), face, middle and upper chest and back, and any other areas with a large number of sebaceous glands. Seborreheic dermatitis can present in the form of patchy, yellow scaling or thick crusts.

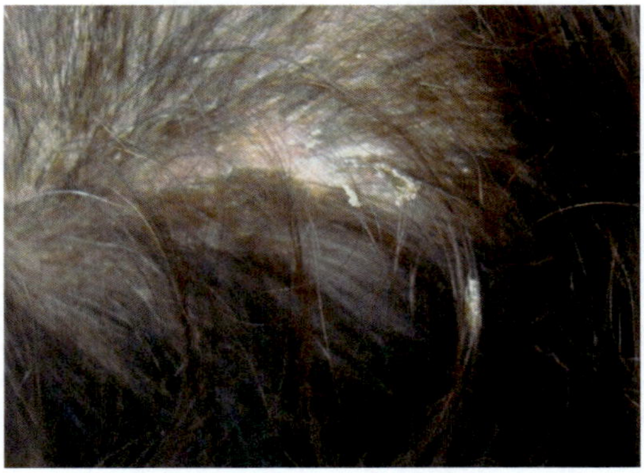

Figure 8.12. Scalp Seborrehic Dermatitis.

Soreness and severe itching rarely occur. One of the most classical locations of seborrheic lesions is the side of the nose and between the eyebrows, as these patches have no well demarcated borders and the lesions are confluent with the surrounding normal skin. In addition to these classical locations, other locations can also be involved. Seborrheic dermatitis may co-occur with psoriasis; therefore, in these combination disorders, it is very hard to make the correct diagnosis. Otherwise, signs of psoriasis should be checked in order to rule out seborrheic dermatitis, such as other locations of psoriatic lesions located at the predelicted areas, nail pitting (although pitting is not a pathognomonic sign), and oil spots. The psoriatic plaques on the scalp are usually much thicker and well-demarcated.

Seborrheic dermatitis of the scalp may in certain circumstances mimic several types of tinea capitis such as the black dot tinea capitis, grey patch tinea capitis, and the diffuse scale tinea capitis.

Differential diagnosis between seborrheic dermatitis located on the scalp and the forehead and tinea capitis can be a great challenge, and the fact that there is no clear demarcation of the lesions adds to the challenge.

It should be stressed that tinea capitis is principally a childhood disease (sometimes adults can be attacked by tinea capitis, too). Regarding the morphology of the scalp between seborrheic dermatitis and tinea capitis lesions, in tinea capitis (black or blond dot tinea subtype), broken hairs combined with easily pulled out hairs should be noted. In seborrheic dermatitis there are no broken hairs and/or easily pulled out hairs.

Differential Diagnosis of Grey Patch Tinea Capitis

A. Atopic Dermatitis

Atopic dermatitis is a chronic inflammatory disorder that causes dry, itchy, scaly skin that may appear on the entire body but mainly appears at the popliteal and cubital fossas. During infancy, it tends to appear on the cheeks, the buttocks, the groin area, and around the neck. Symmetric lesions are typically observed but lesions can also be asymmetric. Concentrating on the atopic lesions, a great variation can be seen regarding the morphologic type of each lesion. In other words, clinical variation exists both within one patient and between different patients. The difference comes from the fact that atopic dermatitis is characterized by waves of improvements and worsening at different times (depending on various factors, such as the severity level of the atopic lesion – acute, sub-acute, or chronic).

Each of the stages has a different severity, and the different clinical manifestations are due to different factors such as secondary infection, lichenification level, skin tone affecting redness level, different climates, and age.

The classic atopic dermatitis chronic lesion is characterized by an irregularly unbounded skin area but can be round (nummular eczema) or reddish unbounded oval shapes with fine scaling with or without lichenification and/or edema.

One of the most important clinical findings compared to fungi is the sharp border of the lesion, which is observed in the fungal layer. In addition, the sharp border is a little more raised and has a more reddish color, which is due to the fungal element progressing centrifugally, dissolving the keratin.

This raised-red border demonstrates the competition between the fungi virulence and the immune system.

Atopic dermatitis of the scalp may sometimes mimic several types of tinea capitis such as the grey patch type and the diffuse scale tinea capitis type, and also may resemble favus. (Figure 8.13)

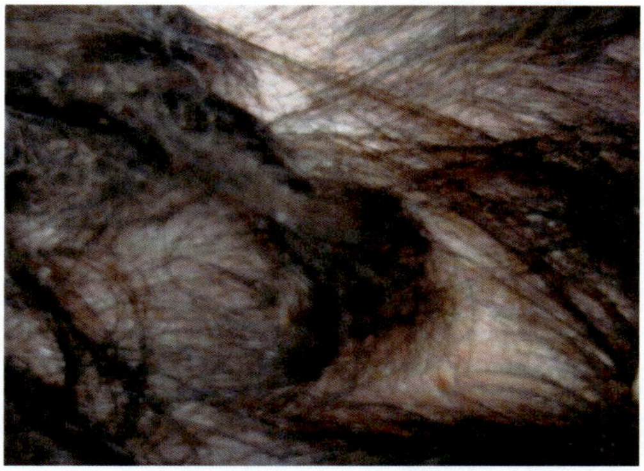

Figure 8.13. Atopic dermatitis involving the scalp.

In atopic dermatitis lesions, there are usually no clear borders or more raised and/or more red borders than in the rest of the lesion.

With respect to lesion morphology, the location and dual sides of the atopic lesions combined with the scalp involvement support the clinical diagnosis of atopic dermatitis.

While the atopic dermatitis lesions in children and adults are located in the classic locations in adults – elbow and knee folds, around the neck, etc., in infants there is an involvement of the cheeks, scalp, around the neck, buttocks, etc.

It is important to emphasize that while patients with fungal infection have the rest of their skin clear, atopic dermatitis patients suffer from dry irritated skin in other regions, too; in relation to the appearance of atopic dermatitis lesions on the scalp, several presentations may be seen. While mild cases may present mild fine scales on different locations of the scalp, the more severe cases may be related to the clinical appearance of tinea amiantacea, which may be a result of atopic dermatitis.

Cradle cap is considered one of the severe presentations of atopic dermatitis, psoriasis, seborrhea, etc. (Figure 8.14). In other words, atopic dermatitis has a wide spectrum of clinical presentations.

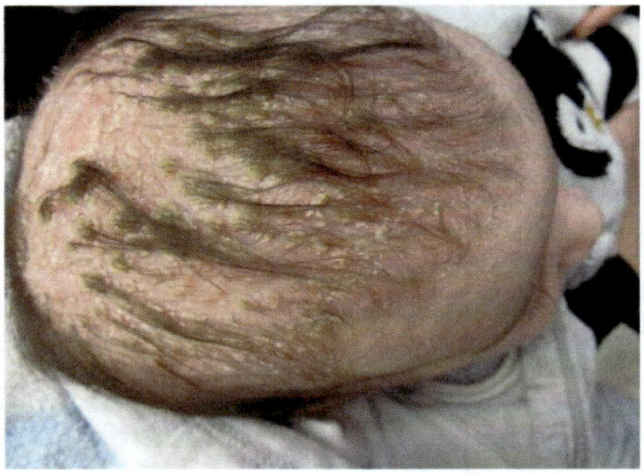

Figure 8.14. Cradle Cap in a baby scalp.

Tinea amiantacea is a skin disorder that manifests in excessive scaling of the scalp, and it can appear as skip lesions or massive confluent lesions. Thick silvery/yellowish scales encircle the hair shafts and may bind tufts of hair (Figure 8.15).

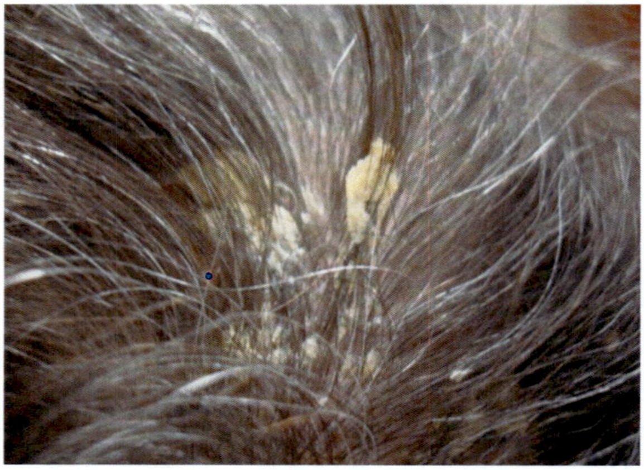

Figure 8.15. Tinea Amiantacea.

Tinea amiantacea can be evoked from one of three disorders: atopic dermatitis, seborrheic dermatitis, and psoriasis, or from unknown origin (Figure 8.15). Pulling a group of hairs once gently in an upward direction, a "shell-like appearance" or "semi roof-like appearance" may be seen.

Atopic dermatitis should be differentiated from seborrheic dermatitis, scabies, psoriasis, and immunodeficiency.

B. Seborrheic Dermatitis

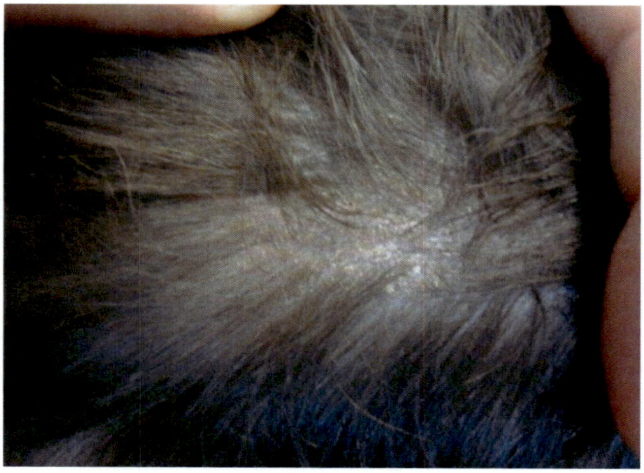

Figure 8.16. Scalp Seborrheic Dermatitis.

In certain circumstances seborrheic dermatitis may resemble the grey patch tinea capitis (Figure 8.16). The scales with the absence of scalp inflammation and the broken hairs above the scalp level support the clinical diagnosis of tinea capitis and not seborrheic dermatitis.

The appearance of grey discoloration is pronounced in the grey patch subtype tinea capitis and not in seborrheic dermatitis patients. However, in dark skin patients the grey discoloration of the scalp may be seen when the seborrheic dermatitis is located on the face or on the upper back/chest, and may resemble sometimes tinea corporis or tinea faciale, respectively.

C. Secondary Syphilis

Due to the fact that this disease has many clinical presentations (thus the name "the great imitator"), it should be ruled out by VDRL/TPHA blood analysis or other available relevant STD analysis. One of the most common clinical presentations of secondary syphilis on the scalp is moth-eaten alopecia. It should be stressed that the moth-eaten alopecia of secondary syphilis is usually seen in adults and very rarely in children. Mycological anaylsis should be done to confirm or reject tinea capitis.

D. Scalp Psoriasis

See more on page 46

Differential Diagnosis of Seborrheic Dermatitis Like/Diffuse Scale Tinea Capitis

A. Atopic Dermatitis

See more on page 48

B. Seborrheic Dermatitis

See more on page 47

C. Scalp Psoriasis (Figure 8.17)

See more on page 46

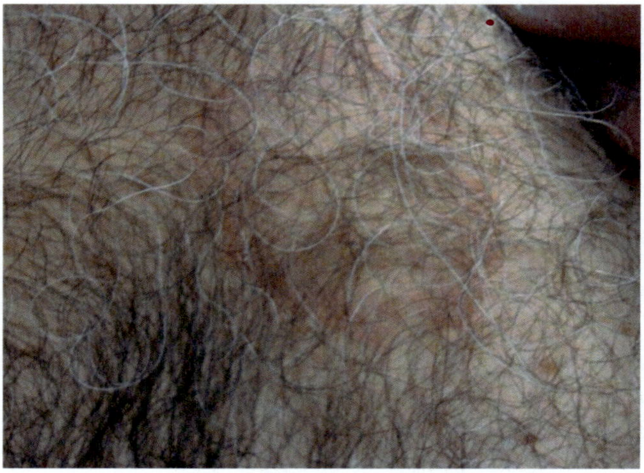

Figure 8.17. Scalp Psoriasis (partially treated).

Differential Diagnosis of Diffuse Pustular Tinea Capitis

A. Folliculitis Decalvans

Folliculitis decalvans (FD) is one of the causes of cicatricial alopecia. It is a rare chronic disorder that presents as pustules and abscesses that involve the hair follicles, which after spontaneous healing resolves in scarring alopecia (Figure 8.18). The cause of this disorder is unknown. Although *Staphylococcus aureus* is found in the pustules/abscesses, it is very important to understand that it is not simply the bacterium itself that is the cause but rather the person's immune system and the bacteria in different relationships. Relevant systemic antibiotics alone will not resolve the problem. No broken hairs or easily pulled hairs are seen; hence kerion celsi may sometimes resemble folliculitis decalvanse, and bacterial analysis should be conducted, relevant systemic antibiotics should be given, and then mycological analysis should be done to confirm the diagnosis of tinea capitis (kerion celsi type).

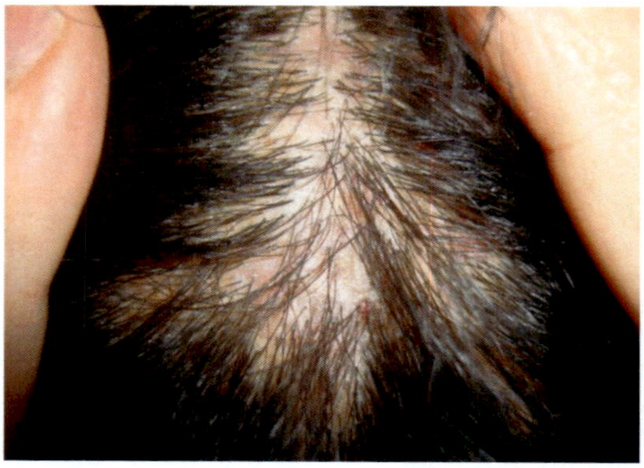

Figure 8.18. Folliculitis Decalvans.

In certain circumstances folliculitis decalvans may resemble several types of tinea capitis, among them diffuse pustular tinea capitis, kerion celsi, variants of tinea capitis, and favus. Since folliculitis decalvans is very rare in infants and young children yet much more common in adults, and on the other hand tinea capitis is rare in adults, folliculitis decalvans is rarely to be considered as a differential diagnosis of tinea capitis. Mycological analysis should be made in the case of any clinical suspicion of tinea capitis.

B. Perifolliculitis Capitis Abscedens et Suffodiens

Perifolliculitis capitis abscedens et suffodiens is a skin disorder that affects the scalp. It manifests as perifollicular pustules, nodules, and abscesses that interconnect with the sinus tracts that drain pus or blood (Figure 8.19). It can be distinguished in differential diagnosis from the diffuse pustular type of tinea capitis, kerion celsi, and favus. This scalp disorder is very rare in infants and young children; therefore the suspicion of perifolliculitis capitis abscedens et suffodiens in infants and young children is doubtful. If there is indeed a suspicion for suffodiens, mycological analysis should be taken.

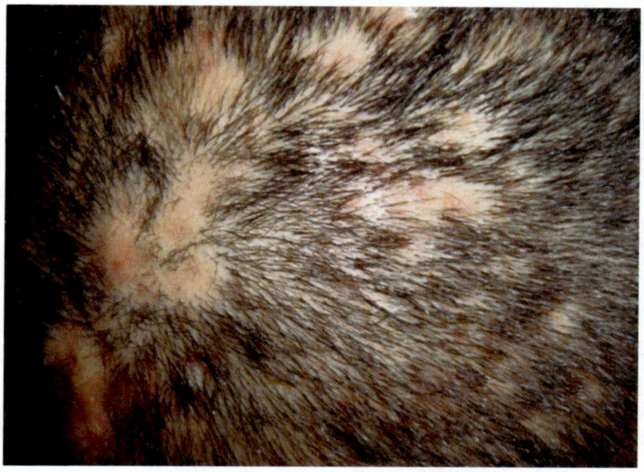

Figure 8.19. Perifolliculitis Capitis Abscedens et Suffodiens.

C. Pustular Psoriasis

Pustular psoriasis is a rare variant of psoriasis. There are several subtypes of pustular psoriasis and the identification of the different types depends on the clinical presentation of the pustules, acute, subacute, or chronic.

The location of the pustule is also variable. In case of acute generalized pustular psoriasis, in the well-known von Zumbusch psoriasis the scalp may also be involved as part of generalized pustular psoriasis. Subacute pustular psoriasis is a rare subtype of pustular psoriasis that is located in the glaberous skin, palms/soles (Figure 8.20) and very rarely on the scalp and manifests as a pustular annular pattern.

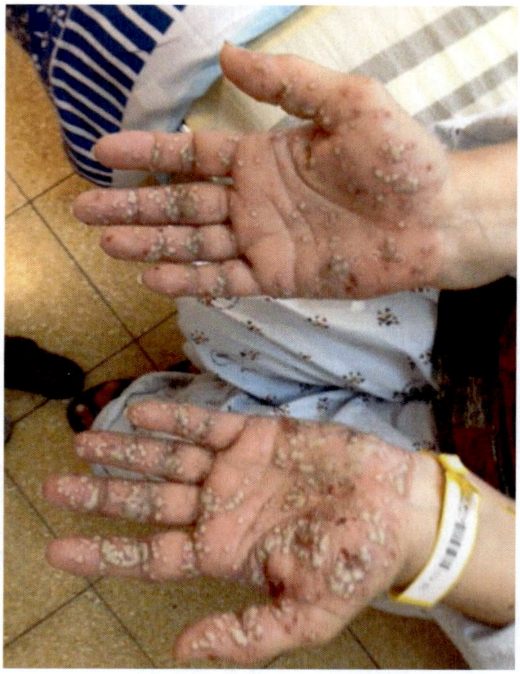

Figure 8.20. Pustular Psoriasis 'palms pustular psoriasis'.

Since tinea capitis is most common in infants and young children, the variant of infantile pustular psoriasis may be included as a differential diagnosis of diffuse pustular tinea capitis.

Differential Diagnosis of Kerion Celsi

A. Folliculitis decalvans

See more on page 52

B. Perifolliculitis capitis abscedens et suffodiens

See more on page 52

C. Impetigo

Impetigo is an acute, highly contagious bacterial infection of the superficial layers of the epidermis. Skin lesions such as cuts, abrasions, and chickenpox may cause secondary infection. Impetigo is a contagious bacterial skin infection that attacks babies and children and is usually caused by *Staphylococcus aureus* or Group A *Streptococcus*. Regarding the location, it could appear at any location on the body but usually attacks exposed areas such as the face, arms, and legs; it rarely occurs on the scalp. The lesion may appear as small vesicles or large bullae or red erosions – which occur as a result of rupture of the vesicles/bullae after a short period of time – such as days. The erosions are covered by moist, golden sticky crusts. (Figure 8.21)

In complicated cases, deeper layers of the skin may be involved. No broken hairs or easily pulled hairs occur, unless the infection invades deeply into the skin; as a result scarring alopecia may occur.

The gravest potential complication of impetigo is post-streptococcal glomerulonephritis, a severe kidney disease that occurs following a strep infection in less than 1% of cases.

Diagnosis of impetigo is usually based solely on the history and clinical appearance.

Bacterial analysis should be taken to establish the diagnosis. In case of clinical appearance that resembles tinea capitis, mycological analysis should be taken after systemic and topical treatment of the secondary infection.

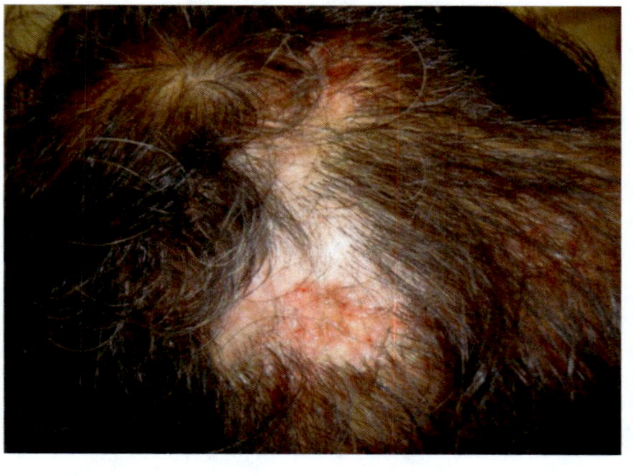

Figure 8.21. Self-inflicted impetiginization: scalp.

D. Scalp Abscess

Scalp abscess is an inflammatory reaction due to different bacteria causing abscesses such as *Staphylococcus* and *Streptococcus* spp. Clinically, abscess is characterized by a collection of pus located in the dermis, and the penetration of the bacteria to that area is due to any type of injury to the skin. Clinically, there is a red, warm, swollen, and tender area ranging in size from several mm up to several cm (Figure 8.22).

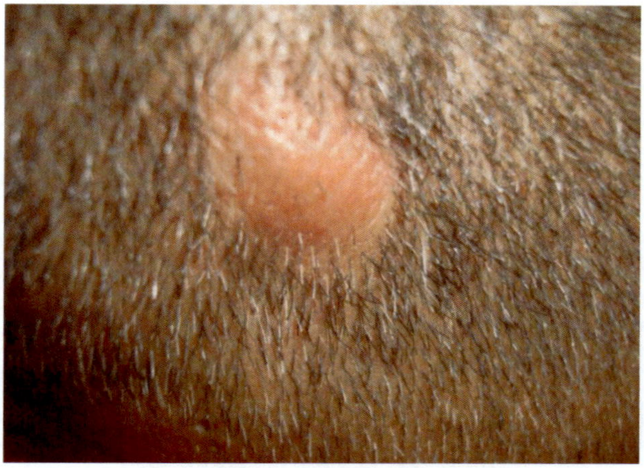

Figure 8.22. Scalp Abscess.

Differential Diagnosis of Favus

A. Seborrheic Dermatitis

See more on page 47

B. Atopic Dermatitis

See more on page 48

C. Scalp Psoriasis

See more on page 46

D. Impetigo

See more on page 54

E. Folliculitis Decalvans

See more on page 52

F. Perifolliculitis Capitis Abscedens et Suffodiens

See more on page 52

G. Secondary Syphilis

See more on page 188

H. Discoid Lupus Erythematosus

Cutaneous lupus erythematosus can be divided into three subtypes: 1) Discoid lupus erythematosus (DLE), 2) Subcutaneous lupus erythematosus (SCLE), and 3) Systemic lupus erythematosus (SLE).

DLE is characterized by inflammation following scarring located on the face, ears, and scalp or other locations on the body and presents as red plaques with a sticky scaling appearance. (Figure 8.23) The center of the lesion is lighter in color with elevated, red, well-demarcated areas. In certain circumstances it may resemble tinea capitis.

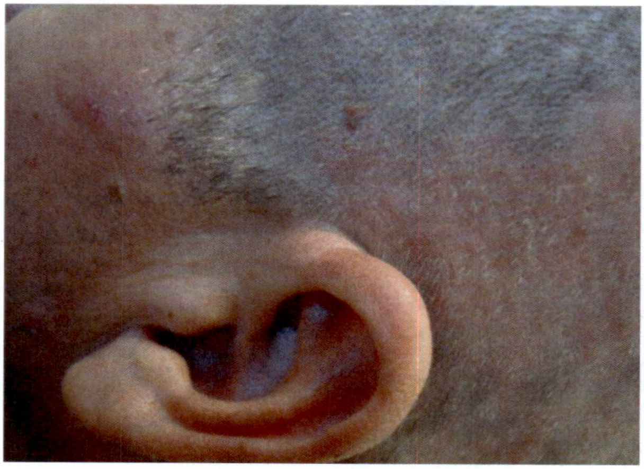

Figure 8.23. Scalp Discoid Lupus erythematosus.

I. Tinea Amiantacea

See more on page 50

Diagnosis

When tinea capitis is suspected, Wood's lamp (filtered ultraviolet light with a peak of 365 nm) should be performed in a dark room. Cases of *Microsporum* such as *M. audouinii, M. canis,* and *M. ferrugineum* will show a bright green fluorescence in the affected hairs. Infection by *Trichophyton schoenleinii* will show a bright/dull green fluorescence. The final diagnosis should be established by direct microscopy and culture. Direct hydroxide microscopy examination of hairs where *Microsporum* infections exist show ectothrix hair colonization with dermatophyte arthroconidia formed and located at the extensor surface of the hair. *T. verrucosum, T. mentagrophytes, T. megninii,* and *T. equinum* also show ectothrix colonization of the hair shaft. Cases of *Trichophyton* infections such as *T. tonsurans and T. violaceum* show endothrix colonization with arthroconidia produced within the hair shaft. [33] Material for mycological examination can be collected using a surgical blade (carefully), toothbrush, or cotton swab from the clinically affected area and placing the specimen onto a glass slide with one or two drops of 10–20% potassium hydroxide (KOH) solution. Since tinea capitis is common in children, extra caution should be taken when obtaining the specimen. A good and painless method to do so, is to very quickly pull a hair bundle from the infected area. The specimen is usually cultured in Sabouraud agar using supplementary chloramphenicol and cyloheximide in order to inhibit co-contaminant culture of bacteria and saprophytic fungi. Usually full length hairs are not infected; however, spores or hyphae may be present at the base of the hair [34].

Additionally, immediate family members of a child who has *T. tonsurans* tinea capitis should also be examined and samples taken for culture whenever possible.

Dermatoscopy can be helpful in the diagnosis of tinea capitis, where the presence of comma-like structures (comma hairs) can be observed when the causative agent is *M. canis*. This can differentiate between cases of alopecia areata where the presence of exclamation mark hairs is characteristic.

Regarding mycological analysis from the scalp, it should be stressed that only dermatophyte infection will be considered as tinea infection of the scalp, because, by definition, tinea capitis is caused by dermatophytes. Non-dermatophyte molds and/or yeast are usually considered to be contamination. In the seborrheic lesions, the so-called *Pityrosporum ovalea/P. orbiculare* exists in large numbers compared to the surrounding area of the scalp.

It is very important to stress that mycological analysis should be interpreted correctly, no over-diagnosis should occur. If non-dermatophyte molds and/or yeasts are found in the mycological analysis, those findings will be considered saprophytes, not pathogens. Sometimes misinterpretation has occurred and systemic treatment is given by mistake.

Treatment

Infections involving hair-bearing skin necessitate oral antifungals, as topical agents fail to penetrate the hair follicle. Hence topical treatment has little place when treating tinea capitis and is only used as adjuvant therapy to systemic antifungals. Patients suspected of having tinea capitis should have a culture performed prior to treatment. Factors that may influence the choice between equally effective therapies include tolerability, safety, compliance, availability of liquid formulation, and cost.

Griseofulvin was the first significant oral antifungal agent available to treat tinea capitis. Since the late 1950s, griseofulvin has been the gold standard for systemic therapy of tinea capitis. It is active against dermatophytes and has a long-term safety profile. The main disadvantage is the long duration of treatment required. The recommended pediatric dose is 10–20 mg/kg/day for 6 to 8 weeks. Griseofulvin is advised to be taken with a fatty meal to facilitate absorption. At this dose, some authors report failure and many experts recommend a higher dose of 20–25 mg/kg/day. Many patients require longer treatment, especially if the infection is caused by *M. canis*. Treatment should be continued for an additional two weeks beyond clinical resolution so that the organism has been eradicated [28]. Data suggest high efficacy rate of griseofulvin for both *T. tonsurans* and *M. canis* for tinea capitis. The reported response rate is 60.7% in a follow-up period of 8 months [34]. The adverse reactions of griseofulvin are headache, epigastric distress, nausea, abdominal cramps, vomiting, diarrhea, hepatic dysfunction, morbilliform eruption, eruption, urticarial, photosensitivity, leukopenia, neutropenia, and lupus erythematous. Because griseofulvin is derived from a species of *Penicillium*, it is expected that patients who are intolerant to penicillin or penicillamine may develop a reaction to griseofulvin; however, this phenomenon is infrequently reported [35]. In most cases, periodic monitoring of the drug's side effects is suggested.

Oral triazole (itraconazole, fluconazole) and allylamine (terbinafine) antifungals also appear to be safe and effective. Fluconazole at a dose of 6 mg/kg/day for 20 days is 89% effective. Other treatment regimens include once-weekly dosing of 8 mg/kg for 8-16 weeks and 6 mg/kg for two weeks followed by an additional week of treatment four weeks later. Fluconazole absorption does not depend on food intake. The most common adverse effects are gastrointestinal problems, cutaneous eruption, and headache. Fluconazole inhibits cytochrome P4503A4 and 2C9 enzyme systems.

The treatment of tinea capitis with systemic itraconazole at doses of 3–5 mg/kg/day for 4 to 6 weeks may be sufficient. Tinea capitis caused by the *Trichophyton* spp. respond effectively in 4 weeks [35], but longer treatment may be required when the causative agent is *M. canis*. Pulse therapy at a dose of 5 mg/kg/day for one week per month for 1 to 3 pulses can be also effective. Itraconazole is better absorbed when taken with a fatty meal. The most commonly reported side effects are headache, skin eruption, gastrointestinal problems, and deranged liver enzymes. The side effects are usually mild and transient in nature; in moderate to severe side effects the systemic treatment should be discontinued. Itraconazole inhibits cytochrome the P4503A4 enzyme system of the liver.

Terbinafine at a dose of 3–6 mg/kg/day for 2 to 4 weeks can be used for eradication of *Trichophyton* spp. Longer treatment periods of 4 to 8 weeks are required for the eradication of *Microsporum* as terbinafine is not as effective as it is against the *Trichophyton* species, and in case of treatment with terbinafine higher doses may be required. An alternative regimen is that of pulse therapy. Terbinafine's absorption is unaffected by the presence of food. The most frequently reported side effects are deranged liver enzymes, epigastric pain, anorexia, and vesiculopustular eruption. Terbinafine inhibits the cytochrome P4502D6 enzyme system and should be kept in mind when prescribing.

In comparative studies of tinea capitis caused by *M. canis*, griseofulvin and itraconazole have shown about the same efficacy [37]. Some studies comparing terbinafine and griseofulvin when the predominant organism was the *Trichophyton* species have shown similar efficacy. Others have shown a higher complete cure rate and a mycological cure rate higher for terbinafine than for griseofulvin (45.1% vs. 39.2% and 61.5% vs. 55.5%, respectively) [39]. In this study, patients who received more than 20 mg/kg per day of griseofulvin were not found to have a higher complete cure rate than those receiving a dose of 10–19.9 mg/kg per day. A study comparing itraconazole and terbinafine when used to treat tinea capitis caused by *T. violaceum* showed similar efficacy [40]. The newer oral antifungal agents, including terbinafine, itraconazole, and fluconazole, appear to have similar adverse effects to those of griseofulvin in children with tinea capitis caused by the *Trichophyton* spp., while requiring a much shorter duration of treatment; [38]; however, they are more expensive.

Scarring can cause significant and extensive disfigurement, especially in the case of inflammatory tinea capitis and kerion. Oral glucocorticoids co-prescribed can potentially reduce the associated inflammation and pain and also reduce scarring. Although there are no randomized trials that provide evidence of an improved cure rate, glucocorticoids have been reported to be beneficial in reducing inflammation [40]. Opinions on this matter appear to be a topic of controversy between expects since some feel that oral glucocorticoids are not beneficial.

It is important when managing patients with tinea capitis to apply preventative measures since the disease is contagious. Individuals who are residing with infected patients should be examined and treated simultaneously in an attempt to reduce re-infection. Household transmission can also be prevented through treatment of infected animals. Attempts at eradication require a strong collaboration between dermatologists and veterinary services for successful treatment. Additionally, articles such as combs, brushes, and hats used by the patient should be either disinfected or discarded or at least the sharing of certain objects should be discouraged. Different shampoos have been shown to help the eradication of dermatophytes and reduce transmission. Selenium sulphide, zinc pyrithione, povidone iodine, and ketoconazole shampoos are commonly prescribed. These shampoos should be used two to four times weekly for two to four weeks and should be applied to the scalp and hair for 5 minutes.

Routine screening in schools (main mode of transmission) can be difficult yet cost-effective, and the screening of children who have infected classmates may be of benefit.

Complications

Fungal infection of the scalp may infiltrate the surrounding area of the scalp such as the forehead, upper neck, and temporal areas. Secondary bacterial infections can complicate tinea capitis, especially if left untreated, leading to kerion formation. Non-reversible patches of alopecia can also affect patients. Id reactions (also known as dermatophytid reactions) can complicate cases of tinea capitis. An id can also be observed before and during treatment with griseofulvin and may resolve with ongoing griseofulvin treatment. Id reactions present at a distant site as symmetrical erythematous papules and plaques, most commonly over the face, neck, and upper trunk, but can also be generalized (Figure 8.24).

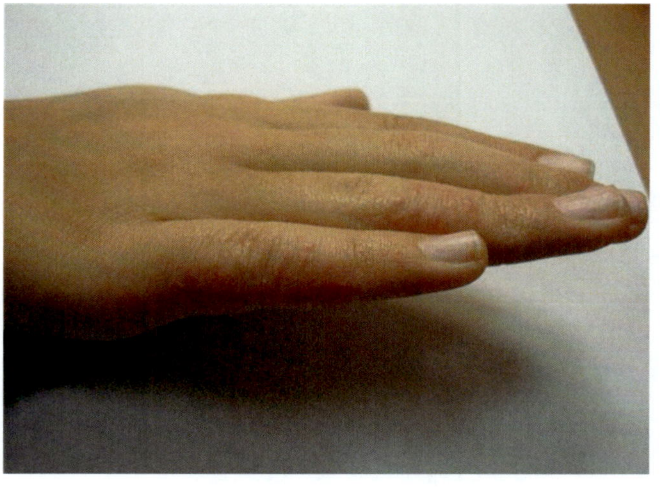

Figure 8.24. Id reaction due to tinea capitis.

The dermatophyte reactions resolve once the original infection has been controlled and can be managed with the use of topical steroid treatment and emollients. Erythema nodosum, hypopigmented scaly lesions, has also been described as a skin reaction to fungal infection of the scalp.

Follow-Up

Clinical and mycological examinations should be conducted at regular intervals of 2-4 weeks. Treatment may be stopped after the culture becomes negative or when hair regrowth is clinically evident. Duration of treatment should be individualized according to response.

Chapter 9

Tinea Faciale

Synonyms: tinea faciei

Definition: Tinea faciale indicates dermatophytos is affecting the glabrous skin of the face, thus excluding the areas of the moustache- and beard-growing regions in adult males, which are named tinea moustache and tinea barbei, respectively.

Tinea faciale is often separated from tinea corporis and regarded as a separate entity in its own right due to the problem of distinguishing it from other photosensitive dermatoses such as lupus erythematosus and polymorphous light eruption, or other dermatoses such as seborrhea and seborrheic dermatitis or psoriasis. In addition, it should be considered as a distinct form because of the distinct facial anatomy and physiology characteristics of the disease.

Epidemiology

Tinea faciale is considered a rare dermatophyte infection affecting the glabrous skin of the face that occurs worldwide.

Tinea faciale seems to represent less than 1% of official dermatoses, and when classified together with tinea corporis, it accounts for 3–4% of all cases of tinea corporis [41]. The true incidence and prevalence of tinea faciale worldwide remains unknown, and though many studies have been undertaken of the epidemiology of dermatophytoses, only a few large case series of tinea faciale have been reported, most of them analyzing data collected over short periods of time [42].

Tinea faciale occurs worldwide but has a predilection for warm, humid climates [43]. Tinea faciale may occur in all age groups, although two major peaks of incidence have been observed– the first in childhood with a primarily male prevalence (Figure 9.1), and the second peak in adults mainly aged 40 and older, with a female prevalence [41, 42].

Tinea faciale and tinea barbei may co-occur. (Figure 9.2)

The occurrence in children often results from direct contact with animals. Children are usually infected during school vacations, being in more frequent contact with pets. The other peak incidence is adults, who commonly have heightened physical activity, especially between 20–40 years [43]. While infrequent, tinea faciale has also been described in infant and neonates, who probably got contaminated by family members [44-47].

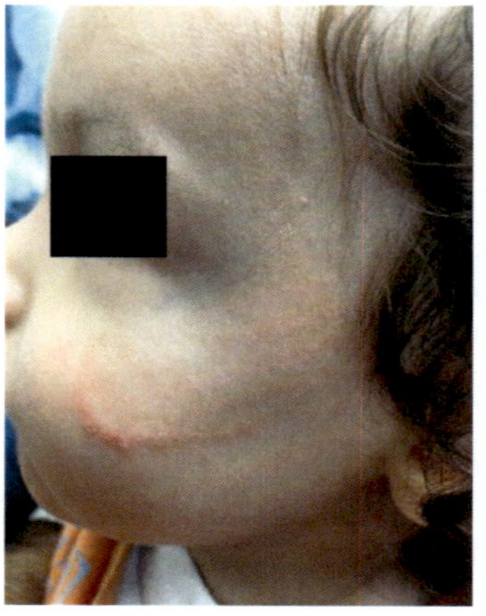

Figure 9.1. Tinea Faciale 1.

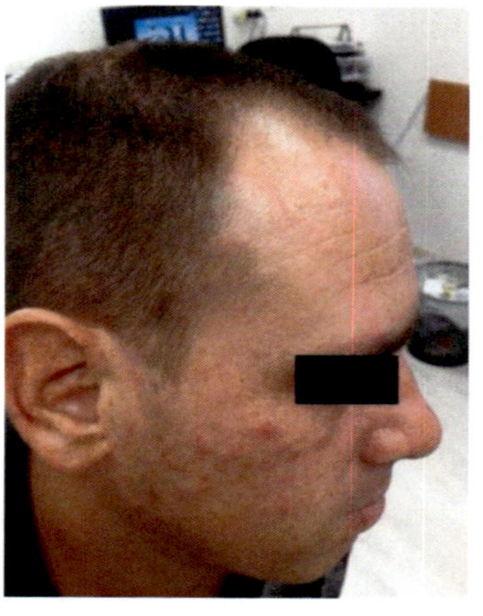

Figure 9.2. Tinea Faciale 2.

It has been suggested that females are affected more frequently than males, but the difference may be semantic, as dermatophyte infections on the bearded areas of males are often diagnosed as tinea barbae, whereas in females they are more likely to be diagnosed as tinea faciale [41].

Pathogens

Tinea faciale infection is frequently the result of professional exposure to infected animals or inter-human contact during leisure activities. It is also acquired from contact with infected animals, including domestic pets and livestock. Infected animals are usually asymptomatic. It can also be spread through person-to-person contact from fungal infections anywhere on the body [48].

The culprit dermatophytes vary according to the geographical location and the potential reservoirs in the environment.

The dermatophytes commonly implicated are: *Trichophyton rubrum* [44], *Trichophyton mentagrophytes* [49], and *Microsporum canis* [43]. In atypical presentations, *Trichophyton mentagrophytes* is the most common organism isolated [50].

Other etiological pathogens implicated in the pathogenesis of tinea faciale include *T. tonsurans, Epidermophyton flocossum, T. violaceum, M. canis, Microsporum gypseum, Trichophyton violaceum,* and *Trichophyton erinacei.* The frequency of these fungi varies according to the geographical prevalence.

In the United States, *Trichophyton tonsurans, T. rubrum*, and *M. canis* are the most usual causative species [41], whereas in Croatia and Spain, *T. mentagrophytes, T. rubrum,* and *T. granulosa* are the most frequently identified dermatophytes In Italy, *M. canis* is the most reported causative agent of tinea faciale and tinea corporis in several regions. [49]

Zoophilic dermatophytes, such as *T. verrucosum* and *M. canis,* are found around the globe in association with livestock and pets.

Tinea faciale is extremely rarely seen among infants. Up to the present, *T. rubrum, T. violaceum, Microsporum gypseum, M. canis,* and *T. tonsurans* have been reported to cause tinea faciale and tinea corporis among neonates aged 2 to 28 days [46, 51].

The concurrence of tinea capitis and tinea faciale is well known, and this association is especially marked in regions where *T. tonsurans* is predominant and is the major cause of tinea capitis [42].

Contributing Factors

The main factors that favor tinea faciale infection in children and adolescents are promiscuity, crowded places such as schools and sports centers, and increased contact with domestic animals and play [41].

Contributing factors that increase mycotic infections in adults include life-style changes, gyms, swimming pools and sports centers, and also exposure to zoophilic dermatophytes in farmers during work, or in taking care of rabbits, sheep, and cattle.

Tinea faciale occurs more frequently in subjects who reside in tropical climates [52].

Outbreaks have occurred in wrestlers or individuals who experience fair amounts of skin-to-skin contact and/or trauma [53].

It is also acquired from contact with infected animals, including domestic pets and livestock that are usually asymptomatic. Tinea faciale has also been noted to occur more frequently after holidays and vacations [54].

Repeated washing, exposure to the sun and pollution, and use of creams and cosmetics often contribute to a modification of the clinical picture and result in an atypical presentation, which may lead to misdiagnosis.

Clinical Presentation

Typical manifestation of tinea faciale is one or more fine circular or oval erythematous plaques covered by very fine scales tending to be clear in central areas. Tinea faciale most often begins as flat, scaly plaques that develop a raised border that may advance outwards in all directions, and may or may not develop papules, vesicles, and crusts. The central area becomes hypopigmented or brown and less scaly as this occurs.

Tinea faciale can occur in single or multiple scaly, fine plaques with or without an annular structure with central clearing [41,42]. This clinical manifestation is similar to tinea corporis.

Lesions may produce a burning or tingling sensation and be mildly pruritic or asymptomatic. Sunlight often exacerbates symptoms. Tinea faciale can clinically mimic other facial dermatoses and is often initially misdiagnosed and treated as other skin conditions.

Many lesions tend to progress with time, and it often requires more than 6 months and even up to 2 years before they are diagnosed [55].

Tinea faciale occurs simultaneously with other dermatophytic infections, especially with tinea corporis, tinea capitis, and onychomycosis; hence other possible involved areas need to be examined [40]. One study showed that in 85% of tinea faciale patients the nails, especially the toenails, were also infected by the same agent that was isolated from the face [56]. In cases of persistent tinea faciale infection and frequent relapses, alternative sources of infection need to be checked.

Atypical Forms

Tinea faciale is a dermatophyte infection of the face that may consist of very polymorphic lesions, which can be atypical as there is a broad range in size, degree of inflammation, and depth of invasion. Atypical presentations are more frequently observed in adults than in children and may be characterized by patches of erythema without scaling, simple popular lesions, or pustules [50] (Figure 9.3).

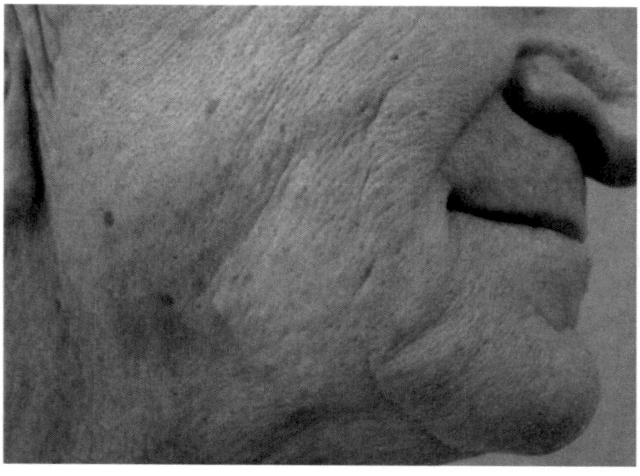

Figure 9.3. Atypical Tinea Faciale.

The use of topical steroids on undiagnosed mycotic lesions favors a pathomorphosis, losing their more characteristic features and symptoms. In addition, exposure to sunlight, repeated washing, and use of cosmetics often determine atypical clinical presentation that may lead to incorrect diagnosis. These factors certainly contribute to the pathomorphosis of the lesions, thus changing the clinical pictures of the dermatophytosis so that they mimic other dermatitises such as the photo-induced forms.

Zoophilic dermatophytes, such as *T. verrucosum* and *M. canis*, are associated with more severe inflammatory reactions than those caused by anthropophilic fungi. More severe inflammatory plaques are round, intensely inflamed, and can have a boggy, pustular surface. Pustules may result from the infection of hair follicles. Secondary bacterial infection or bacterial folliculitis can also occur.

Tinea faciale located at the periocular area is rare condition. Several cases of this rare condition were reported [57]. Due to the fact that periocular tinea, may resemble other skin diseases such seborrheic dermatitis, contact dermatitis etc., the correct diagnosis is often missed . Well demarcated borders of the perioccular tinea usually located at the glabrous skin rather than at the scalp areas may help for the suspicious of fungal infection. Sometimes severe inflammatory reaction may be seen at the perioccular tinea as may be seen in tinea capitis complicated with kerion celci [58-60].

The following clues can be of help in diagnosing atypical tinea faciale:

- Key features that should arouse suspicion for tinea include the presence of scaling, and exacerbation with the use of topical corticosteroids.
- Small follicular papules and vesicle-pustules with brittle or fragmented hairs inside.
- Serpiginous if not semi-annular borders with constant scaling, even if a central clearing is absent and desquamation seems diffused.
- Indolence and very slow progression of disease, especially compared with diseases such as discoid lupus or polymorphous light eruption.
- Less symmetrical onset and progression of the lesion.
- Tinea is not a common skin disease for neonates and infants, which may be a clue that their parents or other intimate contacts have encountered similar dermatophytosis.
- In periocular tinea, the loss of eyelashes or eyebrows can be a helpful clinical feature.

In case the lesions are located around the eyes towards the forehead, look for sharp edges at the edges of the lesions.

Diagnosis

Tinea faciale can mimic many dermatological skin conditions; hence, mycological investigation is essential for diagnosis. This includes direct examination (KOH) and culturing. Direct mycological examination with potassium hydroxide (20% KOH) preparations made with scrapings at multiple sites within the affected area can confirm the diagnosis in the majority of cases.

Direct microscopy in addition to detecting dermatophyte hyphae can be used to identify parasites such as demodex. Surface scrapings should be obtained from the border, where there are more fungal elements. Scrapings are placed on a slide in 10–20% KOH solution with the addition of dimethyl sulfoxide (DMSO). The latter dissolves background keratinocytes to enhance the visualization of fungal elements. If DMSO is not used, the slide should be warmed. The specimen is then examined with a light microscope. Microscopic examination of potassium hydroxide (KOH) preparations is the simplest, most rapid and most sensitive test. It should be performed in every case of possible mycotic infection.

Fungus detection can be followed by mycological culture to determine the species but does not need to be performed routinely.

If one has a high degree of suspicion for tinea but the KOH preparation is negative for fungal elements, then rapid response to antifungal therapy is most probably due to improper sampling of the area or a mistake that was made by the mycologist. There could be other options; for example, there is only skin dryness and no fungus, and what assists the dryness is the moisturizer – of which the antifungal cream mainly consists. The antifungal ingredient did not have any influence on the dryness, but the moisturizer did.

When diagnosis is in doubt, cutaneous biopsy can be helpful in establishing the correct diagnosis. The histopathological features of tinea faciale can be variable. These can range from simple chronic hyperkeratosis to a different degree of epidermal spongiosis with infiltration by mononuclear cells and neutrophils [61]. The common intermediate presentation is that of chronic dermatitis with hyperkeratosis, parakeratosis, hypergranulosis or hypogranulosis, infliltration of mononuclear cells, spongiosis, and mild to moderate acanthosis [62]. The dermal infiltrate is perivascular in principle, rather than periadnexal [41, 63-65].

A Periodic Acid Schiff (PAS) stain is appropriate in the setting of dermatophyte infection as well [66-67]. PAS staining can aid in detecting hyphae in the stratum corneum [43].

False negatives can occur in fungal culture for a number of reasons, including prior use of antifungal drugs and sampling error. Polymerase chain reaction (PCR) is more accurate than traditional culture (beware of over-diagnosis), and the results are rapid, available within days. PCR is not widely available and not routinely used [55].

Differential Diagnosis

Tinea faciale is frequently mistaken for other infections because of its pleomorphic appearance and broad spectrum of differential diagnosis.

Tinea faciale may clinically resemble several skin diseases such as seborrheic dermatitis, polymorphous light eruption or other photosensitivity and as a result it was found that 50% of patients with tinea faciale were misdiagnosed as having a photosensitive skin disorder [69].

Misdiagnosed tinea faciale often leads to a delay in appropriate therapy. Tinea faciale treated with topical steroids or calcineurin inhibitors may lose some of its characteristic features and can result in a change in the clinical appearance and resultant tinea incognito.

It is important to consider tinea in the differential diagnosis of all facial eruptions.

A. Discoid Lupus Erythematosus

Discoid lupus erythematosus (DLE) is a type of skin lesion usually located on the face, scalp, ears, and other exposed skin areas. DLE is an autoimmune disorder in which autoantibodies attack different locations at the dermis–epidermis junction and cause skin lesions.

Clinically there is an erythematous plaque covered with sticky scales, and in certain circumstances may resemble tinea capitis or tinea barbae. The DLE lesions have well-circumscribed borders and the center of the lesions is flattened somehow. The attached scales in DLE are different from the point of view of the attachment to the underlying skin. In tinea faciale/corporis the scales are usually fine and pull off easily. In any case of suspicious fungal infection, mycological analysis should be taken.

See more in page 56

B. Polymorphous Light Eruption (PLE)

Polymorphous light eruption is a type of eruption that is caused by the sun, usually located at the areas exposed to sunlight as a result of photosensitivity. This type of rash has several forms, hence the name polymorphous. The same patient would experience one form of the rash. PLE appears much more commonly in females than males (Figure 9.4). Some children may be affected. The classical clinical presentation of PLE is red to pink raised papules located at the outer side of the face, neck, or other exposed areas. These papules may converge to form a type of plaque that may sometimes resemble tinea faciale.

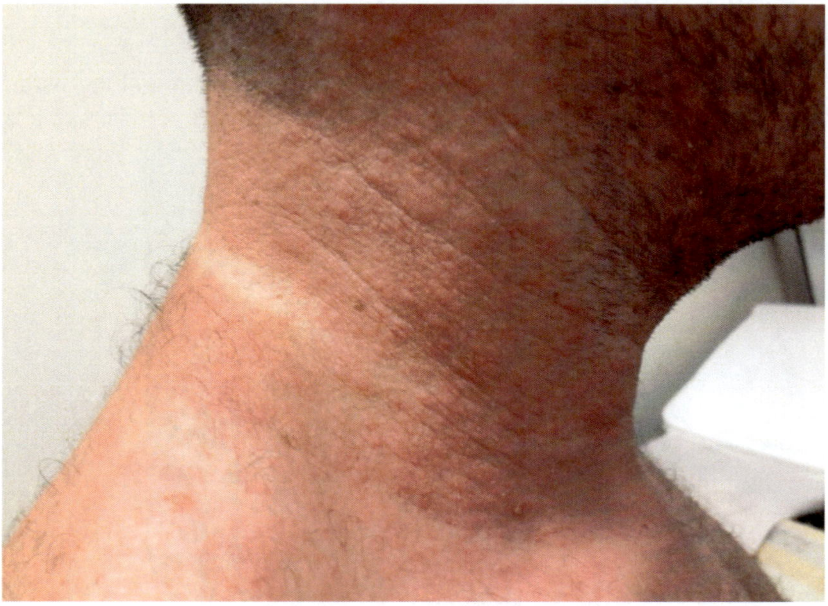

Figure 9.4. PLE-Polymorphous Light Eruption.

C. Lymphocytic Infiltration

Lymphocytic infiltration is a type of T-cell benign lymphocyte that infiltrates the skin, causing the appearance of red spots with a diameter of several mm up to 2 cm and located in different areas of the body, but may also appear on the face (Figure 9.5). The appearance of these papules may be arranged in an annular pattern that resembles tinea faciale. Lymphocytic infiltration usually has no scales. Biopsy with specific stains should be applied for final diagnosis.

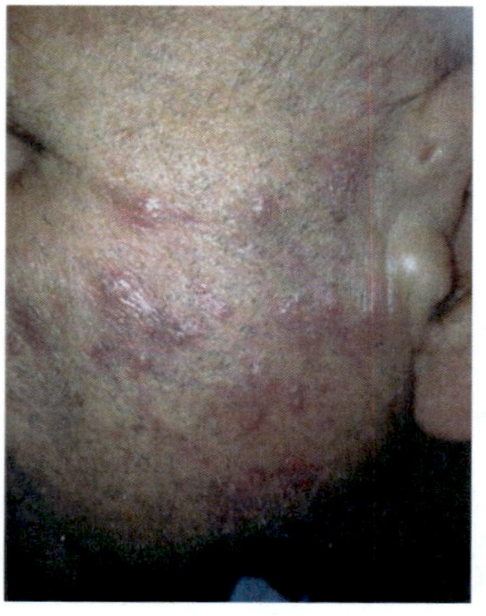

Figure 9.5. Lymphocytic Infiltration.

D. Rosacea

Rosacea is a relatively common rash that involves facial flushing along with a stinging, itching or burning sensation. Its variable clinical signs include erythema, telangiectasia (Figure 9.6), papules and/or pustules which in certain circumstances may resemble acne vulgaris (Figure 9.7).

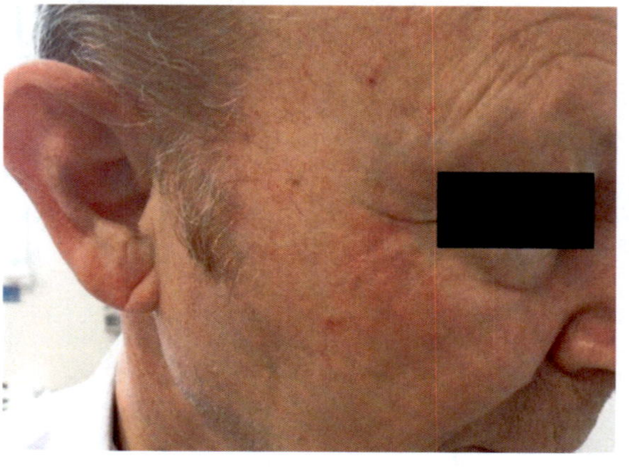

Figure 9.6. Telangiectatic rosacea.

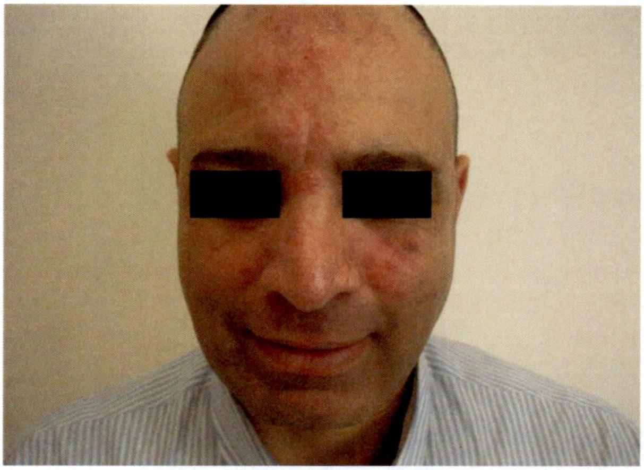

Figure 9.7. Papulo Pustular Rosacae.

Rosacea is usually diagnosed clinically, although skin biopsy from rosacea lesions is not fully pathognomonic but sometimes it is done just to rule out other skin disorders such as lupus erythematosus, sarcoidosis or other granulomatus. Rosacea lesions may sometimes arrange in an annular pattern having the clinical presentation of tinea faciale, but the classical distribution of rosacea may lead to the diagnosis of popular rosacea. With any suspicions for tinea faciale, mycological analysis should taken.

E. Seborrheic Dermatitis

See more on page 47

F. Atopic Dermatitis

See more on page 48

G. Contact Dermatitis

Regarding the morphologic parameters of contact dermatitis, the condition may sometimes resemble tinea corporis simply because of the fact that both contact dermatitis and tinea capitis have well-demarcated borders; allergic contact dermatitis (usually) has no well-demarcated borders. This kind of disease is not considered one of the differential diagnoses of tinea corporis. The distribution of the lesions is very important. The distribution of tinea corporis is located on the buttocks (above and/or beneath the buttocks) and the sides of the abdomen or other parts of the body. Allergic contact dermatitis usually appears on the hands and also (less frequently) at the locations mentioned above regarding tinea corporis. Allergic contact dermatitis located on the face areas usually has no well-demarcated borders and is located more often on the sides of the neck and around the eyes but could occur on any location. In cases in which allergic contact dermatitis might have a clinical picture of well-circumscribed borders, somehow the suspicion of tinea faciale will be taken into account and mycological analysis should be taken.

H. Perioral Dermatitis (Periorificial Dermatitis)

Perioral dermatitis is a common rash usually located around the mouth and consists of small red dense or sparse papules (Figure 9.8). One of the major characteristics of this rash is that there is no involvement of the lips and around them. This rash could occur around the nose and eyes.

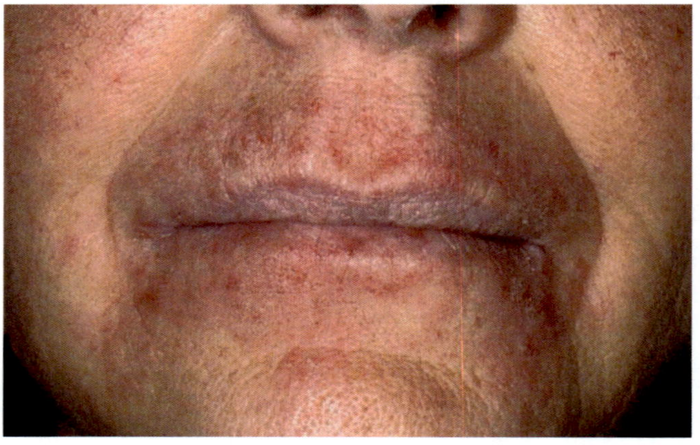

Figure 9.8. Perioral Dermatitis.

Another type of perioral dermatitis – granulomatous perioral dermatitis – causes inflamed papules and pustules. It occurs more often in women between the ages of 25 and 40 and rarely in men. The cause of this is unknown but could happen by using high potency steroid cream for an unknown reason, by neglecting facial hygiene, or using makeup that contains Vaseline. Sometimes several papules flow together, making a circinate configuration that may mimic tinea faciale.

I. Pityriasis Alba

Pityriasis alba is one of the minor criteria of atopic dermatitis (Figure 9.9). Pityriasis alba appears as whitish papules covered by very tiny scars, round or elliptical in shape, 1–5 cm, but could be smaller or larger (Figure 9.10). Pityriasis alba occurs more often in children and is more pronounced in dark-skinned children. Clinically, these fine white plaques have well-demarcated borders, but there is no central healing appearance.

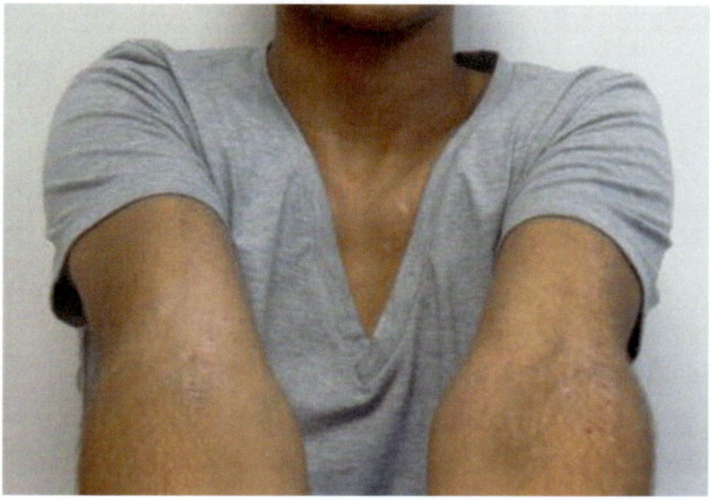

Figure 9.9. Atopic Dermatitis.

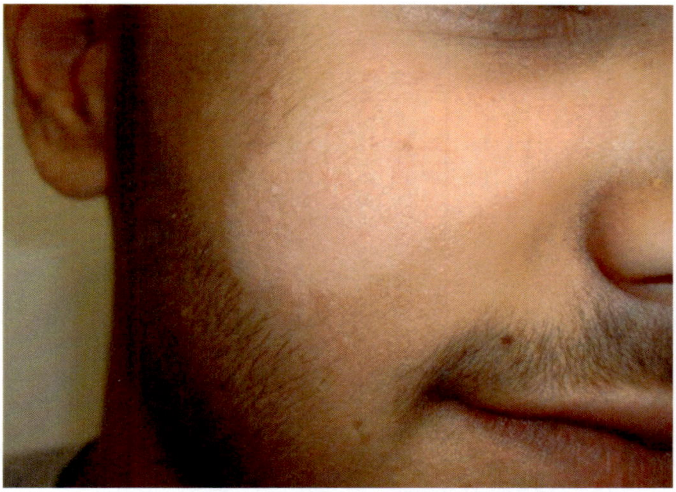

Figure 9.10. Pityriasis Alba in a child with Atopic Dermatitis.

J. Impetigo

In case the impetigo is located on the face and might have an annular pattern, the differential diagnosis of tinea faciale might be considered. In such a case the bacterial cause (if one exists) should be treated properly, after which mycological analysis should be taken (Figure 9.11).

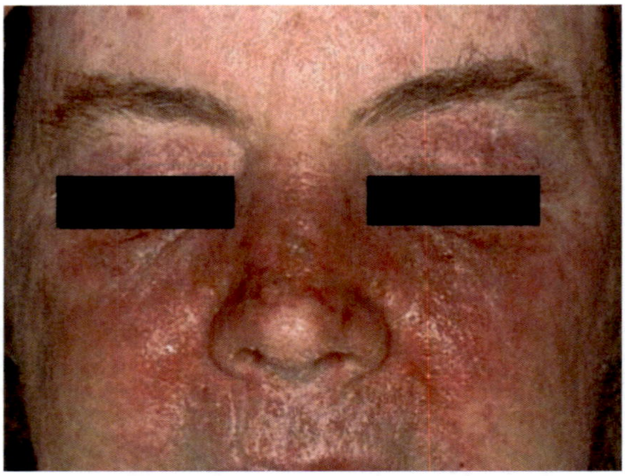

Figure 9.11. Impetignization of the face.

K. Granuloma Annulare

Granuloma annulare is a common benign inflammatory dermatosis of unknown cause.

Granuloma annulare is clinically characterized by the appearance of little dense beads, which have a bit of a glaze on the side.

The main characteristic of these lesions is that their edges are well-defined, raised, and stand out more than the center of the lesion or the outer uninvolved skin around it.

Granuloma annulare usually appears bilaterally on the dorsal side of the hands, chest, shoulders, and rarely on the face (Figure 9.12). If there is involvement of the face combined with involvement on the hands and shoulders, etc., it should be stressed that rarely will one find a fungal infection that is confined to the arms and/or the chest and not in any other locations.

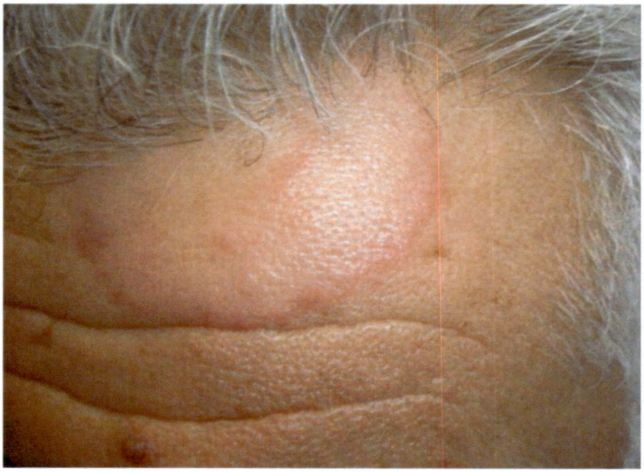

Figure 9.12. Granuloma Anulare Face.

One of the parameters helping in diagnosis is the lack of scaling in granuloma annulare, which is found in fungal infection.

Granuloma annulare may cause mild or a more severe itching, similarly to fungal contamination.

A biopsy should be taken in order to diagnose the granuloma culture.

L. Lichen Planus

Lichen planus is one of the most common papulosquamous disorders. It presents as an inflammatory dermatitis that affects less than 1% of the population. Clinically, there are erythematous/violaceous papules or plaques covered with fine sticky scales; the papules/plaques are typically polygonal but could have other shapes. Many subtypes of lichen planus exist. Hence, we are dealing with tinea faciale lichen planus, which is different than tinea faciale. The color and shape of lichen planus papules and especially the sticky scales can help to differentiate it from tinea faciale.

M. Borderline Lepromatous Leprosy

Borderline lepromatous leprosy is a chronic bacterial disease caused by *Microbacterium leprae*. The disease can attack the skin, mucus membrane, the nervous system, etc. There are several clinical presentations, beginning with indeterminate leprosy with a very mild presentation, and lepromatous leprosy, which is the most severe case. The borderline tuberculoid leprosy and borderline leprosy are considered as mid-strength leprosy disease. The lesions also have elevated well-demarcated borders, which sometimes mimic tinea faciale or tinea corporis. The clinical presentation is determined by the strength of the specific immune response against the bacterium.

Clinically, 3 of the 6 clinical subtypes of skin leprosy may sometimes resemble tinea infection, and it is due to one of these 3 subtypes: 1) Borderline tuberculoid leprosy (BT), 2) Borderline leprosy (BB), and 3) Borderline lepromatous leprosy (LL). Their plaques may have well-demarcated borders with fine scales, and sometimes central healing may occur (Figure 9.13).

Loss of skin sensation (temperature and touch) is one of the major keys to differentiate it from fungal infection.

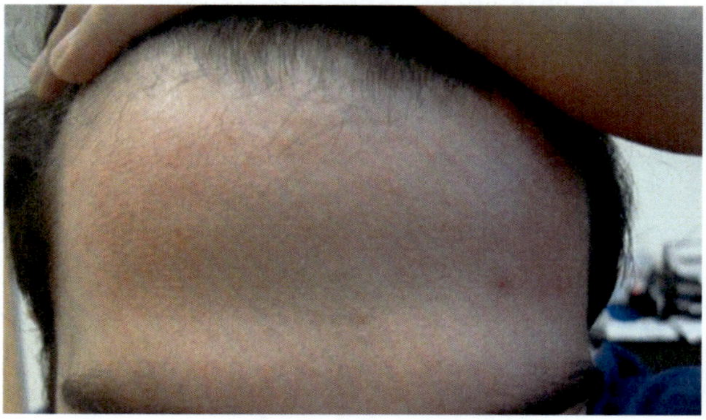

Figure 9.13. Lepromatous Leprosy Face Borderline.

N. Demodex Folliculitis (Demodicosis)

Demodex folliculitis is a type of folliculitis located at the hair follicle, caused by the mite demodex. This mite, considered a saprophyte on the body of the hair follicle, is most commonly found on the face, namely the forehead, nose, cheeks, eyelashes, chin, and external ear canal. There are two types of demodex that exist in human beings: *Demodex folliculorum* and *Demodex brevis*. *D. folliculorum* is usually located at the small hair follicles, such as the eyelashes; *D. brevis* is located near the sebaceous glands that are connected to the small hair follicles. *D. folliculorum* is twice as big as *D. brevis*. Clinically, there is a red, rough, irritated skin rash, sometimes with well-demarcated borders, which is responsible for the following skin disorders: pityriasis folliculorum, rosacea, perioral dermatitis, and blepharitis. Each form may resemble fungi.

O. Psoriasis vulgaris

See more on page 91

Treatment

Most cases of tinea faciale are superficial and curable with topical antifungals. The two classes of antifungal medication most commonly used are azoles and allylamines. Most of these are applied to affected areas once or twice daily. Azoles should be continued for 3–4 weeks and at least 1 week after resolution of the lesions [70].

Topical allylamines, such as terbinafine, are usually effective in a week-long regimen. A cost-effective drug such as miconazole is an acceptable first line choice.

Other antifungal drugs may be used for resistant infections. An added benefit of using ciclopirox and terbinafine is their anti-inflammatory effect. Topical terbinafine is more often prescribed because of its fungicidal properties. To prevent relapses, topical therapy needs to be continued for a minimum of 2 weeks after the eruption has cleared clinically.

Resistant strains, long standing infections, extensive disease, multiple plaques, and lesions affecting the vellum hairs may require oral antifungal therapy [41, 45, 49, 71].

Oral terbinafine has been shown to exacerbate psoriasis and should therefore not be used as a first line drug if the patient has psoriasis [72].

Secondary bacterial infections may require antimicrobials. Therapy with terbinafine or itraconazole, associated with topical anti-fungal therapy or without the topical antifungal, leads to healing within 3–6 weeks without relapse or side effects. The topical antifungal may help in the duration of the system therapy and the clinical presentation of the lesions. Therefore, tinea faciale therapy cannot be standardized but must be selected on a case-by-case basis taking into consideration all the above-mentioned variables. Terbinafine, itraconazole, and fluconazole have been shown to be superior to griseofulvin because they concentrate at the level of the skin [73].

Patients with highly inflamed lesions may benefit from a short course of oral prednisone [74].

Follow-Up

The prognosis for patients with tinea faciale is good. Tinea faciale usually responds to azoles within 4–6 weeks and to allylamines within 1–2 weeks. Re-evaluation of the diagnosis is important if improvement does not occur after 4 weeks of therapy. Complications of tinea faciale are unusual, but can include scarring and abscess formation.

Identification of the source and treatment of infected pets are important in preventing recurrent infection.

Complications such as scarring and abscess formation are rarely reported. These are more likely to occur after treatment with topical steroids because of modification of the clinical picture and possible delay in correct diagnosis.

Close collaboration with veterinary services and educational programs, especially with infants, are required in the prevention of infection from zoophilic dermatophytes.

Chapter 10

Tinea Barbae

Synonyms: Tinea barbae/tinea moustache

Definition: Tinea barbae/tinea moustache is a fungal infection of the skin located at the beard and/or the moustache. It affects only adult males (Figure 10.1).

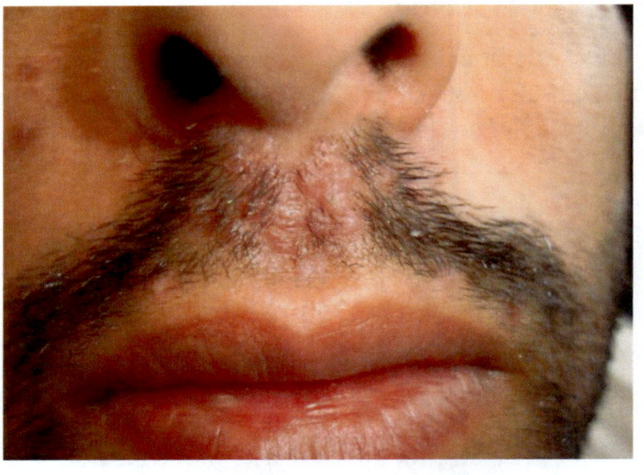

Figure 10.1. Tinea Moustache.

Epidemiology

Tinea barbae is not a common fungal infection, but sometimes it can be seen, especially in farm workers.

Pathogens

The most common pathogenic organisms causing tinea barbei/moustache are Trichophyton verrucosum, Trichophyton rubrum, and Trichophyton mentagrophytes.

The involvement of the hair shaft is an ectothrix infection.

The contamination is usually from animals (cattle, horses, etc.) to the person, and it is uncommon for people to contaminate each other.

Clinical Presentation

Clinically, there are several erythematous inflamed plaques of different sizes (1–5 cm in diameter), but the plaque size could be smaller or larger. These plaques may discharge mild sticky serous fluid, causing the plaque to be wet. In more severe cases, papules and/or pustules are located around the inflamed plaques.

Because of the presence of the hair shafts within the inflamed plaque, these hairs can be pulled out easily. Although these lesions look terrible, they are usually not painful.

Differential Diagnosis

A. Acne Vulgaris

Acne vulgaris is a very common skin lesion located on the face, including the beard area. The lesion may contain closed or open comedones, papules (small or large), and nodules that can be huge and even reach 2–4 cm in size. Usually the nodules are somewhat elevated from the level of the skin and also feel fluctuated or firm by gentle touch (Figure 10.2).

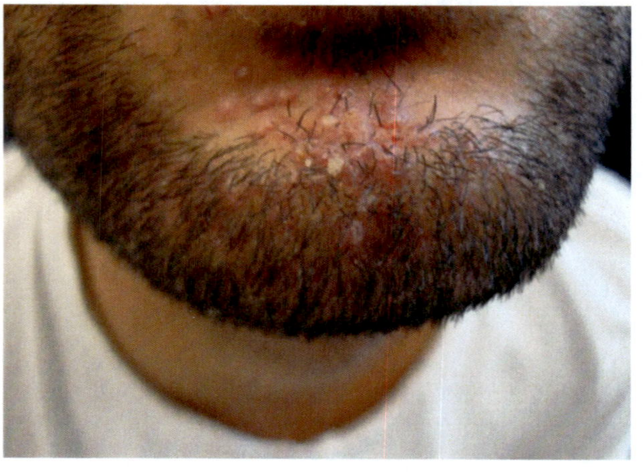

Figure 10.2. Tinea Barbae mimicking acne vulgaris.

B. Actinomycosis

Actinomycosis is a bacterial infection caused by various bacterial species of the genus *Actinomyces*. The most common subtype is *Actinomyces israelii*, which is anaerobic Gram-positive bacterium. Usually the penetration of this bacterium to the subcutaneous tissue is through the oral or other mucosa. After penetration of the *Actinomyces* to the soft tissue, it proliferates, and as a result there is an inflammatory reaction that causes the soft tissue to be swollen, mimicking abscess formation with or without sinus tract formation – to various degrees; once the sinus tract ruptures, a discharge of serous fluid to the overlying skin occurs. Sometimes *Actinomyces* spread to other tissues, such as the pulmonary and/or gastrointestinal systems. Clinically, in certain circumstances it may resemble tinea barbae because of the inflammatory process of the host against these bacteria (Figure 10.3).

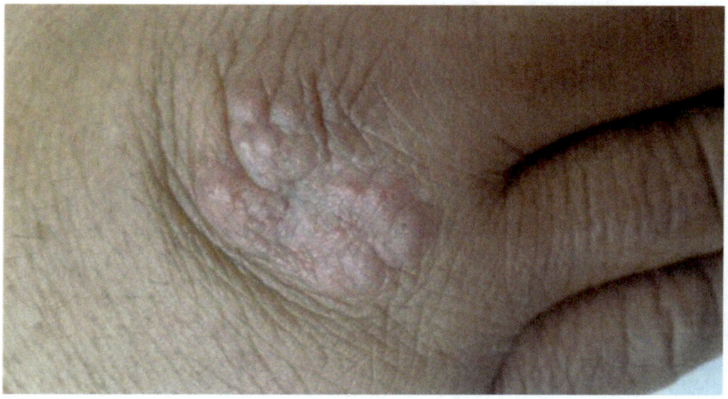

Figure 10.3. Actinomycosis on the dorsal hand..

For final diagnosis, specific bacterial smear and culture should be taken, and if it is positive, the proper systemic antibiotic should be given. In the case of not achieving complete cure, mycological analysis should be taken from the superficial and the deep lesions, including the hair follicle itself.

C. Folliculitis

Folliculitis is a type of inflammatory process of the hair follicle. Folliculitis may be caused by different types of bacteria or fungi. Wherever there are follicles, folliculitis might occur. There are several ways for the bacteria or fungi to penetrate the skin: mechanically (by wearing tight clothes or underwear), which irritates the hair shaft causing a microscopic gap and allowing the bacteria/fungi to penetrate this gap (between the hair shaft and the surrounding skin), or by shaving the beard hairs and by this action the bacterium/fungus may penetrate to the deeper parts of the skin. Cosmetics and/or chemicals or different oils may also be the cause of folliculitis. Clinically, there are red pimples that may turn to pustules, and within the center of the pimples/pustules the hair shaft can be seen. If the folliculitis is superficial, the hair shaft cannot be pulled out easily, but if there is a deep folliculitis, meaning that the folliculitis itself is located around the hair follicles, the hair shaft can be pulled out easily.

The relevant bacterial smear and culture should be taken and then the relevant topical and/or systemic antibiotic should be recommended. Sometimes tinea barbae may be contaminated by bacteria that may be masking the fungus; therefore, the bacterial elements should be treated first, and then afterwards mycological analysis should be conducted if the suspicion of tinea barbae exists.

Several close follicles may contaminate together and present a clinical picture that resembles tinea barbae.

D. Rosacea

Rosacea is a chronic inflammatory condition located on the face area and resembles acne. Since this disorder occurs much more in adults than in childhood, it is often called adult acne-like skin disorder. It is more common in women than men, with a peak onset in 30–60-year-old patients. Rosacea usually starts as redness (flushing and/or blushing) of the central face, the forehead, the nose, around the cheeks, and less often at the ears, chest, and scalp. Rosacea tends to be a chronic disorder with waves of exacerbation and remission. Several factors may flare the skin condition, such as hot and/or spicy food, alcohol, exposure to heat, environment, and emotional stress. Rosacea has different degrees of severity and four different subtypes, as follows:

Erythematous rosacea_– erythemato telangiectatic rosacea that contains telangiectasia, which expresses as redness and telangiectatic blood vessels on the skin.

Papulopustular rosacea – contains papules and pustules of different sizes.

Phymatous rosacea – the red skin becomes thickened and develops a bumpy texture.

Ocular rosacea – the eyes become red and irritated, combined with edema of the eyelids.

Once the papules and pustules merge to create a plaque-like erythematous lesion, it may resemble tinea barbae. But the classical clinical picture of rosacea is presented as telangiectasia, papules, and pustules – and there is not a skip between lesions as can be noted in tinea barbae (there is normal skin appearance between the tinea barbae lesions).

In any clinical suspicions of tinea barbae, mycological analysis should be conducted not only from the superficial areas of the lesions but also from the deeper parts of the hair follicles by pulling out the shaft.

If mycological analysis is positive, the relevant systemic antifungal should be recommended.

E. Cutaneous leishmaniasis:

Leishmaniasis can be divided to 3 groups

1. Visceral leishmaniasis
2. Cutaneous leishmaniasis
3. Mucocutaneous leishmaniasis

Regarding the differential diagnosis of tinea barbae, we will focus on the second subgroup, cutaneous leishmaniasis.

Cutaneous leishmaniasis is one of the most common sub groups of leishmaniasis. The protozoa parasite is transmitted to the human skin from female sand flies (phlebotomine sand flies).

There are more than 20 species of leishmania and the clinical presentation of the infected skin depends on the type of the leishmania protozoan and on the immune system of the patient. Clinically there are one or more ulcerated (or not ulcerated) plaques sized 0.5–5 cm (rarely more than 5 cm in diameter), usually oval in shape, covered by dry or wet crusts (Figure 10.4).

There is an irregularity of the surface of the lesions. Once the lesions reach complete cure scars will remain for life. Lesions located at the beard areas in certain circumstances may resemble tinea barbae. In a suspicion of tinea barbae a mycological analysis should be taken in order to find the mycological organism. In case of negative results, bacterial analysis should be taken first and after precise antibacterial treatment for 7–10 days mycological analysis should be taken again. If the results are negative again, biopsy should be advised to determine the type of the lesions.

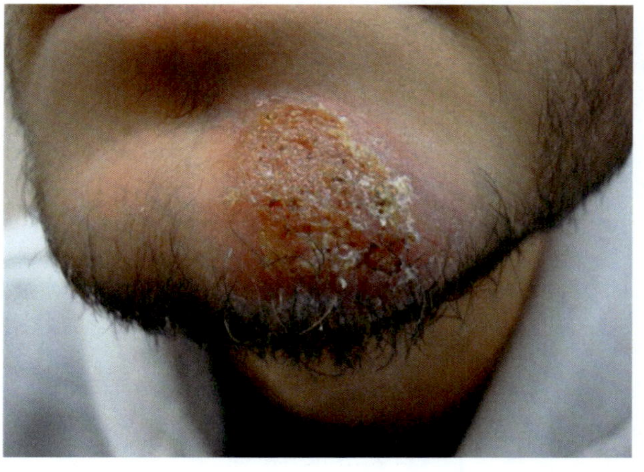

Figure 10.4. Cutaneous Leishmaniasis.

Diagnosis

Sometimes secondary infection may be involved in such a case. A fungal smear and culture should be taken after the relevant topical and systemic antibiotic has been given for 7–10 days.

After treating the bacterial infection, mycological analysis (direct microscopy and culture) should be conducted, including from the deepest part of the hair shaft.

The diagnostic approach to tinea barbae is as for tinea capitis – the inflammatory subtypes such as kerion celsi should be identified.

Treatment

As tinea barbae involves the hair follicles, systemic administration of oral antifungals is often needed. The correct treatment – systemic antifungal – should be given according to the mycological analysis results.

The systemic treatment is terbinafine 250 mg/d or itraconazole 200 mg/d for 1–2 months.

Chapter 11

Tinea Corporis

Synonyms: Tinea circinata, ringworm of the body

Definition: Tinea corporis refers to all dermatophytoses of glabrous skin except the palms, soles, scalp, and groin.

Epidemiology

Tinea corporis is a very common infection worldwide and its epidemiological features vary according to geographical area. This can be attributed to several factors, such as migratory streams, lifestyle, socioeconomic conditions, and incidence of peculiar comorbidities.

According to epidemiological data, 20–25% of the world population suffers from skin mycoses. Tinea corporis is considered to be the third most prevalent superficial mycosis of the skin preceded by tinea pedis and onychomycosis. Although dermatophytic infections are frequent afflictions in adults and children, it is quite uncommon to find these infections in the neonatal age group [75].

Tinea corporis can be acquired from infected humans or animals or via autoinoculation from reservoirs such as different facilities inhabited by different fungi (e.g., showers, swimming pools). Different populations are known to have high incidence of tinea corporis, such as athletes participating in combat sports. Tinea corporis gladiatorum has been described in 11–14% of judo fighters and occurs even more frequently among wrestlers, from whom it gets the name tinea corporis gladiatorum [76,77] (discussed in more detail in the special form section). Epidemics of tinea corporis can also occur in the setting of geriatric wards.

Tinea imbricata, a variant of tinea corporis, is commonly caused by *Trichophyton concentricum* and has a distinctive epidemiological distribution as it is frequently limited to areas of the Far East, South Pacific, and South and Central America.

Pathogens

All known dermatophytes can potentially produce lesions of the glabrous skin, hence tinea corporis. The most common causes worldwide are *Trichophyton rubrum*, *Trichophyton mentagrophytes*, *Microsporum canis,* and *Trichophyton tonsurans*. Because tinea corporis' epidemiological features vary according to the geographical area, for any part of the world the causes of tinea corporis can be assessed by reference to the prevailing dermatophyte flora of the region.

Natural infection is acquired by deposition of viable arthrospores or hyphae on the surface of the susceptible individual. Tinea corporis can be transmitted directly from infected humans or animals or via autoinoculation from reservoirs such as *Trichophyton rubrum* colonization of the feet. Infection may also spread from the scalp down the neck onto the upper trunk, or from the groin onto the buttocks and the lower trunk. Zoophilic pathogens are more likely to affect children, especially *M. canis* from dogs or cats. Although the most common source of infection is an active lesion on an animal, contamination from another human may also occur. Fomite transmission and infection from soil is also well-established.

Tinea capitis and tinea corporis are the predominating superficial mycoses among the pediatric population with *T. violaceum*, *M. canis,* and *T. rubrum* being the most predominant predop fungi [78]. In young children infected with *T. rubrum* or *Epidermophyton floccosum*, half of the cases may have originated from their parents.

Tinea incognito refers to a dermatophytosis characterized by modifications to the clinical picture following the use of topical steroids and is most often caused by *T. rubrum*. Majocchi granuloma is an infection frequently caused by *T. rubrum* that occurs when fungal hyphae invade hairs and hair follicles. In the case of follicular involvement, *T. rubrum* and *Trichophyton verrucosum* are the most likely pathogens involved.

Tinea corporis gladiatorum, a common infection among athletes, is mostly caused by *Trichophyton tonsurans,* an anthropophilic dermatophyte spread by close skin-to-skin contact. Tinea imbricata is caused most commonly by *Trichophyton concentricum* and is frequently limited to areas of the Far East, South Pacific, and South and Central America.

Contributing Factors

Occlusive clothing (use of tight, occlusive, synthetic material) and warm, humid climates are frequently associated with more frequent and extensive eruptions. In addition, frequent skin-to-skin contact and minor trauma from competitive wrestling create an environment in which dermatophytes multiply.

Diabetes mellitus, immunosuppression, atopic dermatitis, poor hygiene, and the poor nutritional state of people together with high temperatures and humidity are some of the predisposing factors that favor pathomorphosis of fungal infections.

Immunosuppression plays an important contributing role in tinea corporis and often results in infections that tend to be widespread and exhibit unusual clinical features [79]. In particular, immunosuppressive drug therapy is the major cause of immunocompromised status, which results in impaired host defense mechanism and occurrence of opportunistic infections such as tinea corporis [80] and predispositions to a variety of cutaneous complications [81].

Systemic immunosuppression or localized immunosuppression, most commonly due to a potent topical steroid, can significantly impair cell-mediated defense. Impaired cell-mediated immunity reduces the number of epidermal antigen-presenting Langerhans cells. Furthermore, corticosteroid-induced thickening and delayed desquamation of the stratum corneum have also been suggested as contributing to the development of fungal infections [82]. Not only topical corticosteroids, but also topical immunomodulators including pimecrolimus and tacrolimus, have also been reported to induce tinea incognito.

Genetic predisposition does not correlate with cases of tinea corporis infections; it has only been described in tinea imbricata and may be inherited in an autosomal recessive character. On the other hand, onychomycosis due to *T. rubrum* is also inherited genetically.

Majocchi granuloma is a deep fungal infection, usually caused by *T. rubrum.* Practically, the fungus incade the hair shaft and the hair follicles. Majocchi granuloma occurs frequently in woman who shave their legs or in men around their wrists, usually at the hairy area, normally the distal part of the wrists. Histologically suppurative folliculitis combined with dermal granulomatous response may be seen. Majocchi granuloma may be seen more often in immusupression hosts, clinically inflamed folliculitis combined with papules and/or pustules or even nodular lesions [83, 84]. (Figure 11.1, Figure 11.2)

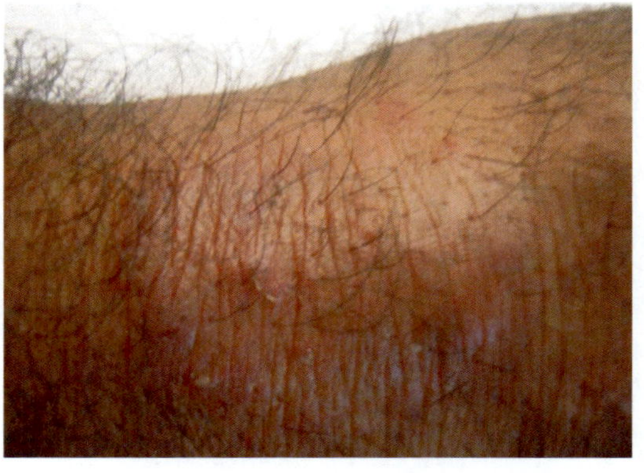

Figure 11.1. Majocchi Granuloma: localized.

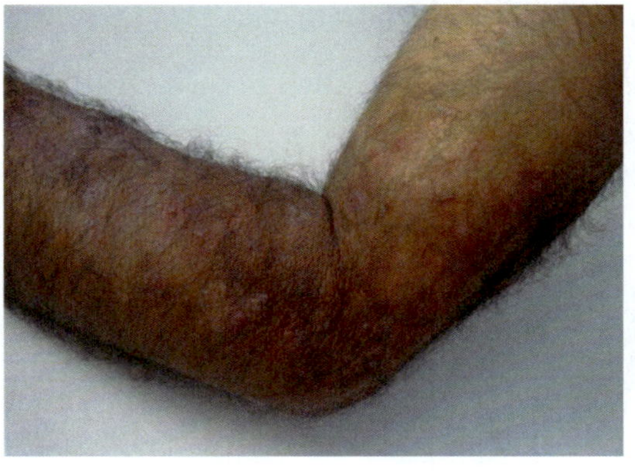

Figure 11.2. Majocchi Granuloma: widespread.

Presentation

The site of infection is typically on exposed skin, unless the infection represents an extension from a pre-existing infection. The clinical manifestation of tinea corporis results from invasion and proliferation of the causal fungus to the stratum corneum. Terminal hair in the affected area can also be invaded. After an incubation period of 1–3 weeks, the infected skin becomes prominent.

Tinea corporis can clinically present with many variants, but the classic presentation consists of an annular lesion, usually sharply marginated with scale and with a raised active erythematous border. Single lesions may occur, or there may be multiple plaques that may remain discrete or become confluent. The classical annular pattern of ring worm infections is a result of the centrifugal immigration of the fungus from the center of the lesion combined with the local inflammation host response. Lesions may be serpiginous and/or annular (Figure 11.3, Figure 11.4). However, many lesions lack any tendency to central clearing.

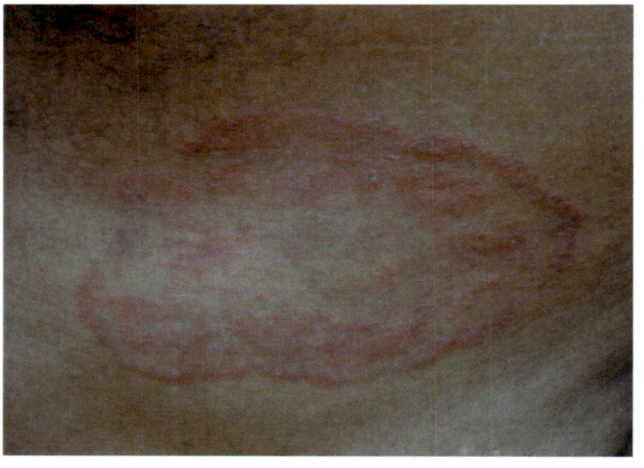

Figure 11.3. Tinea Corporis.

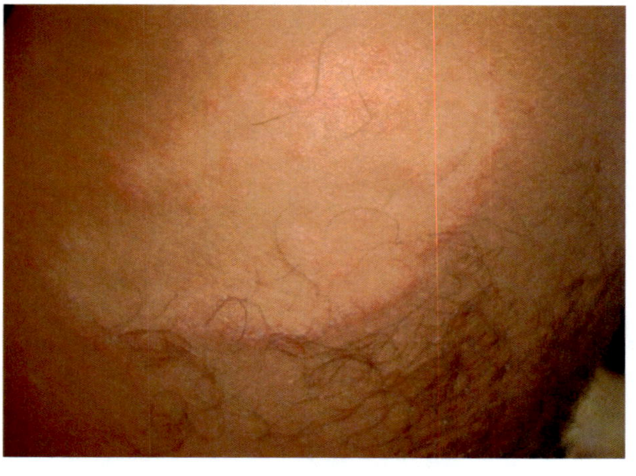

Figure 11.4. Tinea Corporis.

The border can often be vesicular and advance centrifugally. The typical plaque of tinea corporis is characterized by elevated red, well-defined borders compared to the surrounding area, combined with central healing, due to the fungus leaving the central area and its activity with keratine on the borders. In other words, once the fungus has "finished" with the central area, it moves centrifugally to look for more keratine, giving the center time to heal. The center of the lesion is usually scaly and during remission exhibits clearing from the center of the lesion towards the periphery. Central resolution is a common but not invariable feature of tinea corporis and is considered a more common finding in inflammatory lesions.

The clinical pattern may be modified in patients with an altered degree of immune response. Atypical presentations of dermatophytosis include cases of tinea incognito, tinea in immunosuppressed patients, and tinea in patients with chronic cutaneous diseases such as atopic dermatitis. Atypical mycotic infections are also observed more frequently in HIV-positive patients and should be kept in mind when coming across atypical and extensive tinea corporas [85].

Special Forms

Tinea corporis is a dermatophytic infection that was treated (by mistake) with topical steroids for a lengthy period of time and, as a result, the clinical picture may look different without the classical clinical presentation of dermatophytic infection of the skin. The more potent the topical steroid is and the longer the duration of using the cream, the less characteristic the classical mycotic infection appears. The classical clinical presentation of tinea corporis is a result of the immune system's reaction to the violence and, as a result, the uppermost layer of the epidermis is damaged. Once the local immune system is disturbed, the balance between the immune system reaction and the fungi violence is disturbed in favor of the fungi. The unclassical clinical presentation may lead to misdiagnosis. The topical steroid depresses the local immune system and, as a result, the violence of the fungus increases, so the balance of the depression of the immune system and the fungus violence is disturbed due to the use of the topical steroid in favor of the fungal violence. After discontinuation of the topical steroid, rebound of the fungus may be seen.

Lesions tend to spread and lose their peculiar patterns, taking on different clinical features that mimic other pathologies. Concentric vesicular rings are sometimes suggestive of tinea incognito. Even though topical corticosteroids are considered the main causative agent for tinea incognito, topical immunomodulators, including pimecrolimus and tacrolimus, have also been reported to induce tinea incognito.

Tinea corporis gladiatorum refers to the epidemic type of tinea corporis among wrestlers as a result of contamination fo the fungus from the close skin-to-skin contact of athletes. Among wrestlers, tinea corporis gladiatorum often presents as well-defined, erythematous, plaques covered by fine scales located usually around the neck, arms and head, consistent with the typical areas of skin-to-skin contact prevelant in their sport [78,86].

Tinea purpurica refers to the purpuric variant of tinea corporis and is considered a rare manifestation. The predisposing factors are not well established. Effected patients have a history of topical or systemic steroid therapy that reduces cell-mediated inflammatory response.

Tinea imbricata is most commonly caused by *T. concentricum* and clinically appears as a plaque consisting of concentric erythematous rings. Lesions of tinea imbricata demonstrate minimal to absent vesiculation. Centrifugal spread within an area of central clearing followed by a second wave of scaling can soon arise and can be repeated to grow into numerous concentric rings. Pruritus that is intense may lead to lichenification, and lesions may resolve to postinflammatory hypopigmentation.

T. equinum results from exposure to horses and clinically presents as plaques of tinea corporis that do not have a severe inflammatory reaction and have a tendency for spontaneous resolution.

Lesions caused by *M. canis* to the glabrous skin can occur and are characteristically annular or oval.

Tinea corporis due to *M. canis* presents differently compared to tinea corporis due to other dermatophytes such as *T. rubrum* or *T. mentagrophytes*. The lesions are usually oval or elliptical in shape, with or without central healing (Figure 11.5); there are no impresive circinate borders. The whole lesion has the same color and the same texture. Usually there are no elevated borders, but sometimes this can be seen. The entire lesion is evaluated in the same way as nummular eczema lesions or guttate psoriasis. The size of the lesions is from several mm to 2–3 cm. Children are much more effected than adults.

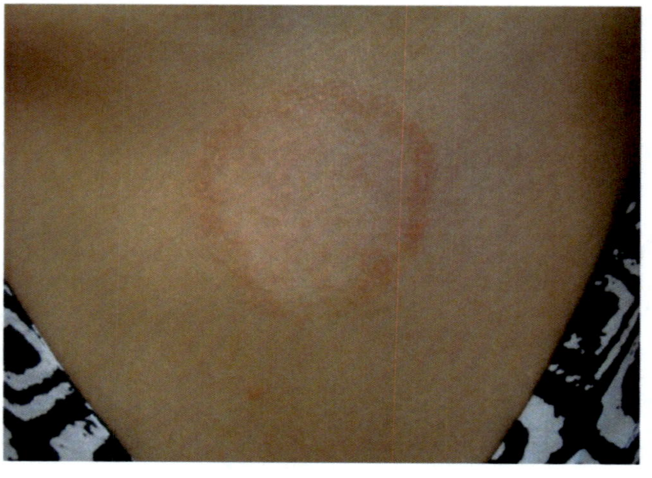

Figure 11.5. Tinea Corporis due to M.Canis.

M. audouinii produces short-lived lesions of tinea corporis.

Infection with *T. verrucosum* occurs from exposure to cattle, *T. mentagrophytes* var. *erinacei* is obtained from hedgehogs, *T. mentagrophytes* var. *mentagrophytes* are likely to cause inflammatory lesions of tinea corporis.

Lesions related to tinea capitis caused by *T. verrucosum*can lead to extensive annular lesions on the neck and upper trunk.

Tinea corporis caused by *T. rubrum* can be extensive and the inflammatory margin difficult to distinguish. *T. rubrum* infections may also present as large, confluent, polycystic or psoriasiform plaques. Lesions can present on the buttocks, lower back, and at distant sites of the trunk as an extension to from tinea cruris. Extension of the lesions to the legs can also occur from tinea pedis caused by *T. rubrum*. Extensive lesions of tinea cruris can also occasionally be observed in cases of *Epidermophyton floccusum* and *Trichophyton mengninii* infections.

Rarely, deep forms of tinea corporis can occur that are atypical and present with dermal or subcutaneous involvement. A few reported cases of dermatophyte infections invading the bone, central nervous system, and lymph nodes have occurred.

Carrier Stage

Tinea corporis can result from repeated autoinfection with pathogenic dermatophytes from the patient's scalp, which serves as a reservoir for the pathogen. Tinea capitis due to *T. tonsurans* often has a subtle noninflammatory appearance resulting in asymptomatic covert carriage, which makes diagnosis difficult; such asymptomatic carriers with the dermatophyte on the scalp may act as vectors of infection [85]. Lesions can present on the buttocks, lower back, and at distant sites of the trunk as an extension from tinea cruris. Extension of the lesions to the legs can also occur from tinea cruris. Lesions of tinea cruris can also occasionally proceed to infect areas in the buttocks and trunk.

Differential Diagnosis

A. Pityriasis Rosea

Pityriasis rosea is one of the papulosquamous disorders characterized by a mild inflammatory skin disease that is expressed by red- and pale-pink-colored papules and plaques covered with unique scales arising from the center of the lesion and pilling off centrifugally (like the rose flower – hence the name rosea) (Figure 11.6).

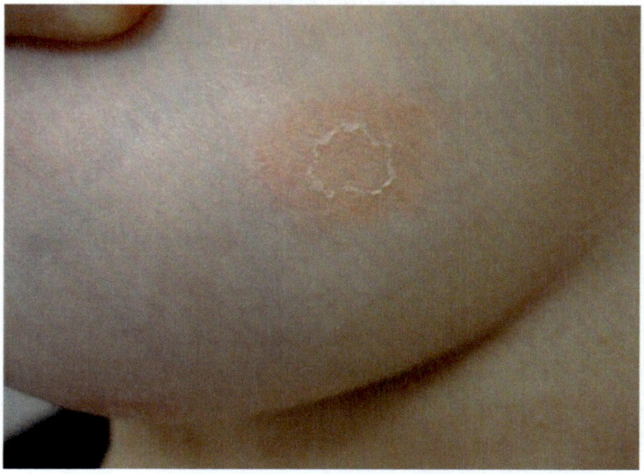

Figure 11.6. The so-called herald patch (or "mother patch") of Pityriasis Rosea.

The rash usually begins with the appearance of a first relatively big lesion – the so-called herald patch (or "mother" patch), and after a few days or weeks there is a widespread eruption (smaller than the mother patch) usually located at the torso and the proximal areas of the lower and upper extremities, with an approximate duration of 6–8 weeks and spontaneous disappearance of the lesions, without any residual effects.

This kind of rash is usually asymptomatic, but sometimes itching or tingling sensation scan occur.

The disease is said to be caused by a viral agent, but some investigators have suggested a fungal exception is involved; so far no definite fungal agent has been found.

Pityriasis rosea usually disappears by itself without treatment.

B. Atopic Dermatitis

Clinically, atopic dermatitis lesions usually have no well-demarcated borders, and the sides of the atopic lesions merge gradually with the adjacent normal skin. The transition of atopic lesions (redness, lichenification, edema, and scales) to normal skin decreases gradually, usually in all parameters, concluding with normal skin with no well-demarcated lines (Figure 11.7).

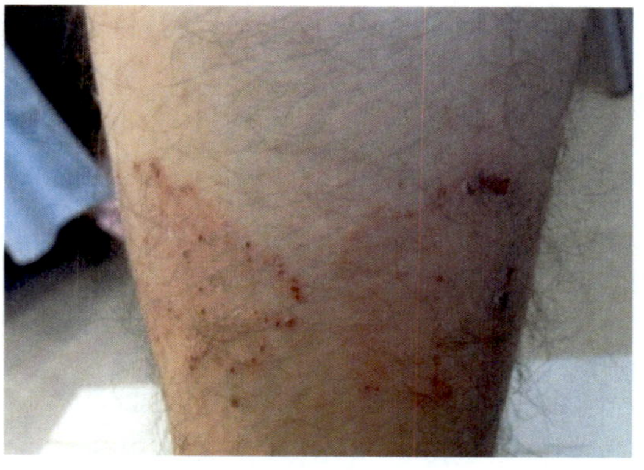

Figure 11.7. Atopic Dermatitis on the shin.

Looking at the distributions of the lesions on the body surface, bilateral distributions (must not be symmetrical), and the clinical morphology of untreated lesions, namely red and well-demarcated elevated borders, central healing may contribute to having the suspicion of tinea corporis, which can be confirmed by mycological analysis (direct smear and mycological culture).

Sometimes the well-demarcated lesions of atopic dermatitis may be seen (usually not around the whole lesion) concentrating at the well-demarcated area and may resemble tinea corporis lesions. Tinea corporis lesions treated with topical steroids – by mistake of course – may obscure the classical clinical appearance of tinea corporis and may resemble the clinical presentation of atopic dermatitis lesions.

C. Erythema Multiforme

Erythema multiforme (EM) is an acute, usually self-limiting, type 4 hypersensitivity reaction. There are two subtypes: erythema multiforme minor and erythema multiforme major, and its severe stage – the Stevens-Johnson Syndrome (SJS).

Erythema multiforme minor presents as one or several papules with the pathognomonic iris lesions, "the target lesions", which gradually disappear after several days or weeks. Sometimes the erythema multiforme lesions may emerge and create an annular or arcuate pattern that in certain circumstances may resemble tinea corporis. Erythema multiforme is usually the result of external causes such as viruses (herpes simplex, mycoplasma, Epstein-Barr virus, etc.), different drugs, or unknown reasons.

The relatively rapid resolution of the lesions combined with the rapid appearance of the target lesions strongly supports the diagnosis of erythema multiforme. In case of the annular/arcuate lesions lasting for more than 10 days with no clinical change, mycological analysis/biopsy should be taken for final diagnosis. Skin eruption is characterized by atypical target lesions (Figure 11.8), usually located on the palms and soles and could occur on any location of the body. On the glablous skin, this kind of rash may mimic tinea corporis due to *M. canis*.

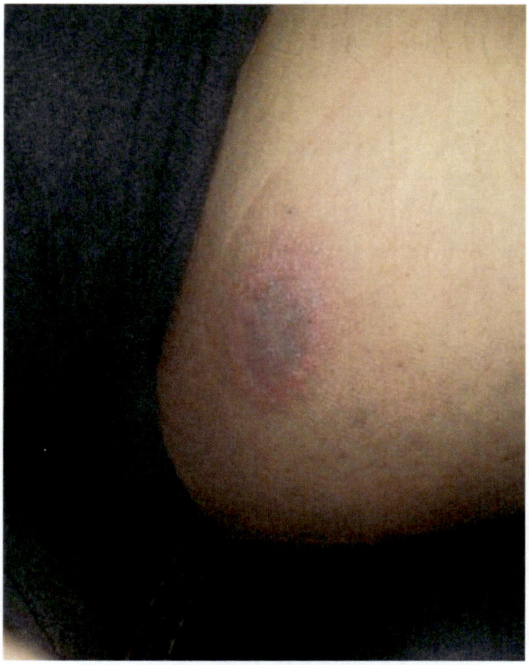

Figure 11.8. Atypical Erythema Multiphorme.

D. Psoriasiform eruptions (e.g., psoriasis)

Annular psoriasis is one of the subtypes of psoriasis vulgaris. This unique pattern is presented as annular plaques with red well-circumscribed elevated borders with or without central healing-like appearance and are covered by fine silvery-white scales. Despite the lack of circinate borders, the well-demarcated borders combined with the central healing might mimic tinea corporis. However, in annular psoriasis the plaques are less pronounced than in tinea corporis (Figure 11.9).

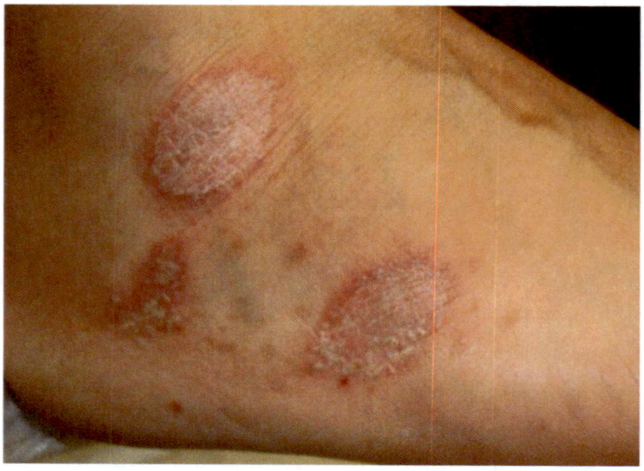

Figure 11.9. Plaque Psoriasis mimicking Tinea Corporis.

E. Guttate psoriasis

Guttate psoriasis is a unique type of psoriasis vulgaris that occurs during childhood and adolescence several weeks after strepococcal or viral infections, usually in people with a genetic predisposition to psoriasis (Figure 11.10). A third of this population will develop psoriasis vulgaris, and in the majority of them the guttate psoriatic rash will disappear in time with or without treatment. This typical psoriatic rash has a tendency to recur after re-exposure to streptococcal or viral infections. Clinically, this rash is composed of small reddish purple plaques that are elevated from the body surface with circumscribed lesions and covered by white crusty scales round/oval in shape. This clinical presentation may mimic tinea corporis due to *M. canis* in childhood.

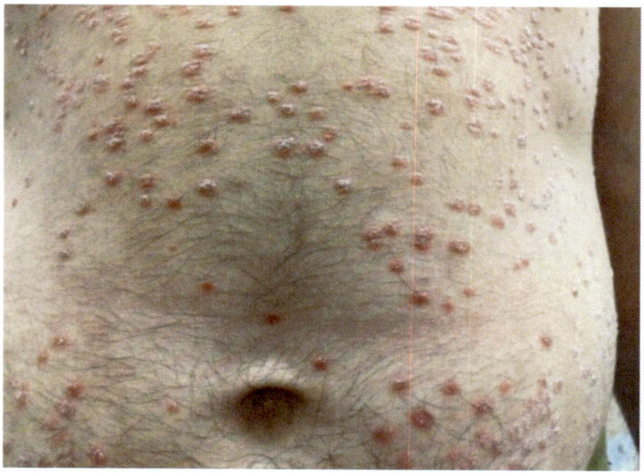

Figure 11.10. Gutate psoriasis.

F. SCLE – Sub-acute Cutaneous Lupus Erythematosus

SCLE is one of the three types of Lupus Erythematosus and presents as solitary or several erythematous plaques. The plaques have well-circumscribed borders and the centers of the lesions are not as pronounced as the borders; therefore there is a resemblance to tinea corporis (Figure 11.11). Mycological analysis or skin biopsy should be taken for final diagnosis.

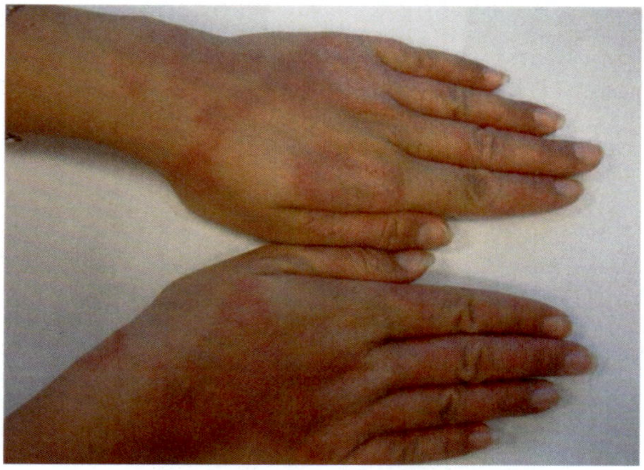

Figure 11.11. SCLE-Sub-acute Cutaneous Lupus Erythematosus.

G. Nummular Eczema

Nummular eczema is a type of or variant of atopic dermatitis that manifests in coin-shaped plaques of one to several cm or even less, covered by scaling, usually located on arms and/or legs, and trunk.

This type of atopic dermatitis is more common in children but could occur at any age. Regarding tinea corporis, nummular eczema may resemble unique fungal infection caused by *Microsporum canis*. Atopic dermatitis/nummular eczema that is located on the face, in certain circumstances may resemble tinea faciale. Lesions of nummular eczema partially treated with topical steroids may camouflage the classical picture of the nummular eczema, and may mimic tinea faciale (Figure 11.12).

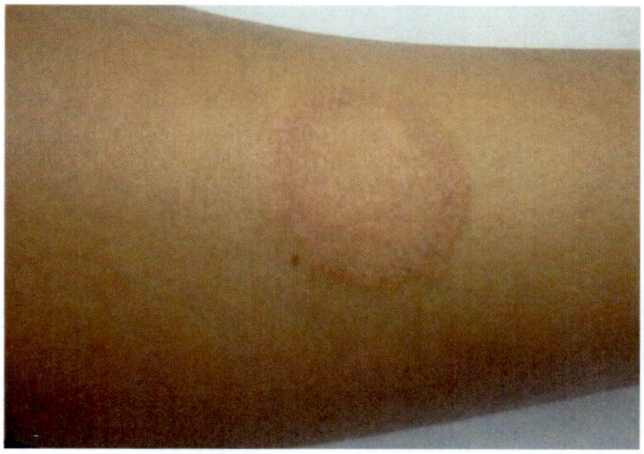

Figure 11.12. Nummular Eczema.

Sometimes, the difference between tinea faciale and nummular eczema is very difficult to notice because in most cases both diseases have well-circumscribed borders and do not show central healing. In the case of atopic background, atopic dermatitis with an additional rash such as nummular eczema should be considered as nummular eczema. However, in case the diagnosis is not clear enough, mycological analysis should be taken for final diagnosis.

H. Lichen ruber planus

See more on page 73

I. Granuloma annulare

See more on page 72

J. Lymphocytic infiltration of the skin

See more on page 68

K. Seborrheic dermatitis

See more on page 47

L. Rosacea

Rosacea is a relatively common skin rash that involves facial flushing along with a stinging, itching or burning sensation. Its clinical signs include erythema, telangiectasia and papules/pustules.

The diagnosis of rosacea is made clinically, although a skin biopsy is sometimes performed to exclude other cutaneous diseases, such as lupus or sarcoidosis.

M. Secondary syphilis.

See more on page 188

N. Pityriasis versicolor

See more on Chapter 16

O. Erythrasma

See more on Chapter 20

P. DASP – disseminated actinic superficial porokeratosis

DASP is a rare inherited skin condition (autosomal dominant) expressed by small papules and plaques of 5-20 mm.

Those lesions are usually located on the legs and arms; the papules gradually enlarge up to 10 mm or more. The color of the lesion is brown or red-brown; while the center area of the lesions is pale brown the borders of the lesions are red-brown, elevated, and well-demarcated (Figure 11.13).

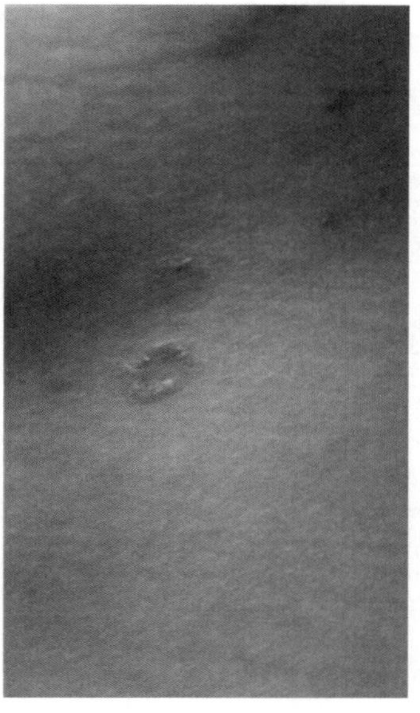

Figure 11.13. DASP - Disseminated Actinic Superficial Porokeratosis.

Circumscribed from the normal skin, DASP almost never occurs at the scalp and rarely occurs at the face.

The well-circumscribed borders with the central depressed flat area (compared to the raised borders) may resemble tinea corporis. But the lesions in DASP are small in size, and the shiny elevated borders are much more pronounced compared to tinea corporis.

In contrast to tinea corporis caused by *T. rubrum* or *T. mentagophtes*, the lesions in tinea corporis caused by *M. canis*, are relatively uniform in shape; in other words, the borders are well-circumscribed but usually there is no difference between the well-demarcated borders to the rest of the lesion.

Another difference is that in DSAP there are mild tiny scales, while in tinea corporis caused by *M. canis* the scales are stuck somehow to the underlying gentle crust.

Mycological analysis should differentiate between these diseases.

Q. Parapsoriasis

Parapsoriasis is a group of skin disorders that present as macules and/or plaques covered with fine scales that may mimic psoriasis; hence the name. In 1902 Brocq [87] was the first to use the term parapsoriasis and three types of diseases were included under the name:

1. Pityriasis lichenoides et variceliformis (acuta and chronica)
2. Small plaque parapsoriasis
3. Large plaque parapsoriasis (parapsoriasis en plaque).

There is a new classification of parapsoriasis, adding lymphomatoid papulosis to the above.

Each of the above skin disorders presents differently, but the large plaque parapsoriasis may in certain circumstances resemble tinea corporis, especially if the plaques have well-circumscribed borders with more or less normal central skin appearance (Figure 11.14)

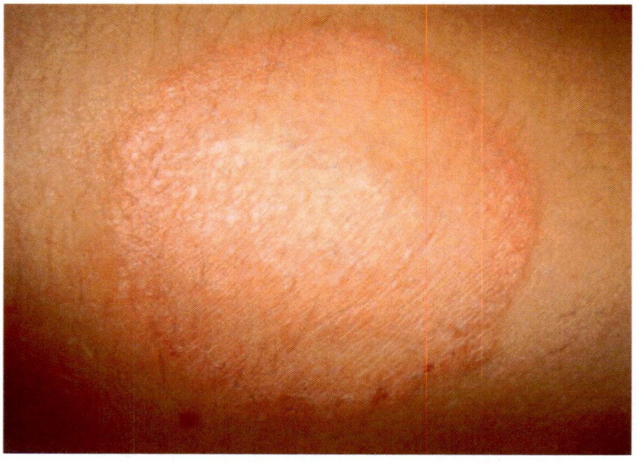

Figure 11.14. Parapsoriasis.

If mycological analysis is negative, repeated biopsies should be taken to rule out the possibility of progression to Cutaneous T-cell Lymphoma of the skin (CTCL; mycosis fungoides). Repeated biopsies are necessary because it is not common to find specific histological indications of mycosis fungoides in the first biopsy, and several biopsies may be needed before the final diagnosis is established. The disease mycosis fungoides has no connection to fungal disease, but the name was applied because the clinical presentation may look like fungal infection of the skin (well-circumscribed circinate borders, central healing, fine scales, itching sensation, etc.).

The other subgroup of parapsoriasis, namely pityriasis lichenoides et varioliformis (acuta and chronica) and small plaque parapsoriasis, are rare to non-existent.

Diagnosis

Even though tinea corporis can masquerade as a large number of cutaneous diseases, in clinical practice it is quite simple to diagnose because of its peculiar presentation in roundish erythematous-scaling blemishes expanding from the center (ring-worm).

Treatment

The first choice of treatment for dermatophytoses of glabrous skin and tinea corporis is topical therapy with azoles, hydroxypyridones, allylamines, and morpholines.

If topical therapy fails or an inadequate effect is suspected or more diffuse lesions and hair infection occur, systemic therapy with oral antifungal agents is recommended.

Topical and/or systemic antifungal therapy is used in tinea corporis caused by *T. tonsurans* [76].

Morishita et al. reported that the penetration speed of *T. tonsurans* to the human stratum corneum was faster than that of other dermatophytes [88]. Kasai reported that *T. tonsurans* easily invaded the hair roots from the early stage of infection and that systemic antifungal administration was necessary [89]. Before deciding on treatment, look for another location of fungal infection such as onychomycosis.

In the case of tinea corporis and onychomycosis, which is not a rare scenario, the duration of treatment should be calculated according to the onychomycosis, which is longer.

For the systemic treatment of patients with tinea corporis, a 7-day treatment regimen of 100 mg itraconazole daily was able to achieve a mycological cure rate of 90% [90].

Complications

Tinea corporis is not a serious skin disorder, but it constitutes a serious problem for patients' quality of life in view of the considerable discomfort and/or cosmetic deformity it causes. Lesions of tinea corporis can resolve spontaneously or may persist for years. In the center of the lesion, healing can resolve to post-inflammatory hyperpigmentation, change of texture, or erythematous dermal nodules; lichenification may be presented due to chronic scratching.

Pruritus in lesions of tinea corporis are rarely intense and may lead to lichenification (Figure 11.15). Overuse of potent topical steroids may lead to permanent stria (Figure 11.16).

Rarely, deep forms of tinea corporis can occur that are atypical and present with dermal or subcutaneous involvement. A few reported cases of dermatophyte infections invading the bone, central nervous system, and lymph nodes have occurred.

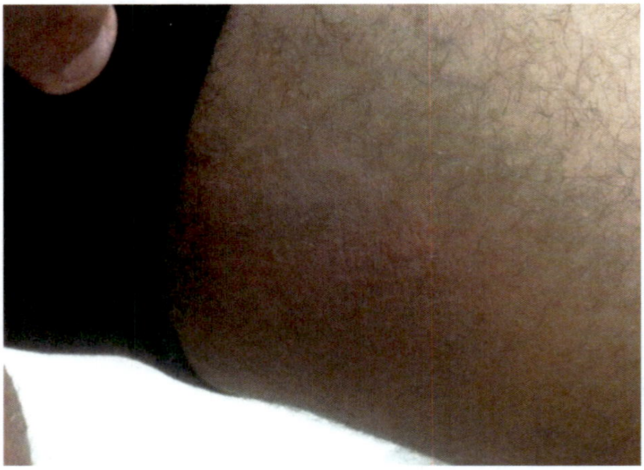

Figure 11.15. Lichenification.

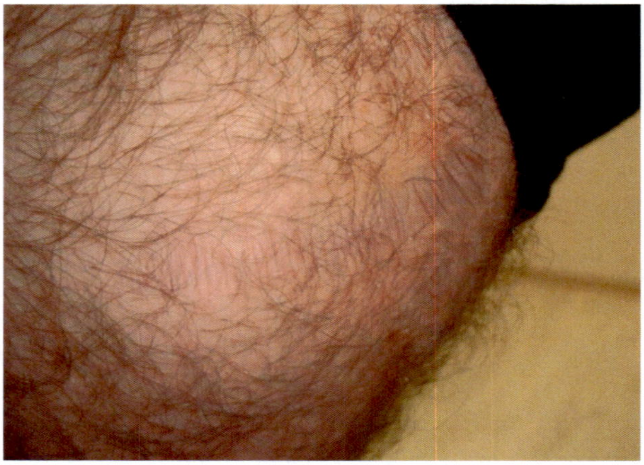

Figure 11.16. Permanent Stria.

Follow-up

The natural history of tinea corporis is considerably variable. Some inflammatory cases of animal infection have resolved spontaneously in a few months, while typical cases of tinea corporis caused by *T. rubrum* infection may persist for years.

Chapter 12

Tinea Cruris

Synonyms: Jock itch, eczema marginatum

Definition: Tinea cruris is a superficial dermatophyte infection of the proximal medial thighs and buttocks characterized by inflammatory and non-inflammatory lesions that rarely invade the hair follicles (Figure 12.1).

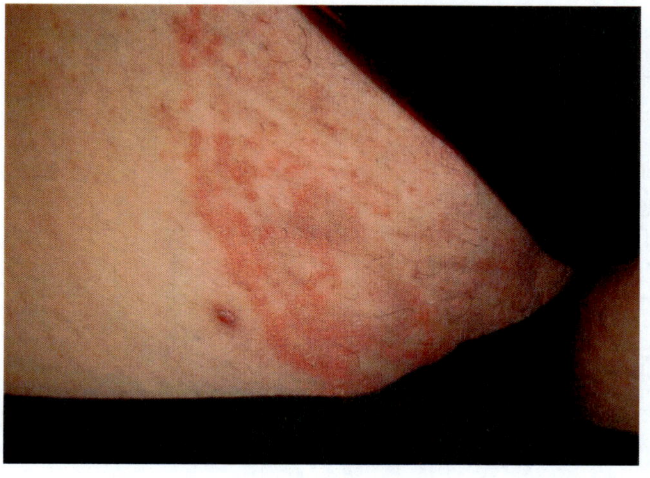

Figure 12.1. Tinea Cruris.

Epidemiology

Dermatophytoses are by far the most prevalent of the three major classes of superficial fungal infections; the others are superficial mycoses and candidiasis. The prevalence of superficial mycosis infections has increased gradually. Up to date, more than 20–25% of the world's population suffers from one or more different types of the fungal infection. Tinea cruris has a worldwide distribution with a preference for adolescents and adults. The range of frequency of tinea cruris varies between 2.5% and 52% [91, 92].

This dermatophytosis appears to be up to three times more frequent in men than in women [93-96]. Elderly patients are also more likely than the general population to have tinea cruris due to structural changes, altered immunological response, and different environmental influences. Mechanical and functional changes, as well as the reduced immunological capacity of aging skin predispose the elderly to a variety of skin diseases including fungal skin infections.

The prevalence of tinea cruris in children and adolescents appears to be underestimated. In a study in Hong-Kong, the prevalence of tinea cruris in school children and adolescents showed it to be one of the most common skin diseases [97]. Underdiagnoses may be attributed to the fact that children and adolescents frequently do not seek medical advice, mainly because of the embarrassing anatomical location.

Tinea cruris is frequently associated with other superficial mycoses. Tinea pedis, tinea corporis, and tinea cruris frequently occur together or in close succession. Infection from autoinoculation from a reservoir on the hands or feet (tinea manuum, tinea pedis, and tinea unguium) is three times more common in men than in women [93-96].

The frequency of fungal infections varies with seasons, with the largest number of cases of tinea pedis and tinea cruris occurring in the summer months [97].

Pathogens

Tinea cruris spreads by direct contact: with other people (anthropophilic organisms), animals (zoophilic organisms), or soil (geophilic organisms), as well as indirectly from contaminated fomites (e.g., towels, sheets, clothes, upholstery, hairbrushes, and hats).

Direct inoculation through breaks in the skin occurs more often in individuals with depressed cell-mediated immunity. Dermatophytes invade and persist in the stratum corneum and rarely penetrate below the surface of the epidermis and its appendages.

Mycotic infection of the skin can be caused by dermatophytes, yeasts, and nondermatophyte molds, although dermatophytes are the most frequently encountered causative agent.

The causes of dermatophytoses are classified into three anamorphic genera, *Trichophyton*, *Microsporum*, and *Epidermophyton*, depending on their conidial structures. Anthropophilic dermatophytes are the main agents of tinea cruris throughout the world, in particular *Trichophyton rubrum*, *Trichophyton mentagrophytes*, and *Epidermophyton floccosum* [98]. In particular, *T. rubrum* is considered the most common source of tinea cruris [99].

The causative dermatophytes for tinea cruris change over time and their distribution varies in different geographical locations depending on social and environmental factors. A study in India has shown that the most common pathogens identified were *T. rubrum* (22.6%), *Epidermophyton flocossum* (2.8%), and *Microsporum gypseum* (1.4%) [100]. Another study in India, using direct microscopy and culture, has identified *T. rubrum*, *Trichophyton mentagrophytes*, *Candida ablicans*, and *Candida tropicalis* as the most common pathogens causing tinea cruris [101]. In Western Europe, *T. rubrum* was the most frequently isolated dermatophyte in cases of tinea corporis and tinea cruris [102]. An epidemiological study from the US has identified the most common pathogens causing tinea cruris/corporis as *T. rubrum* (38.9%), *T. tonsurans* (38.9%), *M. canis* (7.2%), *T. mentagrophytes* (2.9%), and in descending order *T. verrucosum* and *C. albicans* [103]. In

Brazil *T. rubrum* was diagnosed in 45 (90%) cases followed by *T. tonsurans* in three (6%) and *T. mentagrophytes* in two patients (4%) [104].

Predisposing Factors

Multiple factors may predispose the development of tinea cruris. These include heat, humidity, excessive sweating, occlusive undergarments, climate, and immunocompetence of the host [97, 99, 100].

Obesity is considered a risk factor in tinea cruris. Obese adult men are affected more frequently with tinea cruris than women, and it is rarely seen in children. Because excessive perspiration is the most common predisposing factor for tinea cruris, patient education on proper hygiene makes intuitive sense for successful treatment, yet it has not been studied [105].

Tinea cruris typically occurs under conditions of high ambient temperature and humidity. Occlusion of the scrotum from wet or tight-fitting synthetic clothing and physical exercise provides a humid and warm ambient atmosphere that favors fungal growth and facilitates an optimal skin-surface environment for infection [106].

Localized immunosuppression, such as topical use of corticosteroids, or systemic immunosuppression such as HIV infection and consumption of systemic immunosuppressive medication, can lead to more extensive and atypical forms of tinea cruris.

Clinical Presentation

Tinea cruris (or "jock itch") is an extremely pruritic infection of the groin and surrounding area. It often affects the groin aera and may extend to the buttocks (Figure 12.2) and abdomen (Figure 12.3). The scrotum tends to be spared. Patients with tinea cruris suffer from itching and burning sensation.

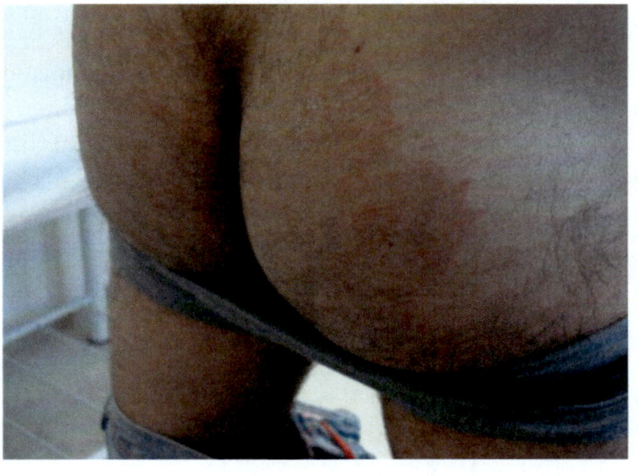

Figure 12.2. Tinea Corporis on the buttocks.

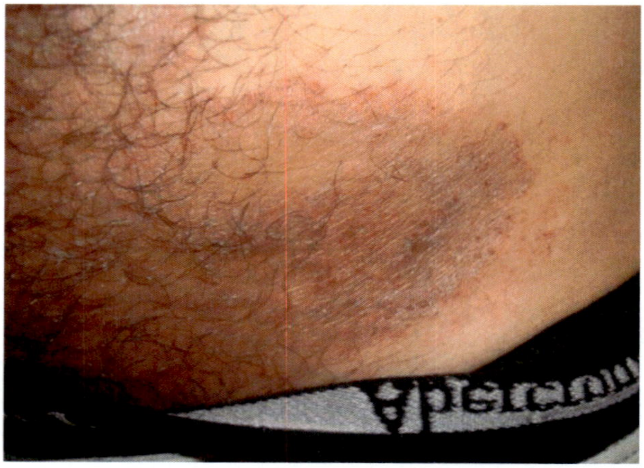

Figure 12.3. Tinea Corporis on the abdomen.

The clinical presentation may show a characteristic pattern of inflammation, called an "active border" [104]. The inflammatory response is usually characterized by a greater degree of elevated erythema covered by fine scales pronounced usually at the edge of the lesions.

Papules/pustules or vesicles located at the active edge of the fungal plaque, along with different degree of maceration, are usually located at on an erythematous lesion with well circumscribed boreders. Central clearing of the lesion may be present, due to the centrifungal immigration of the fungus, which distinguishes dermatophytoses from other papulosquamous eruptions, but it is not a rule.

Clinical diagnosis of tinea cruris is often easy and straight forward but one should always evaluate the lesions during physical examination; the feet and nails should always be considered a possible reservoir [106].

Special Forms

Immunosuppression

Immunodeficient patients are at increased risk for opportunistic fungal infections, including those with any organ transplant, those who take immunosuppressant or myelotoxic drugs, and patients with HIV lymphoma, leukemia, diabetes, a primary immunodeficiency, or an autoimmune disorder [97]. In this patient group tinea cruris may have extensive and atypical presentation (Figure 12.4). Patients with locally compromised immunity resulting from the use of topical steroids are also at risk for mycotic infection. Fungal lesions that are mistaken for eczema or dry skin and treated with topical steroids tend to become more severe, just because of the decrease of local immunity due to the topical steroids.

Mucocutaneous manifestations in patients with HIV are very common. In a study with an HIV population, the most common lesion was oral candidiasis (36%); dermatophytosis was the second common infection (13%) along with gingivitis.

Tinea lesions tend to present more frequently with lower levels of CD4 count [107].

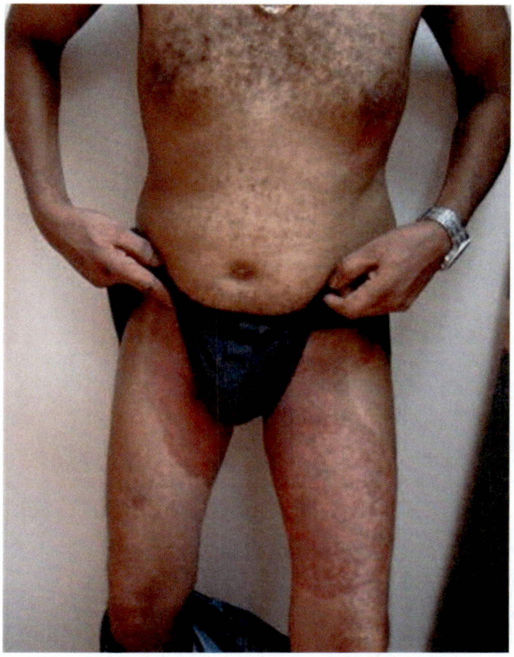

Figure 12.4. Widespread Tinea Cruris.

In HIV patients tinea cruris often presents with truncal involvement and may follow tinea pedis and onychomycosis in frequency; it presents as an expanding scaling plaque of the upper thighs and groin, with central clearing and a red elevated border.

HIV patients who have tinea corporis might also have tinea cruris that was spread from the groin area to the trunk [108]. This extensive form of tinea occurs in hot, humid climates and may be seen at all levels of immunosuppression. In severely immunosuppressed patients with AIDS, lesions may have little inflammation and often lack the elevated border and central clearing typical of tinea (anergic tinea). They are recognized as sharply marginated areas of hyperkeratosis resembling dry skin. The penis and scrotum may also be involved; this is not noted in non-HIV-infected patients [109].

Dermatophytoses have been detected in 42% of renal transplant patients, with tinea cruris and tinea corporis being the most frequent clinical types observed. *T. rubrum* was the most commonly isolated pathogen [110]. Tinea cruris in this patient group can be widespread because renal transplant patients are in constant immunosuppression from the intake of combined immunosuppressive drugs such as prednisone, azathioprine, cyclosporine, and tacrolimus; increased thickening and delayed desquamation of the horny layer produced by the steroids could favor infection and chronicity.

Hair Follicle Involvement

When the hair follicles become involved in a tinea cruris infection, the presentation can be atypical (Figure 12.5). Lesions may mimic acne, rosacea, bacterial folliculitis, pyoderma, or herpes.

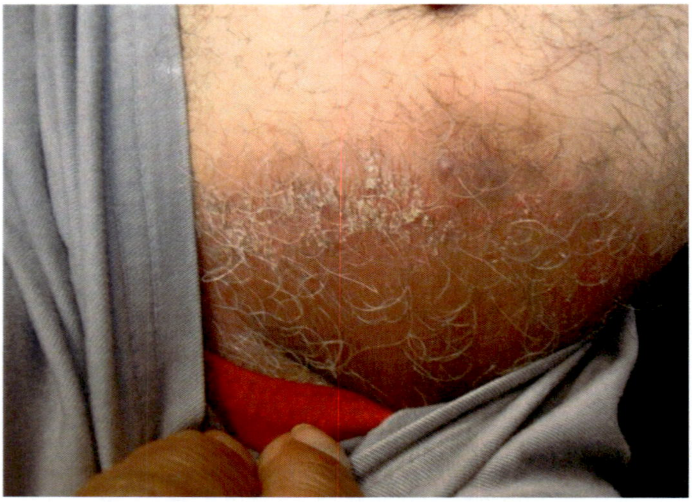

Figure 12.5. Tinea Corporis with involvement of the hair follicles.

Occult Disease

Asymptomatic dermatophyte infection may present in uninvolved intergluteal folds up to 6 cm from positive lesions and has been postulated to act as a reservoir for the recurrence of tinea cruris [98].

Diagnosis

Tinea cruris is generally easy to diagnose because of its characteristic, sharply defined peripheral scale; areas of skin from the inguinal folds and perineum to the inner thighs and even the buttocks may appear reddened and inflamed.

When there are diagnostic difficulties or for confirmatory purposes, potassium hydroxide (KOH) microscopy aids in visualizing hyphae and confirming the diagnosis of tinea cruris. Scrapings are taken with a scalpel. They are examined in potassium hydroxide or a fluorescent stain. Skin scales can be sent to a laboratory folded in a card (transport packs are available).

Other diagnostic modalities that can also aid in the differential diagnosis include Wood's lamp examination, fungal culture, and skin or nail biopsy.

The advent of molecular biology technologies has enabled the development of methods like the polymerase chain reaction (PCR) that are highly sensitive and specific and can be used for diagnosis of fungal pathogens. Recently, other techniques such as restriction fragment length polymorphism (RFLP) [111], real time PCR [104], and multiplex PCR assay [100] have been adapted for detection of dermatophytes from clinical specimens. This approach is very effective for detecting dermatophytes, but these methods still need to be compared to the standard clinical laboratory tests.

Differential Diagnosis

The differential diagnosis of tinea cruris has a broad spectrum. Often the clinical diagnosis is straight forward but occasionally can be challenging.

Central healing (clearing) combined with the well circumscribed/demarcated borders helps to distinguish tinea cruris from other papulosquamous/plauqes disorders.

A. Psoriasis Inversa/Flexular Psoriasis

Plaque psoriasis is a chronic inflammatory disease. It involves raised plaques that are usually oval or irregular in shape, sized from one to several cm. The plaques have a distinctive red color and are well defined, with sharply demarcated borders (Figure 12.6). They usually appear on the scalp, trunk, and limbs, with a predilection for extensor surfaces, such as the elbows and knees. Plaque psoriasis may also involve the nail as well as the joints causing arthralgia/arthritis. The psoriatic plaques and tinea corporis both have well-defined borders, but plaque psoriasis does not have elevated borders or central healing as can be seen in tinea corporis.

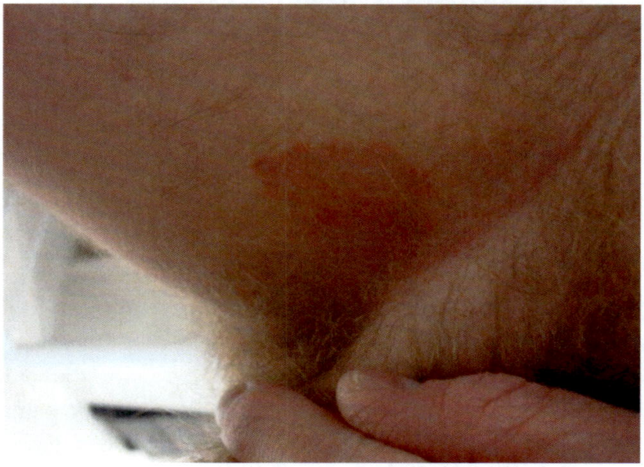

Figure 12.6. Psoriasis Inversa.

The diagnosis of psoriasis is almost always made on the basis of clinical findings. Laboratory investigations are rarely used. A skin biopsy may confirm the diagnosis of plaque psoriasis.

One of the clinical subtypes of psoriasis is psoriasis inversa. This subtype involves the body folds such as groin, axilla, and gluteal cleft. The location of psoriasis inversa causes decreasing or absence of scales, which is a very characteristic feature as it appears due to friction of the skin folds and the moisture in those areas. Clinically, there are well-demarcated borders and the borders are somewhat elevated and more pronounced than the center of the lesion. It may resemble tinea corporis in certain circumstances.

Having these lesions at other intertrigene locations, and of course if the classical clinical presentation supports the clinical diagnosis of psoriasis, there is no complete central healing of the intertriginous psoriasis lesion; usually there is an erythematous moist plaque with well-demarcated borders.

B. Intertrigo

Schematically intertrigo can be divided to 3 subtypes – mechanical, biological, and chemical.

1. Mechanical intertrigo refers to a type of dermatitis located at intertriginous areas such as the groin (Figure 12.7), axilla, under the breasts, abdominal folds, and buttocks.

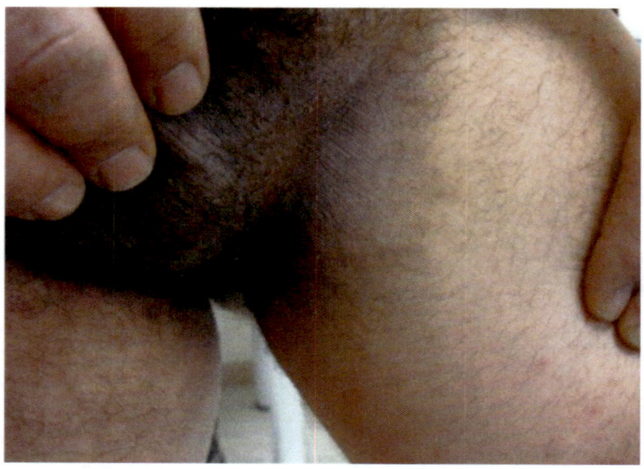

Figure 12.7. Groin Intertrigo.

It is caused by several factors such as maceration, moisture, friction activity, lack of ventilation, and exposure to heat.

Mechanical intertrigo is usually seen in obese people with diabetes, especially after sweating and/or after exercise. Clinically, there are erythematous patches with no well-demarcated borders, moist, and oozing. The center of the patch is more inflamed than its unclear border.

2. Biological intertrigo refers to bacterial, viral, or yeast infection at the intertriginous areas. The pre-existing moist erythematous patch is caused by one of the above biological infections. Clinically, secondary infection may be revealed by relevant lab tests. Candida intertrigo is a *Candida* infection located at the intertriginous skin folds, especially the groin area. It is much more common in infants who wear diapers, which supply ideal surroundings for the candida.

3. Chemical intertrigo may refer to any type of chemical irritation, alkali or acid. Clinically, the erythematous patches occur on the top of the skin folds since the folds themselves are in first contact with the irritant. Separating the folds reveals that there is no involvement of skin irritation, similarly to allergic contact dermatitis. In contrast, in psoriasis inversa, seborrheic dermatitis, or atopic dermatitis there is involvement between the skin folds.

4. Seborrheic dermatitis in the groin area is not that common and it may occur in infants. In adults, the involvement is mainly on the scalp, sides of the nose, eyebrows, eyelids, behind the ears, and central upper trunk. The lower the part of the body is, the smaller the concentration of sebaceous glands present.

The groin area is not a common area but clinically, erythematous moist patches covered by yellowish sticky scale may be seen in the skin folds in case of obese people, or at the groin sulcus, which spreads centrifugally. The further away you get from the center the less red the skin is; the borders are unmarked.

C. Erythrasma

Erythrasma is uniformly brown and scaly, with no active edge; it fluoresces a brilliant coral red.

See more on Chapter 20

D. Seborrheic dermatitis

Seborrheic dermatitis consists of greasy scales, with scalp (dandruff) and sternal involvement.

See more on page 47

E. Allergic Contact Dermatitis/Irritant Contact Dermatitis

Allergic contact dermatitis (ACD)/irritant contact dermatitis (CD) is a reaction of the skin to different agents that the patient is allergic to, hence the name allergic contact dermatitis, or irritation of the skin by different irritants such as strong acid or base or other irritation agents.

Textile contact dermatitis could appear at any location with which it had been in contact. Regarding the groin area, textile contact dermatitis may cause an erythematous skin covered with mild scales, itching, and sometimes a burning sensation. Textile contact dermatitis can be caused by synthetic, natural, or both fibers. The fibers themselves rarely cause contact dermatitis but the clothes contain ingredients other than fibers, such as formaldehyde resin (prevents wrinkles on clothes), PPD (para-phenylenediamine), and different types of dyes that may cause an allergic reaction by allergic contact dermatitis or irritant dermatitis (Figure 12.8).

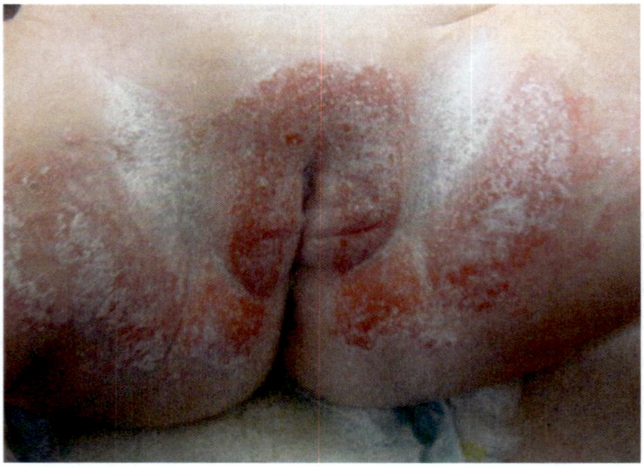

Figure 12.8. Irritant Contact Dermatitis.

Different washing powders, fragrances, etc. may also cause contact dermatitis. In case of suspicion of ACD due to clothes (textile dermatitis) the dermatitis should appear not only at the groin area (unless the patient wore new underwear or only this underwear was washed with a certain washing powder). It could appear at any location of the skin that was in contact with the clothes.

Clinically, in allergic contact dermatitis there are no well-circumscribed borders of the erythematous patch. In addition, there is no central healing. In irritant contact dermatitis there are well-defined borders but there is no central healing. Usually, depending on the irritant, the central part of the lesion has more inflammatory processes compared to its peripheral borders.

It is not common to have atopic dermatitis only at the groin area but it could appear in this location in addition to other locations such as cubital fossa or popliteal fossa around the neck.

In case of AD at the groin area, no well demarcation of the borders should be seen, nor central healing.

Relevant patch test is advised in order to determine its cause.

F. Lichen planus

See more on page 73

Treatment

Generally speaking, tinea cruris responds well to topical treatment with an antifungal solution or cream. Several topical preparations are approved for the treatment of tinea cruris.

Selection should be based on patient compliance (duration of treatment), overall cost, and tolerability. The two main classes of antifungals are allylamines and azoles.

However, in more severe presentations or when there is follicular involvement it may require the use of a more efficacious oral treatment. The disadvantage of an oral treatment is that there is a greater potential for adverse events and drug–drug interactions. 1 The length of treatment with an oral antifungal determines the degree of toxicity and clinical tolerance.

The Guidelines of Care published by the American Academy of Dermatology suggest that oral therapy may be necessary for hyperkeratotic lesions, especially on the palms and soles, for disabling or extensive disease, for chronic infections, in immunosuppressed patients, or in patients who are intolerant of or unresponsive to topical agents [112].

Refractory tinea cruris infections may occur even in patients who are seemingly immunologically intact. Although a response may be obtained with topical or systemic therapy, there is recurrence in 60% to 70% of patients. Frequently these infections require prolonged therapy with systemic and topical agents.

Usually an active immune system is critical to achieve a mycologic cure; in patients with an immune deficiency, especially those infected with human immunodeficiency virus (HIV), fungal infections and specifically tinea cruris can be severe, aggressive, and persistent, and usually require systemic administration of an antifungal agent [97].

Topical Agents

Tinea cruris is managed most frequently with administration of topical imidazoles or allylamines for 2 to 4 weeks; generally, more than 80% of patients are cured.

One of the more popular azoles is clotrimazole (Lotrimin, Mycelex), one of the oldest antifungal treatments. One RCT compared cure rates for 139 patients for clotrimazole 1% cream compared with ciclopirox olamine 1% cream when both were applied twice daily for 28 days. By the end of the 4-week period, 69% of the clotrimazole group was clinically and mycologically cured compared with 64% of the ciclopirox group. 11 Miconazole 2% cream (Micatin, Monistat) (used twice daily for 2 weeks by inmates in a Florida prison) demonstrated 75.5% clinical clearing (against tinea cruris, pedis, or corporis, or *Candida* cutaneous infections) when compared with placebo (NNT=1.57). Of the 99 patients evaluated, 48 were diagnosed with tinea cruris; however, results were not broken down into diagnostic category. The length of follow-up for these patients was not disclosed [113].

The results of two multicenter, double-blind, parallel group trials reported the effectiveness of ciclopirox in the treatment of tinea corporis/tinea cruris [114]. In one study, ciclopirox olamine cream 1% (ciclopirox 0.77%) was compared with the cream vehicle, and in the other trial ciclopirox olamine cream 1% was compared with clotrimazole cream 1%. Treatment consisted of twice daily applications for 4 weeks followed by a 2-week post-treatment period during which the patients were evaluated while off antifungal therapy. After the first week of treatment, and through to the end of the trial, ciclopirox olamine cream 1% was significantly more effective than the vehicle alone. At the final post-treatment visit (either 1 or 2 weeks post-treatment), the mycologic response rates in the ciclopirox olamine 1% and vehicle groups were 47/66 (71%) and 26/66 (39%), respectively. The overall response rates in the two groups were 40/66 (61%) and 10/66 (15%), respectively.

In the group of patients with tinea corporis/tinea cruris treated with either ciclopirox olamine 1% or clotrimazole 1%, at the final post-treatment visit (either 1 or 2 weeks post-treatment), the mycologic response rates in the ciclopirox olamine and clotrimazole groups were 25/33 (76%) and 27/36 (75%), respectively. The overall response rates in the two groups were 20/33 (63%) and 26/36 (71%), respectively [115].

Topical terbinafine is the one of the most common topical agents used for the treatment of tinea cruris. Terbinafine is available in several 1% formulations (emulsion-gel, cream, and solution/spray), and dosed once daily for 1 week. When terbinafine is applied topically it rapidly penetrates the stratum corneum.

Several studies have assessed the efficacy of terbinafine and compared it to other topical agents. In a multicenter, double-blind RCT bifonazole 1% cream for 3 weeks was compared with terbinafine 1% cream used daily for 1 week (followed by 2 weeks of its vehicle cream). Mycological and clinical cure rates were greater than 95% in both groups at 3 weeks. At the 8-week follow-up, no statistically significant differences were seen in KOH positivity rates (20.24% of patients in the bifonazole-treated group were KOH-positive vs. 11.76% in the terbinafine group). Symptom relapse rates at 8 weeks were not available [116].

Butenafine (Mentax), a benzylamine antifungal, was 88% to 93% mycologically effective in a noncomparative study when used twice daily for 2 weeks. 9 Similar results were found in a study of 76 patients with tinea cruris; after 2 weeks of daily application, 78% (modified intent-to-treat group) were mycologically cured. Mycological cure plus "cleared" or "excellent" clinical evaluation remained 73% at day 42 vs. 5% of the placebo group (NNT=1.47) [117].

Ajoene 0.6% gel (isolated from garlic) can be used as an alternative treatment option. In an RCT study ajoene was as effective as terbinafine 1% cream (both applied twice daily for 2 weeks) in 60 Venezuelan Army soldiers. 13 Sixty days after treatment, 73% of the ajoene-treated patients and 71% in the terbinafine group were asymptomatic. An open-pilot study of 14 patients with tinea cruris demonstrated 71% mycological cure with a honey, olive oil, and beeswax (1:1:1) mixture, applied 3 times daily up to 3 weeks, likely due to honey's inhibitory effect on fungus and beeswax's anti-inflammatory properties [105].

Systemic Agents

Tinea cruris often responds to topical agents. However, when the infection is extensive or when topical treatment fails, an oral antifungal agent is required.

Fluconazole, itraconazole, and terbinafine have all been shown to reach effective and persistent levels in the stratum corneum for treating cutaneous fungal infections.

Treatment

One-week treatment with itraconazole capsules 200–400 mg/day or for 2 to 4 weeks with terbinafine 250 mg/day is usually effective.

Terbinafine levels in skin were investigated after oral administration of 250 mg/day for 1 and 2 weeks. Rapid delivery of the drug to the stratum corneum was noted, principally by sebum and diffusion [118].

One to four weekly doses of 150 mg of fluconazole were assessed with tinea corporis/cruris in a smaller study 11 that examined once-weekly fluconazole at a dose of 150 mg for tinea corporis or cruris. The authors reported a cure rate of 95% overall, and noted that 70% of patients required double doses for cure, 20% of patients required 3 doses, and 10% 4 doses. No serious clinical side effects or laboratory abnormalities were found [119].

Complications

Tinea cruris generally responds promptly to topical agents without any further complications, although refractory tinea cruris infections may occur even in patients who are seemingly immunologically intact. Recalcitrant tinea cruris infections often may invade beyond the stratum corneum to involve the follicles, progressing to form chronic inflammatory lesions (Figure 12.9). Once this organism becomes established, it tends to spread and become chronic. Although a response may be obtained with topical or systemic therapy, there is recurrence in 60% to 70% of patients [97].

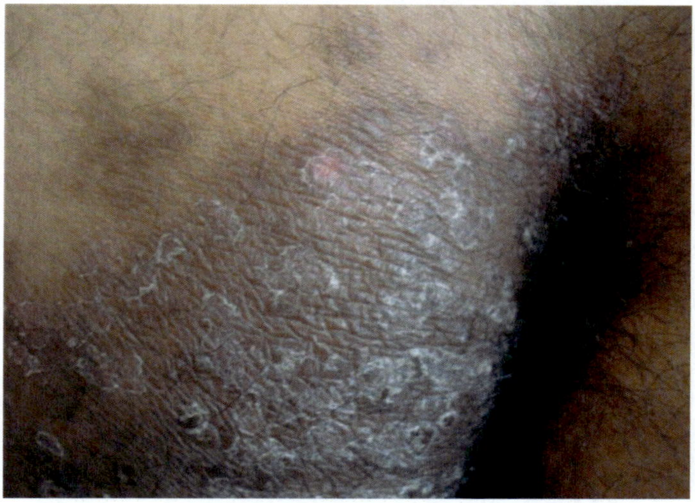

Figure 12.9. Chronic Recalcitrant Tinea Corporis.

In order to ensure that no relapses occur, measures for prevention of these fungal infections should be based on the maintenance of local resistance to infection by prophilatic treatment combined with hygiene.

Follow-up

Tinea cruris is usually straight forward when diagnosing and responds promptly with various topical agents. It may require follow-up when relapses do occur and occasionally may necessitate the use of oral antifungal agents.

It is of significant importance that all the predisposing factors are addressed in order to eliminate relapses. Excessive perspiration and obesity are the most common predisposing factors for tinea cruris and patient education on proper hygiene and weight reduction [111] makes intuitive sense for successful treatment [105]. The affected areas should be kept dry and free from occlusion. Although dermatophytoses do not cause mortality, they do cause morbidity and pose a serious public health risk. In those patients who have repeated tinea cruris, prophylactic treatment for several organisms may be needed.

Chapter 13

Tinea Pedis

Synonym: Athlete's foot

Definition: Tinea pedis refers to all dermatophytoses of the interdigital toe-web space as well as the skin of the feet.

Epidemiology

Tinea pedis is a very common disease in the community and is the most frequent dermatophytosis [120]. Upward of 70% of the general population may have the disease sometime in their life [121].

The age groups between 16 and 60 years are affected more frequently by the disease, with a slightly higher incidence in the 16–45 age group. This may be explained by the fact that the age groups mainly affected involve those working full-time and/or who frequent sports societies and are thus more exposed to the contagion [122]. The prevalence of tinea pedis and onychomycosis has been also shown to increase with age, ranging from 0.7–3.8% in children and adolescents, respectively (age 1–20 years), 15.2–20.1% in adults (age 21–60 years), to 33.7% in older subjects (age >60 years) [123].

It was found that tinea pedis is found only rarely in children; only 4.7% of cases observed involved prepubescent patients [122].

The prevalence of tinea pedis in males has been reported to be slightly higher than in females, but sex has not been extracted as a risk factor [124]. Males were infected approximately three times as frequently as females [122]. This is probably due to the fact that women engage less often in sports activities, wear different types of footwear that allow the circulation of air, and are less subject to contagion by reason of their work environment [122].

Pathogens

Trichophyton rubrum, *Trichophyton mentagrophytes* var. *interdigitalis*, and *Epidermophyton floccosum* are responsible for the most common cases of tinea pedis throughout the world. This dermatophyte profile follows the pattern seen world-wide in past years for tinea pedis. Among the keratinophilic organisms, *T. rubrum* is considered to be the most common fungi pathogen causing chronic symptomatic tinea pedis [120].

Transmission of these dermatophytic pathogens are dependent on the origin of the fungal infection, namely anthropophilic contamination (from human to human), zoophilic (from animal to human), or geophilic (from soil to human). The most common dermatophyte – world wide – causing tinea pedis is *T. rubrum*, which is transmitted in an anthropophilic transmission pathway [125]. A recent study showed that *T. rubrum* accounted for 76–85% of all dermatophyte infections, among them onychomycosis and tinea pedis [126] and may account for over two-thirds of all tinea pedis infections [127,128].

Studies have shown that the most commonly isolated dermatophyte in tinea pedis is *T. rubrum* (17%), followed by *T. interdigitale* (13%), *T. violaceum* (6%), *T. mentagrophytes* (2.4%), and *E. floccosum* (2.4%), while the most commonly isolated yeast was *Candida parapsilosis* (20.4%), followed by *C. albicans* (13.3%) and *Trichosporon* spp. (7%). Other etiological pathogens are due to other *Candida* and *Trichosporon* species (13.3%) and non-dermatophytic filamentous fungi of the genera *Aspergillus* (3.3%), *Scopulariopsis* (1.4%), and *Fusarium* (0.5%) [120].

Epidemiological studies have reported *C. albicans* as the major causal yeast agent of fungal infection involving tinea pedis and onychomycosis. Other studies have shown that the predominant yeast species involved is *C. parapsilosis* [120].

Tinea pedis per definition is a dermatophyte infection of the interdigital toe–web space and/or the skin of the feet. Yeasts and/or non-dermatophyte molds are rarely the only cause of tinea pedis.

Sometimes the existence of non-dermatophyte molds and/or yeast may be revealed at the tinea pedis skin areas not as the only causative agent but as a saprophyte, or as another infection that is not discovered in the laboratory mycological analysis. There are several reasons for having the non-dermatophyte mold/yeast as the only pathogen in tinea pedis. Among the reasons is the technique for taking the scales samples. This sample should be taken from several locations that are clinically suspicious for tinea pedis.

In the case of having non-dermatophyte mold/yeast infection causing tinea pedis, another mycological analysis should be taken and the culture should be obtained on sabouraud–dextrose agar with and without cyclohexamide.

It is not rare that in repeated mycological analysis from feet with tinea pedis combined with choosing suitable culture media, the causing dermatophyte will be found. On the other hand, onychomycosis may be caused by dermatophyte or non-dermatophyte molds or yeast. In a paper published in 2009 [129] in the *British Journal of Dermatology* regarding onychomycosis, it was found that onychomycosis may be caused by one or more dermatophytes. If non-dermatophyte mold was revealed in a mycological analysis the recommendation is to repeat the mycological analysis two more times; if the same non-dermatophyte mold is found and no dermatophyte is found (in relevant mycological culture media) and the clinical presentation is suitable for onychomycosis, only then can the diagnosis of onychomycosis be established, all the more in tinea pedis, that per definition is caused by dermatophytes caused by molds only.

More cases of tinea pedis have been reported to be seen during winter and summer. The increased number of cases of tinea pedis in winter may be due to individuals soaking their feet coupled with occlusive footwear, leading to hyperhidrosis and maceration.

The predominant species identified in athletes is *T. rubrum,* and *T. mentagrophytes* in non-athletes [124].

Tinea pedis occurs in all athletes; the factors that place the athlete at increased risk are darkness, warmth, increased CO_2 tension, and moistness associated with athletic shoes. Recurrence is common in athletes.

Contributing Factors

Many risk factors for contracting tinea pedis have been reported, including predisposing diseases, community living, communal showers and bathing, occlusive shoes and sports practice, as well as a person who works with closed shoes many hours of the day, working in damp areas, working in places with high levels of fungi such as swimming pools and saunas. The prevalence rates of predisposing diseases such as obesity and diabetes were 17% and 8%, respectively, in Europe and 5.3-6% and 5.6–7%, respectively, in Asia [123, 130].

Immune deficiency diseases such as AIDS, have gradually increased with time. Patients having chemotherapy, different types of steroids, organ transplants, and parenteral nutrition, the incidence of tinea pedis has increased [131]. The overall health of the patient is another important risk factor in development of tinea pedis. Obese and older patients with systemic illness such as varicous veins and/or diabetes mellitus are at increased risk for having tinea pedis and/or onychomycosis [132]. Other local factors that may contribute to tinea pedis are trauma, excessive wet/sweating activities such as public showers, swimming pools and wearing occlusive clothes.

A study in Israel showed that repeated foot washing among school children may lead to changes in pH in the stratum corneum, which encourages the fungus to reproduce [133].

Another study on tinea pedis prevalence has attributed 76% to wearing occlusive shoes (with a wearing shoe duration >8 h), followed by 67.6% for frequent communal showers, 54.4% for physical activities, 43.2% for mosque frequentations, 5.8% for diabetes, and 1.2% for obesity [120].

The prevalence rates combining tinea pedis and onychomycosis have been shown to be determined by age, social class, occupation, climate and living environment, and predisposing factorsp [134].

Tinea pedis appears to be associated with socioprofessional status. The prevalence rate of tinea pedis was shown to be higher in blue-collar workers (troop soldiers, guardians, chauffeurs, auxiliaries, manual workers), suggesting that this socioprofessional category might be a population at risk for the occurrence of tinea pedis.

This could be attributed to more traumas probably due to prolonged use of occlusive footwear as reflected by the high rate of this predisposing factor (76%). The increased cases of tinea pedis in winter may be due to soaking of feet coupled with occlusive footwear leading to hyperhidrosis and maceration. However, other contributing factors may be implicated.

Furthermore, significantly higher risk of tinea pedis has been recognized in those engaged in long distance running, swimming, water polo, soccer, and basketball. Several reports have suggested that swimming pools are high risk facilities with respect to infection with the disease [124].

Presentation

Tinea pedis occurs as one of following clinical variants depending on the pathogen, anatomical distribution and location, and may present in a given patient as one of several sympthoms. Typically, three variants are seen, including the interdigital, moccasin type, and vesiculobullous forms of the disease.

Generally chronic, intertriginous (interdigital) tinea pedis is characterized by a erythematous scaling and fissuring of the lateral toe webs (usually between the fourth and fifth toe webs) caused by dermatophyte which penetrate the uppermost layer of the stratum corneum; macerated, erosive infections may follow as a result of secondary overgrowth of commensal bacteria, including Micrococcaceae (usually staphylococci), aerobic coryneforms, and Gram-negative organisms.

Studies have identified the clinical lesions of tinea pedis being maceration in 28.1% of the subjects, erythema in 24.5% of the subjects, desquamation in 19.9% of subjects, fissurations in 13.5% of subjects, vesiculation in 6.7% of subjects, hyperkeratosis in 5.9% of subjects, and pustules in 1.4% of subjects. Pruritus was the most common functional symptom of tinea pedis and was present in 50% of subjects. It was followed by embarrassment (16.3%), pain (10.8%), and smell [120].

Interdigital-Type Tinea Pedis

Interdigital tinea pedis is the most common form, usually manifesting in the interspace of the fourth and fifth digits, and may spread to the underside of the toes (Figure 13.1).

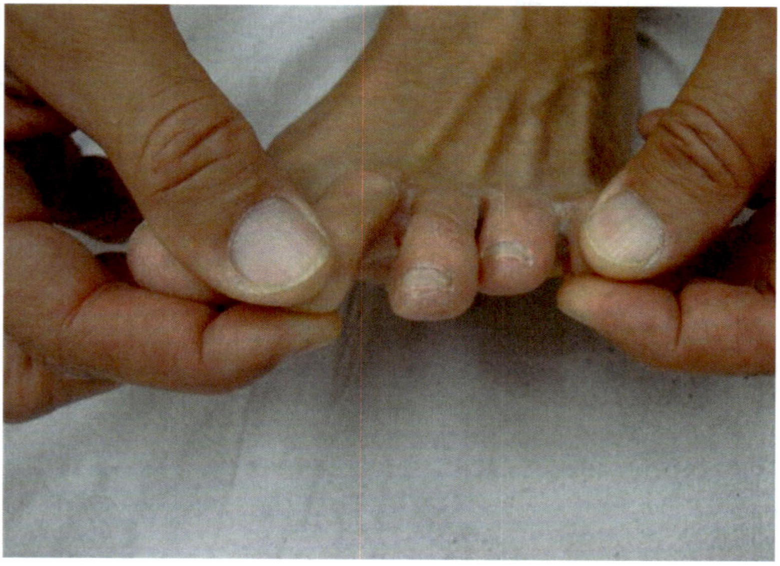

Figure 13.1. Tinea Pedis Interdigitalis.

Nail involvement often occurs and may resemble onychomycosis. In case of a PRP patient with onychomycosis (mycologically) two questions need to be asked. Is the onychomycosis pure onychomycosis? And are there two disorders – onychomycosis and PRP? Hence there is no need to have the skin PRP be close to the nail matrix/nail bed for the involvement of the nails (as in hand eczema). Mycological analysis should be taken followed by proper antifungal treatment (Figure 13.4).

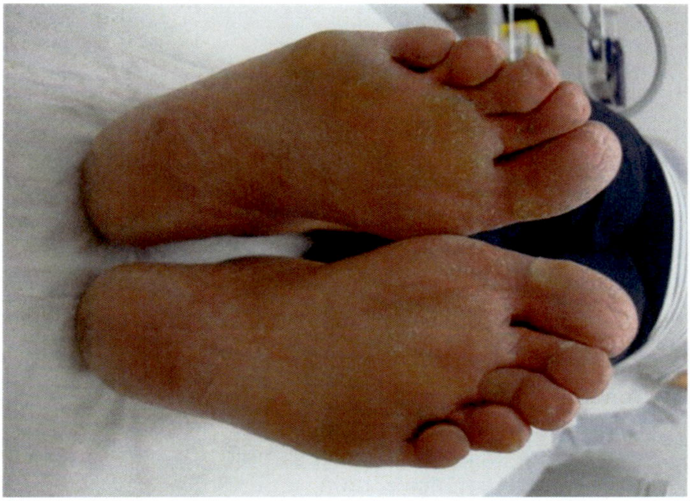

Figure 13.4. PRP-Pityriasis Rubra Pilaris at the soles mimicking Tinea Pedis Moccasin type.

B. Psoriasis

Psoriasis located between the toes is rare. Once it appears there it may emerge to the dorsal and/or plantar part of the foot (Figure 13.5).

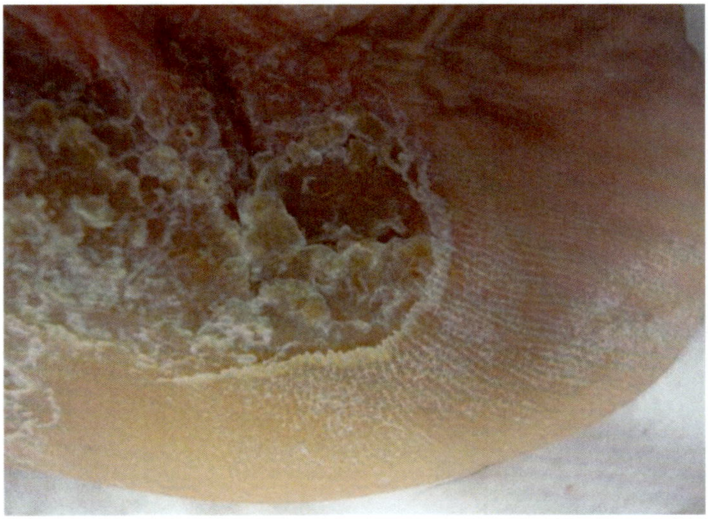

Figure 13.5. Psoriasis Pedis mimicking Tinea Pedis.

Clinically, between the toes the psoriatic plaques tend to be macerated, and while the plaques merge to the dorsal part, circumscribed borders will be seen with no central healing as can be seen in tinea corporis. Other psoriatic plaques are usually seen at other locations of the body, which may support the diagnosis. Sometimes, secondary infection with Gr-/Gr+ bacteria and/or dermatophyte/yeast/non-dermatophyte molds may occur. Relevant bacterial smear and culture should be taken and treated properly.

See more on page 89

C. Secondary Syphilis

See more on page 188

D. Pitted Keratolysis

The location of the pitted keratolysis (immersion foot) is usually at the prominence of the soles, in close contact with the inner side of the shoes. Usually tinea pedis is located between the toes, the central area of the soles (the part that does not have close contact with the inner part of the shoes), and around the soles (sometimes with gradual progression to the glabrous skin, the upper portion of the soles). Besides the location, the clinical appearance of pitted keratolysis is very different. While the clinical picture of tinea pedis may be erythematous, mildly edematous, with or without maceration, and fine or massive scales, the clinical appearance of immersion foot is whitish color, with or without (few or many – depending on the severity) punch out lesions located at the central area of the prominence of the soles (depending on the sub-type).

The smell of tinea pedis lesions (especially when the patient is taking off his shoes) exists at different levels (depending on the severity and the type of fungus), the smell of immersion foot is extremely malodorous.

While tinea pedis usually appears in adults, and less frequently in young adults, immersion foot is present more frequently in children and young adults. (The classic story is of the mother who comes with her son to the clinic and reports an "unbelievably bad smell of my son's foot, especially when he is taking off his shoes." This story is very characteristic for immersion foot.) (Figure 13.6).

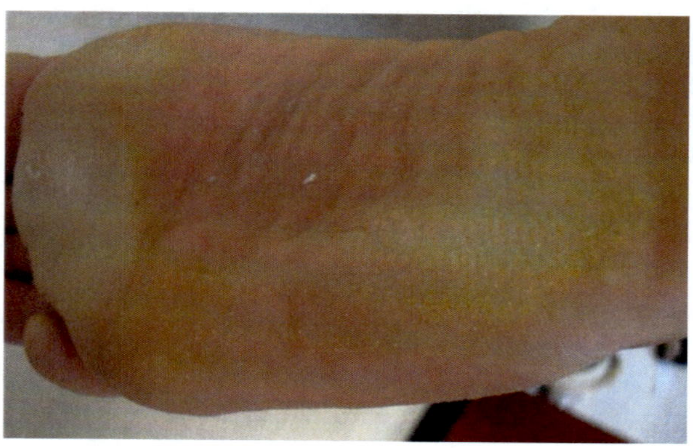

Figure 13.6. Pitted Keratolysis (immersion foot)

Vesiculobullous Tinea Pedis

The third type of tinea pedia is vesiculobullous tinea pedis; it presents the inflammatory type of tinea pedis; vesicles and/or pustules may be seen at the lateral or medial parts of the soles. Fluid-filled vesicles are usually clear but pus usually indicates secondary bacterial infection, most often caused by *Staphylococcus aureus* or group A *Streptococcus*. This form of tinea pedis may be associated with dermatophytid, which will be discussed later in this chapter. Vesiculobullous tinea pedis caused by *T. mentagrophytes* is an acute, highly inflammatory eruption, affecting particularly the arch and side of the foot. Patients with recurrent episodes often have low-grade scaling between bouts of acute inflammation (Figure 13.7) [135].

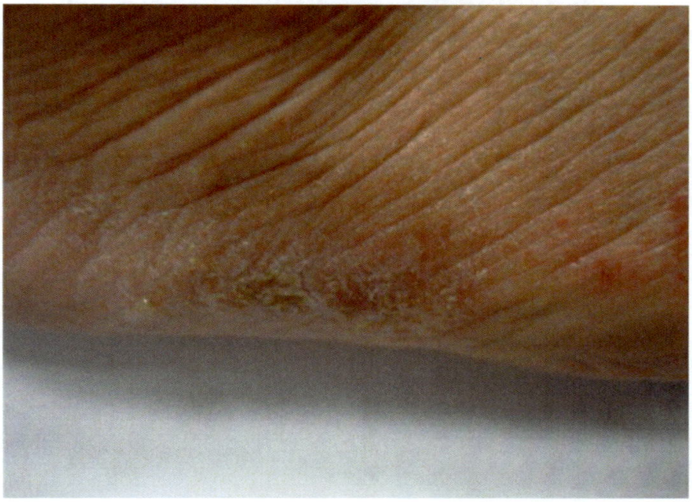

Figure 13.7. Vesiculobulous Tinea Pedis.

Differential Diagnosis of Vesiculobullous Tinea Pedis

A. Dyshidrotic Eczema

Dyshidrotic eczema located on the soles and on the toe web may be differentiated from the vesiculobullous type of tinea pedis (Figure 13.8). With this kind of vesiculobullous rash, which involves the soles only, mycological analysis should be done to rule out/confirm the diagnosis of vesiculobullous type tinea pedis.

In case the vesiculo-bullous rash is located along and/or between the fingernails, palms, along the arms, etc., with or without involvement of the soles, it could be dyshidrotic eczema. In case of severe tinea pedis between and/or around the toenail (erythematous, edematous, macerated, discharge sticky hemorrhagic/serous fluid), severe vesiculobullous eruptions may appear located at the fingernails, palms, along the arms, or even other parts of the upper part of the torso may be involved – this kind of eruption is the well-known "id reaction" (dermatophytid reaction). This vesiculobullous type is the most common subtype of id reaction.

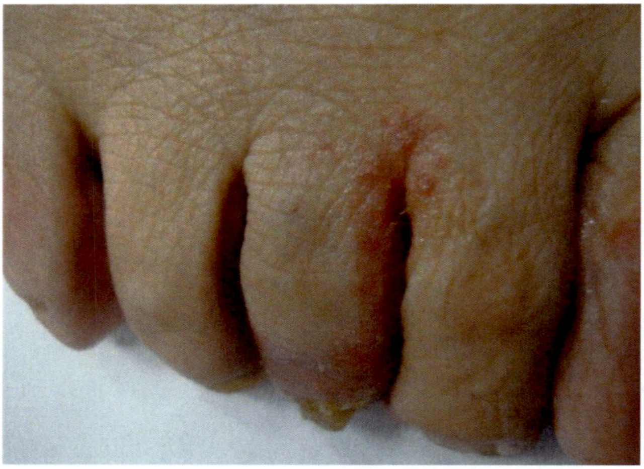

Figure 13.8. Dyshidrotic Eczema mimicking Vesiculobulous Tinea Pedis.

It should be stressed that to have the correct diagnosis of severe tinea pedis with id reaction, the following parameters should exist: the severe tinea pedis began before the id reaction, the fungal analysis is positive from the soles areas, the fungal analysis from id reaction is negative, and once the severe tinea pedis is treated correctly, the id reaction resolves gradually. Regarding the mycological analysis from the soles areas, severe tinea pedis sometimes may be involved with bacterial infection; in this case mycological analysis might be negative – by mistake. Systemic and topical relevant antibacterial medication should be given first and once the bacterial component disappears, mycological analysis should be taken.

B. Erythema multiforme

See more on Chapter 20

C. Friction Blister

Friction blisters are caused by frequent forced friction of the involved skin areas with objects that rub against the skin. The most common locations of these blisters are the feet such as around the heels and the lateral and/or medial sides of the feet (Figure 13.9). Secondary infection (impetiginization) may occur; cellulitis/erysipelas is rare.

Clinically, the blisters may be arranged in different patterns and may mimic the vesiculo-bullous type of tinea pedis.

Mycological analysis and precise anamnesis regarding sports activities may help in final diagnosis. Biopsy for electron microscopy combined with genetic investigation for gene mutation/s from the blister border are rarely needed to rule out epidermolysis bullosa.

D. Pustular Psoriasis

Pustular psoriasis may be located at the soles and palms hence the name palmoplantar psoriasis. This type of palmoplantar psoriasis may appear with or without other locations of plaque-type psoriasis; remission and/or exacerbation may occur.

Palmoplantar psoriasis is seen more often in women. Arthralgia/arthritis may accompany this type of pustular psoriasis.

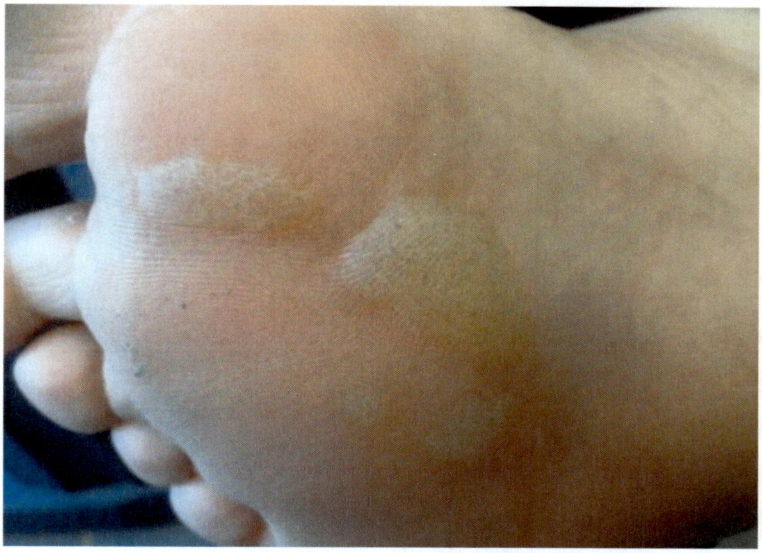

Figure 13.9. Friction Blisters.

E. Gram-Negative Toe Web Infection

Gram-negative toe web infection caused by several Gram-negative bacteria such as *Pseudomonas* spp., *Proteus* spp., *Moraxella* spp., and *Acinetobacter* spp., may be involved in tinea pedis interdigitalis, which is usually caused by fungi. Other bacteria such as Gram-positive and/or anaerobic bacteria may also be involved. Gram-negative bacteria usually produce a greenish–grey color, Gram-positive bacteria cause a moist exudative toe web infection, while the anaerobic bacteria create an extremely malodorous smell.

Gram-negative toe web infection usually occurs in those patients who wear tight shoes combined with extensive sports or physical activities for long periods of time. Usually these Gram-negative infections are secondary to toe web fungal infection. Clinically, the moist exudates combine with discharge of serum/pus exudates, and there is a whitish/greenish/grey color of the moist, macerated toe-web skin (Figure 13.10).

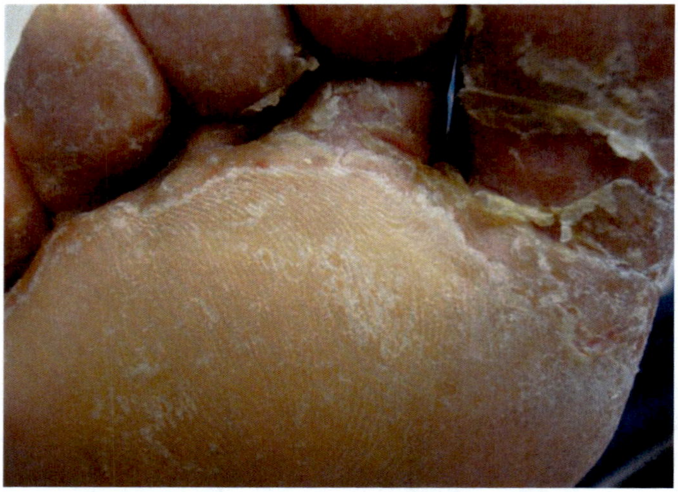

Figure 13.10. Gram-Negative toe-web Infection.

In such cases fungal analysis might be negative because of the superimposed bacterial infection. The first step is to identify the bacterial cause and treat it properly; then mycological analysis should be taken and if fungal infection was also involved, it might be found and should be treated. The Gram-negative bacteria should be treated topically with Castellani Paint combined (depending on the severity) with the relevant systemic antibiotic, and keeping the toe webs ventilated until total cure is achieved. This is done using gauze between the toes at the distal and not the proximal part of the toes.

In case of fluid discharge saline-wet gauze should be applied several times a day until the discharge discontinues. Severe cases should be hospitalized for several days or weeks until complete cure. There is a tendency for the Gram-negative bacterial toe web infection to recur, just like the toe web fungal infection; therefore, after achieving a complete cure preventive topical treatment (anti-fungal and anti-Gram negative bacterial) should be suggested.

Special Forms

When *Trichophyton inlerdigitale* is the causative organism, a vesicular, eczema-like appearance may occur, whereas very persistent, non-inflammatory lesions and dry scaling are characteristic of *T. rubrum* infectionsp [136].

Trichophyton tonsurans is another anthropophilic fungus in North America causing, albeit uncommonly, tinea pedis [125].

Non-dermatophyte filamentous injection molds such as *Scopulariopsis brevicaulis* rarely, if ever, cause infection of the skin of the feet. *Hendersonula toruloidea* and *Scytalidium hyalinum*, on the other hand, can produce lesions between the toes and on the soles that are clinically indistinguishable from those of *T. rubrum*. Infections caused by these two fungi have occurred mainly among patients from tropical and subtropical parts of the world. *H. toruloidea* has been recorded in patients from the Caribbean, Africa, the Middle East, Thailand, Hong Kong, and Fiji.

Scytalidium hyalinum infections have so far been seen only in patients from the Caribbean and West Africa. Many cases of *Hendersonula toruloidea* infection recorded in Europe and Canada have been in immigrants from areas where the fungus is endemic and account for only approximately 2–3% of isolates from cases of fungal foot infections. However, in endemic areas where *H. toruloidea* infections have been studied, the incidence has been found to be high [136].

Yeast infections of *Candida albicans* and other *Candida* spp. may occasionally cause maceration and erosion of the skin of the toe spaces, especially between the 4th and the 5th toes [136].

Carrier stage

Tinea pedis elicits only minor skin changes without any unpleasant odor, which can be represented as an "occult" infection. This can imply that patients with occult disease, even though they are asymptomatic, can still induce transmission. Carrier stage can be considered an early stage for the development of the dermatophytic infection. Hence, it is very important to identify this population in order to reduce the percentage of patients that can be infected with tinea pedis. It has been speculated that immunological factors are involved in those people who harbor dermatophytes while being asymptomatic. In addition, fungal spores can survive in low numbers without germinating and producing invasive hyphal elements. Another factor is the thickness of the stratum corneum at the palmoplantar areas (soles and palms), which is much thicker (30 to 50 times) compared to the stratum corneum of the rest of the body [135].

Further measures regarding public health and personal hygiene must be undertaken in order to reduce the risk of tinea pedis. Public areas that have a high turnover of people, such as gymnasia, farms, factories, swimming pools, changing rooms of sports clubs, and public showers, have a predilection for tinea pedis.

Diagnosis

It is typically easy to distinguish tinea pedis, and the final diagnosis is based on the clinical presentation and mycological analysis (direct microcopy and culture) preparation. Cultures combined with histological examinations are occasionally required. Wood's lamp is not usually helpful in diagnosing tinea pedis but can be used to rule out other mycological diseases such as pityriasis versicolor and tinea capitis caused by *Microsporum* spp. erythrasma are positive fluorescent by Wood's lamp, while common dermatophytes causing tinea pedis do not glow by Wood's lamp. The gold standard diagnostic for tinea pedis is direct microscopy and culture; no partial treatment should begin before the mycological analysis.

Direct Microscopy – Potassium Hydroxide (KOH)

Direct microscopy provides a rapid test for diagnosis of fungal infection of the skin and nails. The areas of samples for mycological analysis should be prepared correctly; cells from the periphery of the affected area are scraped onto a glass microscope slide with a sterile scalpel blade.

One or two drops of 10% KOH solution is dropped onto the collected scales on top of the slide (for rapid result the slides should be gently heated) to dissolve the keratin itself without destroying the hyphea skeleton. Slide preparations should then be examined under a microscope at low or medium power. If a vesicle is being examined, it should be ruptured and the fluid should be examined mycologically. Dermatophytes can readily be distinguished from yeasts and it is possible for a trained observer to differentiate a non-dermatophyte fungus from a dermatophyte. For suspected mold infections, the addition of Parker's blue-black ink (1 part KOH: 1 part blue-black ink) may be helpful [136].

Culture

A glucose/peptone agar (Sabouraud medium) is satisfactory for the isolation of the majority of fungal pathogens of the skin and nail.

Histology

See more on Chapter 4

PCR

See more on Chapter 4

Treatment

The simple cases are solvable by local treatment; in more difficult cases a systemic treatment is also needed.

Tinea pedis usually responds rapidlyto topical antifungal agents such as ketoconazole, terbinafine, econazole, or ciclopirox creams. In the case of interdigital infection, antifungal powder preparations may be more effective.

The duration of the topical treatment is variable and depends on the type of antifungal property; for example, while clotrimazole needs as much as 4 weeks, topical terbinafine needs only one week to eradicate the fungus. "Lamisil once" is a topical terbinafine treatment with a unique vehicle. Its application to the feet creates a "film" that dries very quickly and covers the terbinafine moldes. This treatment is equivalent to 7 days of treatment with lamisil cream, lamisil gel, or lamisil solution. However, the initial clinical response may not be accompanied by a mycologic cure. For refractory cases or stubborn disease, oral antifungals may be required. Oral treatment with griseofulvin, itraconazole, fluconazole, or terbinafine may be effective for this disease. It should be stressed that patient compliance, drug interactions, and less common drug resistance will directly affect the outcome and the percentage of complete cures.

Data show that any topical antifungal treatment does not achieve complete cure about one-third of patients with tinea pedis [137].

Many cases of relapse occur because of the lack of good compliance. It should be stressed that the patient should continue topical treatment at least one week after symptoms have resolved. The treated area should include normal skin about 2 cm beyond the affected area. Different studies show different results by using different topical antifungal agents.

All the antifungal agents may show about the same result over time, although the fungicidal activity of the allylamins/benzylamines and other may show better clinical and mycological results with regard to the period time of the treatment. The fungicidal antifungal afent needs shorter time compared to the fungistatic ones. A comparison study by Suschka et al. between clotrimazole 1% cream once daily and ketoconazole 2% cream twice/day showed that clotrimazole once day is as effective as ketoconazole twice daily [138]. Another randomized, double-blind parallel group study, which compared the effectiveness and the tolerability of topical terbinafine 1% cream twice a day for one week, with clotrimazole 1% cream twice a day for 3 weeks, showed the superiority of terbinafine against clotrimazole cream [120]. The combination of corticosteroid cream/ointment and the antifungal may lead to rapid reaction regarding the aching sensation or discomfort, combined with eradication of the causative agent. Once the clinical symptoms have been resolved, topical antifungal alone may be useful to eradicate the fungus completely. If by mistake the pure corticosteroid will be applied to fungal infection, the clinical symptoms will disappear (not completely), and after discontinuation of the topical corticosteroid a rebound of the fungal infection will occur. On the other hand, the side effects of long-standing topical potent steroids may lead to atrophy of the skin, telangiectasia, hirsutism, etc. These combination agents are relatively contraindicated in children under 12–years-of-age. Steroid therapy is withdrawn once the cell-mediated immune response is curtailed, but continued topical therapy is desirable in an attempt to eradicate residual fungus [135].

The treatment of intertriginous spaces by decreasing the amount of hyperhydrosis and using Castellani's paint (phenolated resorcinol) produces a better response. A novel method using a two-step kit as a topical treatment of tinea pedis was published by Shemer and his collegues. The method was based on soaking the feet in a topical solution for 45 minutes – a single treatment followed by a cosmetic cream resulted in 70% cure rate [139].

Systemic Antifungal Therapy

Once the topical treatment fails, systemic treatment must be taken into account. Systemic treatment may also be the first line therapy in patients with severe disease, such as severe hyperkeratotic lesions or immunosuppressed patients. Oral antifungals penetrate the deeper layers of the skin and have to be administered for a minimum of 2 weeks; in more stubborn cases the systemic treatment should be continued for 12 weeks.

Terbinafine has a rapid and potent fungicidal action that results in a high mycologic cure rate (>80%) and low relapse rate in interdigital tinea pedis with only 1 week of treatment. A study has shown that in patients treated with the l-week clotrimazole regimen only 38% converted from positive to negative mycology (KOB and culture) and did not experience relapse/reinfection [140].

Tinea pedis treated with itraconazole 200 mg twice daily for 1 week showed a cure rate of 85% at week 4 after stopping treatment [141].

A study has shown that systemic treatment with terbinafine for 2 weeks produced significantly higher mycological cure rates and significantly better clinical improvement than itraconazole. At 8-week follow-up 45-50% of itraconazole patients still presented with positive mycology. The fungicidal action produces very high cure rates in all forms of tinea pedis when terbinafine is given orally for short treatment periods [142].

Complications

Tinea Unguium (Onychomycosis)

Tinea unguium is a fungal, usually dermatophyte, infection on the nail matrix, nail plate, or nail bed usually associated with tinea pedis. *T. rubrum* is the major cause of subungual onychomycosis. Onychomycosis accounts for about one-third of fungal skin infections but only about 50% of onychomycoses are due to dermatophitic species.

A study has shown that tinea pedis was associated with onychomycosis in 30.5% of subjects. This rate was lower than that reported in the Hong Kong (37.4%) and Japan (Tokyo; 59%), but higher than that reported in Spain (Madrid; 1.1%) [120, 143].

Lower Extremity Cellulitis

Cellulitis is a bacterial infection of the subcutaneous layers of the skin.

Common predisposing factors forcellulitis include trauma, ulceration, and venous and lymphatic insufficiency. This is because this type of tinea pedis often has fissures between the toenails and plays a role as a port of entry for different bacteria, ending in onychomycosis and peripheral vascular disease. Erysipelas/cellulitis may arise from tinea pedis interdigitalis. Tinea pedis infections, most often interdigital type, may be complicated by cellulitis. Habitual wearing of occlusive shoes may lead to maceration and secondary occlusive conditions developing in the infected interspaces, leading to maceration and fissuring of the skin. This weakens the natural barrier of the skin and may serve as an entry point for several kinds of pathogenic bacteria, e.g., β-hemolytic *Streptococcus* (groups A, B, C, F, and G), *Staphylcoccus aureus*, and/or other *Staphylococcus* spp. Other Gr + and Gr – bacteria may cause cellulitis/erysipelas, but the β-hemolitic *Streptococcus* is the most common bacterial cause of cellulite/erysipelas (Figure 13.11).

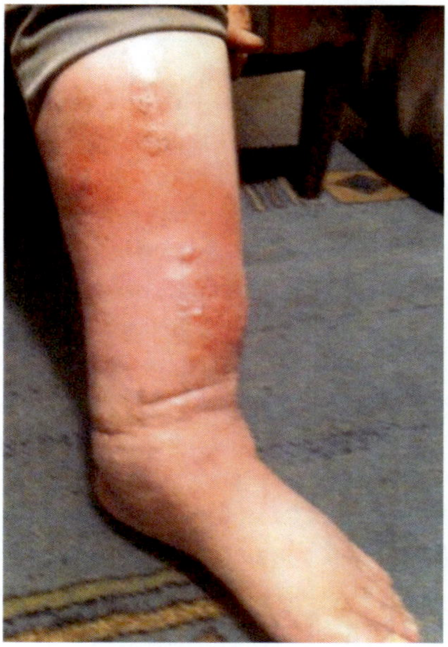

Figure 13.11. Erysepelas.

Complications of Tinea Pedis Moccasin Type

Tinea pedis may arise from the plantar area to the sides of the soles, up to the shin (Figure 13.12).

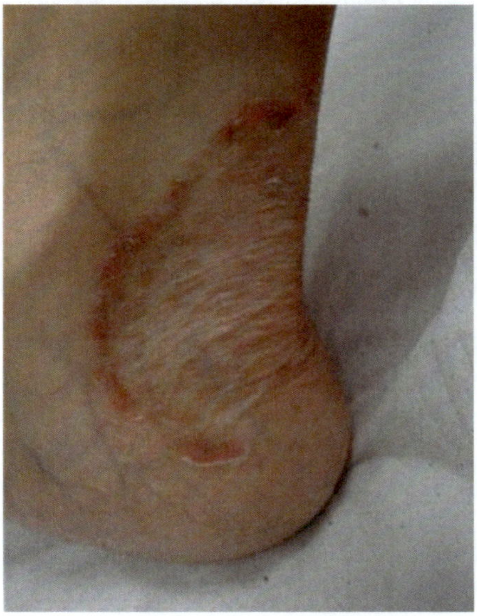

Figure 13.12. Widespread of Tinea Pedis.

Complications of Tinea Pedis Interdigitalis

The most common complaint of patients with tinea pedis interdigitalis is the mild to severe itching sensation. Some patients cannot ignore this disturbing feeling and scratch the toe webs strongly and very often (usually by rubbing the lateral side of the sole and the toe-webs). The more intense the scratching and the more frequent the scratching, the more the lichenification clinical presentation appears. Sometimes, due to the characteristic of the scratching actions, the fungus, which is located between the toes, may emerge to the lichenification site and by mistake a positive fungal smear/culture from the lichenification site could occur. Clinically the lichenification area is thick and hyperpigmented; no well-circumscribed borders or central healing may be seen. In other words, when finding fungus elements or even positive fungal culture at the lichenification areas, treatment with topical and or systemic antifungals is not the only treatment to be given. The patient has to know and understand that the scratching action has to stop (otherwise the lichenification will continue to be present (Figure 13.13). The lichenification area has to be treated properly with a topical low potency steroid with anti-fungal properties applied to the toe web. The caregiver should advise the patient to avoid applying the topical steroid to the webs as it may cause tinea incognito; therefore, parallel treatment with topical and/or systemic antifungal (depending on the severity) is to be given.

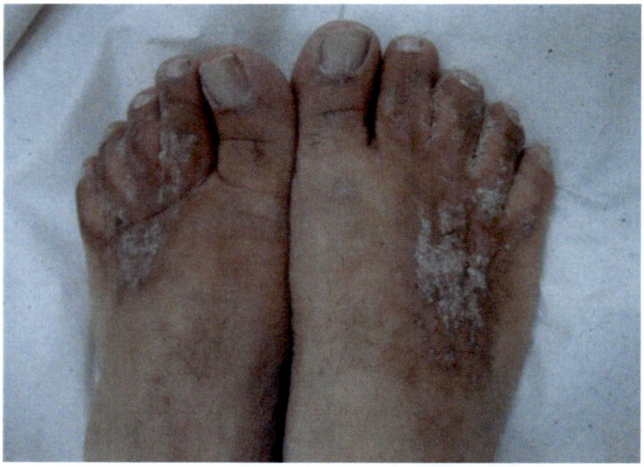

Figure 13.13. Long standing scratching –lichenification.

Dermatophytid

Dermatophytid reaction or id reaction or autoeczematization or disseminated eczema is a unique type of immunological reaction to a fungal infection, usually an acute fungal infection, but after stimulation may evoke the id reaction such as other bacterial infection or non-infectious diseases such as stasis dermatitis. (Figure 13.14)

Id reaction due to fungal infection appears as a rash located in a different area than the fungal infected area.

The following criteria of id reaction must occur:

1. Positive mycological analysis from the suspected location (feet)
2. No fungal elements in the id reaction location (no direct smear and culture)
3. The fungal infection appeared before the id reaction
4. Treatment of the fungal infection caused the id reaction to disappear gradually.

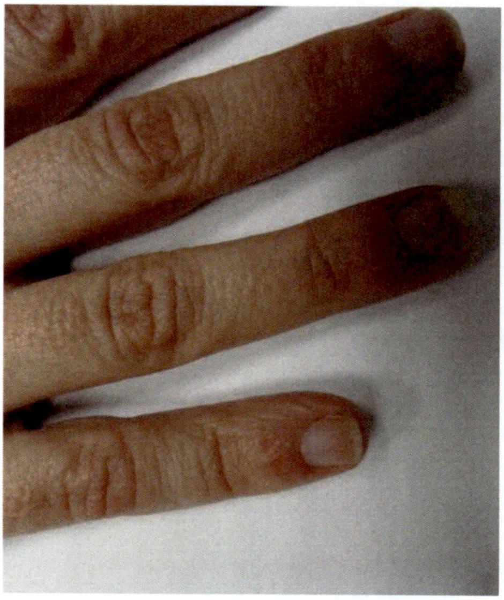

Figure 13.14. id reaction due to severe tinea pedis interdigitalis.

The mycological analysis from the id reaction is negative per definition and once the fungal infection is treated properly the id reaction rash disappears gradually.

Dermatophytid reaction has several clinical presentations:

1) vesicular – bullous eruption on the hand and arms, sometimes indistinguishable from dyshidrotic eczema (pompholyx)
2) follicular papules
3) erythema nodosum
4) erythema annulare centrifugum
5) urticaria
6) erysipelas-like
7) erythema multiform-like eruption

Id reaction usually occurs due to acute tinea pedis; it is more common with *Trichophyton mentagrophytes* but could happen with other dermatophytes.

Tinea capitis may also cause an id reaction due to several acute inflammatory types of tinea capitis. The reaction usually subsides with antifungal treatment. In some patients with follicular invasion, a residual sterile granuloma develops.

Id reactions result from interaction between the circulating antigen and the sensitization of the skin or activated T-lymphocytes that are directed against microbial antigens derived from a nonliving organism [144,145]. The dermatophytic reaction originates from the Greek, denoting a father-son relationship [146]. If a patient experiences an id reaction the primary lesion will demonstrate the presence of the dermatophyte but not in the id reaction. The diagnosis is established with the presence of the mycotic pathogen in the primary lesion, absence of the fungus in the secondary lesion, spontaneous improvement in the secondary lesions after eradication of the primary lesion, and positive reaction to trichophytin [144]. The dermatophytid reactions are most often seen in the hands and feet, usually located far from the location of the fungal infection. There are different types of dermatophyte reactions, the most common are eczematic or dysidrotic, lichenoid, vesicular, follicular, and scaling form.

In adults with tinea pedis, which is usually caused by *T. mentagrophytes*, the most common type of id reaction is seen on the hands and sides of the fingers [147,148]. Some patients with tinea pedis develop acute, symmetrical, vesicular eruptions at a secondary site, usually on the fingers or palmar surfaces and the interdigital spaces. Lesions initially include vesicles and bullae; later papules or pustules can form [147,148].

Generalized follicular papules were rarely observed, and some bacteria, such as β-hemolytic *Streptococcus*, may have been copathogens [149]. Additionally, a case of vesiculobullous tinea pedis with a dermatophytid reaction caused by anthropophilic *T. violaceum* was reported.

Bacterial co-infection

Tinea pedis is commonly co-infected with bacteria. Common bacterial coinfection in descending order of frequency in a study have included β-hemolytic *Streptococcus* (85%), *Staphylococcus aureus* (45%), and Enterobacteriaceae (35%) [125]. Bacterial co-infection can often lead to negative direct microscopy and mycological culture. It is usual prior to initiation of the antifungual treatment to start a course of antibiotic treatment followed by microscopic examination. Once the aetiologic agent is identified the antimycotic agent can be initiated.

Follow-up

Tinea pedis does not often necessitate regular follow-ups. The disease often responds promptly to topical agents but if the infection persists, symptomatic relapse is likely to occur, necessitating repeated courses of therapy and the need for oral agents.

The coexistence of tinea pedis with other types of fungal skin infections is a frequent phenomenon [150]. Many patients with toenail onychomycosis or tinea pedis are not aware that they have a fungal infection, and such patients pose a special challenge for physicians to detect and treat the disease. We should also remember that it was clearly shown that tinea pedis may precede toenail onychomycosis [144].

Fluid-filled vesicles are usually clear but pus usually indicates secondary bacterial infection, most often with *S. aureus* or group A *Streptococcus*. This form of tinea pedis may be associated with dermatophytid or id reaction.

Occult disease should be borne in mind and asymptomatic carriers of the disease should be treated. Further measures regarding public health and personal hygiene must be undertaken in order to reduce the risk of tinea pedis.

Chapter 14

Tinea Manuum

Synonym: Dermatophytoses of the hands/palms, one hand-two feet disease.
Definition: Tinea manuum is a fungal infection of one or both hands/palms.

Epidemiology

Dermatophytic infections of the hands are considered to be rare and occur slightly more often in males than in females. Contagion may take place through contact with another infected individual, with an animal, or, more rarely, with the soil or contaminated objects, or by autoinfection.

Contributing Factors

Patients whose occupations require intensive use of the hands were significantly more likely to develop tinea manuum. Recurring work-related trauma to the hands or picking infected hand nails could result in the development of tinea manuum [151]. In addition, factors favoring tinea manuum other than manual work are hyperhidrosis, existing inflammatory conditions, and frequent use of alkaline soaps.

Pathogens

The most common etiological agents for dermatophyte infections of the palms are *Trichophyton rubrum, Trichophyton mentagrophytes,* and *Trichophyton verrucosum* [152]. Contagion may take place through contact with another infected individual, with an animal, or, more rarely, with the soil or contaminated objects, or by autoinfection. The most frequent infections occur from anthropophilic species of *T. rubrum* [152].

The one hand-two feet syndrome involves dermatophyte infections of both feet, with tinea manuum of the right or left palm; the most frequently identified pathogen involved is *T. rubrum* [151].

Non-dermatophytic filamentous fungi made up 2.3% of the confirmed etiologic agents obtained overall and constituted 3.3% of the agents obtained from nail infections. The most common species were identified are *Scopulariopsis brevicaulis*, *Hendersonula toruloidea*, and *Aspergillus sydowii.*

Only *H. toruloidea* and *S. hyalinum* have been reported to cause palm and sole infections [153].

Clinical Presentation

Tinea manuum is generally unilateral, the right hand being more often affected. On the palms, dermatophyte infection may appear in two forms: dyshidrotic or eczematoid form and hyperkeratotic form (Figure 14.1, Figure 14.2).

Vesicles, in annular or segmental patterns, are present in dyshidrotic form, but bullae are generally infrequent in tinea manuum. The dyshidrotic or eczematoid form tends to be more inflammatory. In its acute stage, it is characterized by 1 or 2 mm vesicles located on the palm of the hand and fingers, arranged in annular or segmental patterns [152]. Occasionally, localized, vesicular patches or erythematous papular lesions may occur, which are usually caused by zoophilic dermatophytes such as *T. mentagrophytes* var. *erinacei* [154].

Tinea manuum usually accompanies tinea pedis or tinea unguium, characteristically involving one palm and both feet (Figure 14.3). The palmar surface is diffusely dry and hyperkeratotic.

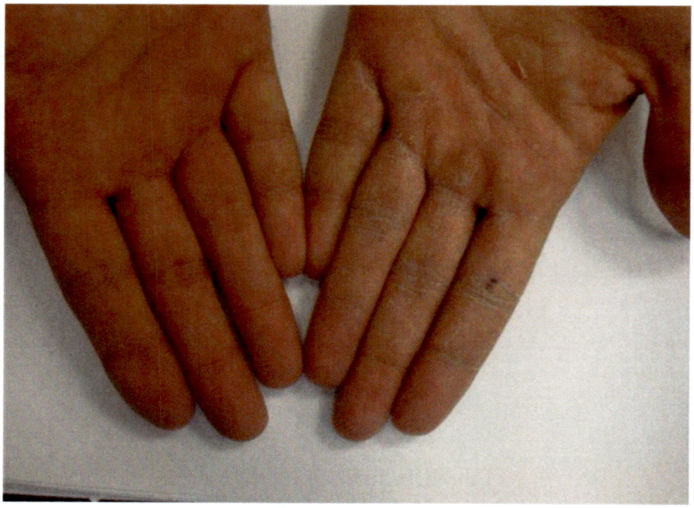

Figure 14.1. Palmar Tinea Manuum.

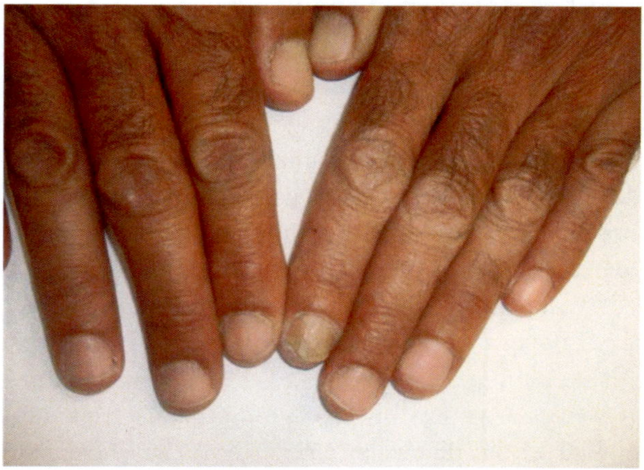

Figure 14.2. Dorsal Tinea Mannum with involvement of the second left nail plate.

When the fingernails are involved, vesicles and scant scaling may be present, and the condition resembles dyshidrotic eczema [106].

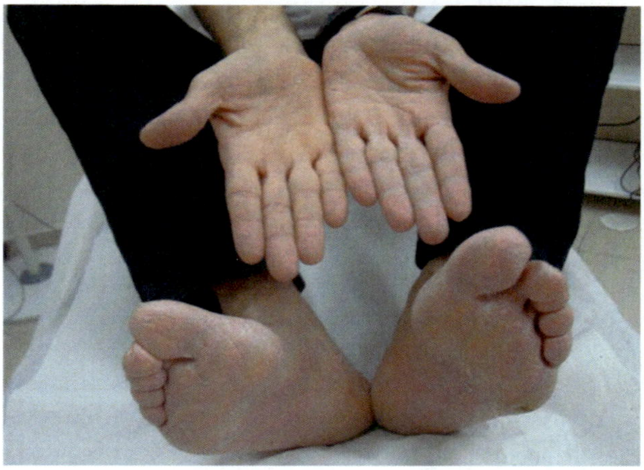

Figure 14.3. Two feet one hand.

Differential Diagnosis

Tinea manuum should be considered in any patient who presents with scaling, fissuring, or erythema of the palms. Tinea manuum may sometimes be misdiagnosed with a number of dermatological conditions such as:

- Irritant or contact dermatitis see more on page 69
- Dyshidrotic eczema or pompholyx

Dyshidrotic eczema is a type of dermatitis of unknown cause characterized by a pruritic vesicular eruption located around the fingers, palms, and soles. The condition affects teenagers and adults and may be acute, recurrent, or chronic. A more appropriate term for this vesicular eruption is pompholyx, which means bubble. The clinical course of dyshidrotic eczema can range from self-limited to chronic, severe, or debilitating. The condition's unresponsiveness to treatment can be frustrating for the patient and physician. Dyshidrotic eczema may be associated with atopy and familial atopy. Of patients with dyshidrosis, 50% have atopic dermatitis. In some patients, a distant fungal infection can cause palmar pompholyx as an id reaction. In one study, one-third of pompholyx occurrences on the palms resolved after treatment for tinea pedis [155]. Patients report pruritus of the hands and feet with a sudden onset of vesicles. Burning pain or pruritus may occasionally be experienced before vesicles appear. Tiny vesicles erupt first along lateral aspects of the fingers and then on the palms or soles. Palms and soles may be red and wet with perspiration. The vesicles usually persist for 3–4 weeks. A variety of factors are possibly related to eruptions: emotional stress, personal or familial atopic diathesis (e.g., asthma, hay fever, sinusitis), certain work exposures (e.g., cobalt) and/or recreational exposures, recent exposure to contact allergens (e.g.,nickel, balsams, paraphenylenediamine, chromate, sesquiterpene lactones), patients allergic to nickel and recently exposed to costume jewelry, recent treatment with intravenous immunoglobulin therapy, and HIV infection. With long-standing disease, patients' fingernails may reveal dystrophic changes (e.g., irregular, transverse ridging; pitting; thickening; discoloration). Interdigital maceration and desquamation of the interdigital spaces are often present, despite the possible absence of a dermatophyte infection. Vesicles and/or bullae may become infected secondarily, and pustular lesions may be present. Cellulitis and lymphangitis may develop. The diagnosis of dyshidrotic eczema is usually made clinically, although bacterial culture and sensitivity tests exclude secondary infection. In dyshidrotic eczema, typical first-line treatment includes high-strength topical steroids and cold compresses. Short courses of oral steroids are the second line of treatment for acute flares, and other immunosuppressants have also been tried.

- Atopic dermatitis-see more on page 48
- Psoriasis

Plaque psoriasis is a chronic inflammatory disease. It involves raised plaques that are usually oval or irregular in shape, of one to several cm. The plaques have distinctive red color and are well defined, with sharply demarcated borders. They usually appear on the scalp, trunk, and limbs, with a predilection for extensor surfaces, such as the elbows and knees. Plaque psoriasis may involve the nail as well as the joints, causing arthralgia/arthritis. The psoriatic plaques and tinea corporis both have well-defined borders, but plaque psoriasis does not have elevated borders or central healing as can be seen in tinea corporis. The diagnosis of psoriasis is almost always made on the basis of clinical findings. Laboratory investigations are rarely used. A skin biopsy may confirm the diagnosis of plaque psoriasis.

Psoriasis may occur also or only at the palms. If the psoriasis plaque appears on the palms and also on other parts of the body such as the knees, elbows, scalp, etc., and the plaques on the palms resemble psoriasis, it should be considered as psoriasis, unless the lesions on the palms resemble tinea manuum – then a mycological analysis should be conducted.

In the case where the psoriasis lesions are only located on the palms, mycological analysis should be taken into account.

It should be stressed that psoriatic lesions are usually more localized and do not tend to appear on the entire palm area. In tinea manuum, there is usually involvement of the entire palm area and there are no plaques per se, but there is a diffuse dryness and thickness of the palms with fine scales. On the other hand, thickness and dryness of the palm could be a presentation of psoriasis, although it is uncommon (Figure 14.4).

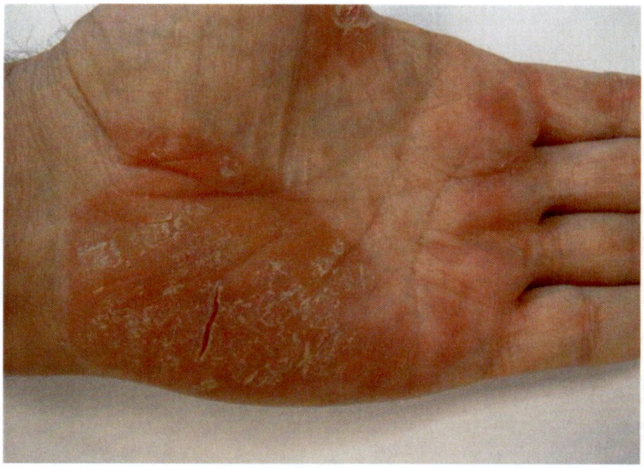

Figure 14.4. Psoriasis of the palm.

Lamellar dyshidrosis (LD)

LD, also known as keratosis, is a kind of disease that is usually due to excessive sweating of the palms and/or soles, causing the skin of the soles/palms to exfoliate (Figure 14.5). Sometimes there is a painful sensation, but usually it is asymptomatic. Usually this disorder is bilateral while tinea manuum is unilateral. LD has occasional or seasonal outbursts, while tinea manuum is usually continuous.

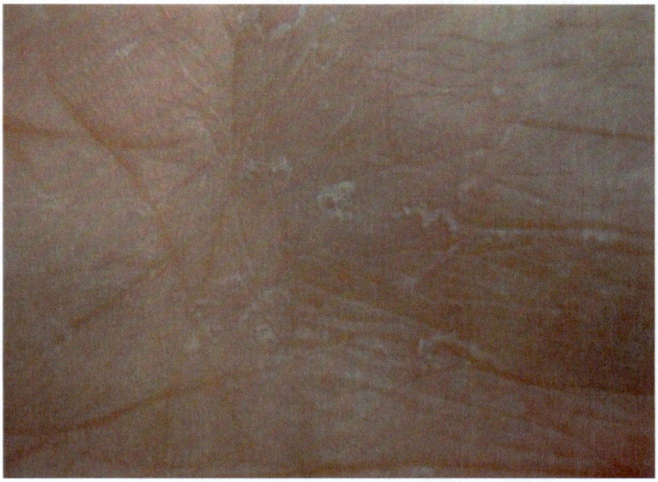

Figure 14.5. LD Lamellar Dyshidrosis.

Scabies

Scabies is a contagious infectious disease caused by the mite *Sarcoptes scabiei*. This mite burrows very tiny "tunnels" in the epidermis, and as a result causes an intense itching sensation. Usually the locations are at the wrist, between the fingers, in the axilla area, and in general where the skin is softer, which makes it easier for the mite to penetrate. In children and in severe cases of scabies, palm involvement occurs (Figure 14.6). The clinical presentation is variable, but solitary or diffuse papules conjoin to plaques up to the hyperkeratosis-like lesions. Usually, if there is involvement of the palm, scabies is also located at other parts of the body.

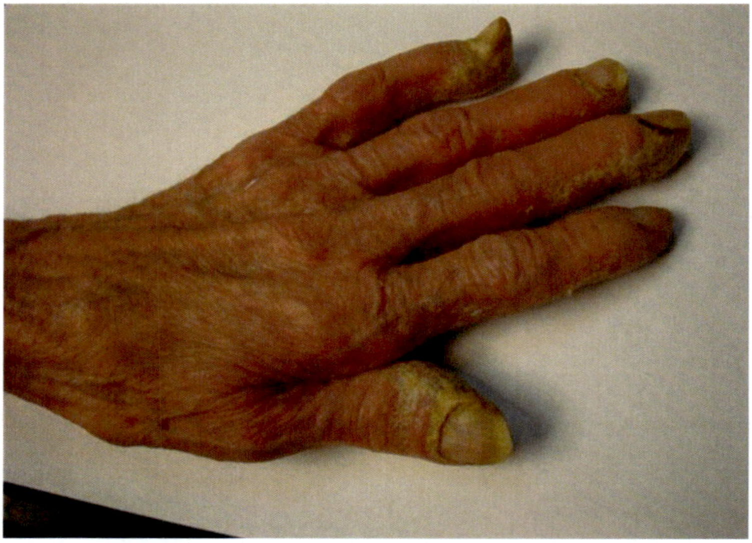

Figure 14.6. Scabies Hand.

Palmoplantar keratoderma

Keratoderma is an acquired autosomal dominant and less frequent autosomal recessive or congenital disorder. There are many different types of keratoderma.

In cases where the disorder is on both the palms and soles and has presented from infancy, it is most likely congenital keratoderma. The acquired cases should be taken into account as a differential diagnosis of tinea manuum, but it should be mentioned that the hypokeratotic plaques are usually not seen in tinea manuum.

Diagnosis

The diagnosis of tinea manuum is confirmed by microscopy and culture of skin scrapings. Occasionally, when diagnostic difficulties occur, skin biopsy and PCR may be required. The laboratory techniques are explained in detail in Chapter 4.

Treatment

The treatment of tinea manuum is systemic in principle, but mild cases can be treated topically. In case the topical treatment has failed, systemic treatment should be given for 1–2 months. If there is onychomycosis involvement of the same hand (not a rare condition) and/or onychomycosis of the toenail, the recommended treatment is systemic, terbinafine 250 mg 1x/d for 3 months, or itraconazole 20 gx2/d for a week, then an interval of 3 weeks and repeated 3–4 times, while having a systemic treatment, relevant blood analysis and CBC and liver function tests should be done every month.

Chapter 15

Onychomycosis

Synonyms: Tinea unguium

Definition: Onychomycosis describes fungal infection of the nail caused by dermatophytes, nondermatophyte molds, and yeasts. Tinea unguium strictly refers to dermatophyte infection of the nail.

Epidemiology

Onychomycosis is a common affliction of toenail disease that is estimated to represent up to 50% of all nail diseases; its prevalence increases with age. It affects up to 14% of the population with both an increasing prevalence among older individuals (nearly 30% of patients are older than 60 years) and an overall increasing incidence [156].

The prevalence of onychomycosis has increased sharply in recent decades, possibly secondary to wearing tight shoes, increasing numbers of individuals on immunosuppressive drugs, an increased use of communal locker rooms, suboptimal immune function, inactivity, and the inability to maintain good foot care [157].

Although infrequent, onychomycoses can affect children 5 and is most likely due to the use of occlusive footwear. There is an increase in incidence among children and adolescents and accounts for up to 20% of dermatophyte infections diagnosed in children [158].

Onychomycosis commonly begins as tinea pedis before extending to the nail bed. This site often serves as a reservoir for local recurrence or for infections spreading to other areas. Up to 40% of patients with toenail onychomycosis show concomitant mycotic skin infections, most commonly tinea pedis (30%).

Many studies have investigated the coexistence of onychomycosis and nail psoriasis [158-166]. Psoriatic patients seem to have increased prevalence of onychomycosis when compared with control groups and literature on healthy populations, even though the final evidence remains lacking [167,168]. It is advisable to rule out onychomycosis in psoriatic patients with nail abnormalities because nail psoriasis is being treated with immunosuppressive drugs, such as steroids, methotrexate, or biologics, which may aggravate mycotic nail infections. Furthermore, specific groups such as people with diabetes have also been found to have a higher prevalence than non-diabetic individuals [169]. Crowded public locations may play a role in the spread of the fungus (anthropophilic contamination such as *Trichophyton rubrum*). Furthermore, factors that increase the prevalence of onychomycosis include increasing age; male sex; genetic factors; underlying conditions such as diabetes, immunodeficiency, peripheral arterial disease, and psoriasis; environmental and behavioral factors such as sports and religious practices; and certain professions such as athletes and swimmers [170].

Pathogens

Most onychomycoses are caused by dermatophytes that belong to three genera: *Trichophyton*, *Microsporum*, and *Epidermophyton*.

Dermatophytes are a homogeneous group of keratophilic fungi. They are transmitted via damp floor surfaces and less frequently via direct person-to-person contact [157]. Several fungi can be causative agents, but three species predominate worldwide: *T. rubrum*, *Trichophyton mentagrophytes*, and *Epidermophyton floccosum* [171,172].

T. rubrum and *T. mentagrophytes* are the first and second most frequent etiologic agents worldwide [171].

T. rubrum is found in 60% of cases, *T. mentagrophytes* in 20%, and *E. floccosum* in 10%. *T. rubrum* is clinically associated with distal lateral subungual onychomycosis [157,173,174].

The genus *Microsporum* is distributed worldwide and *M. canis* is the most common zoophilic species to affect humans, a common cause of tinea capitis in children. *Microsporum* spp. is however an uncommon cause of onychomycosis.

Patients with *M. canis* onychomycosis can be associated with domestic cats or dogs. *M. canis* has been reported to be associated with tinea corporis, tinea capitis, and HIV infection and long-term immunosupressant drug therapy. *M. gypseum* is a soil saprophyte; one source of human infection has been traced to soil with a rising incidence that may be attributable to the domestication of dogs and cats [172].

Nondermatophyte onychomycoses (molds) are more rarely involved and account for 2% to 12% of all nail fungal infections [129,157, 174]. Nondermatophyte onychomycoses are caused by a wide range of fungi, mainly *Scopulariopsis brevicaulis*, *Aspergillus versicolor*, *Aspergillus flavus*, *Aspergillus niger*, *Aspergillus fumigatus*, *Fusarium solani*, *Fusarium oxysporum,* and *Scytalidium* spp. These nondermatophyte fungi are filamentous fungi that lack the keratinolytic capacity of dermatophytes, but they still can infect alone or in combination with the latter. They live on unkeratinized intercellular cement or must take advantage of previous keratin destruction by a dermatophyte, trauma, or another nail disease. For this reason, they are usually secondary invaders and are not primary parasites of the nail plate [175]. The most commonly isolated saprophytic mold is *Scopulariopsis brevicaulis*p [176].

S. brevicaulis, mostly geophilic with a worldwide distribution, and *Avicularia versicolor* are the most frequent nondermatophyte molds found on the feet. The participation of *A. flavus*, *A. niger*, *A. fumigatus*, *A. sydowii*, *A. unguis*, *Fusarium solani*, and *Fusarium oxysporum* as pathogens must be carefully considered because they have a universal distribution and are common laboratory contaminants. *Scytalidium* spp. (previously

Hendersonula toruloidea) cause infection of the toenails and fingernails and can also affect the skin of the hands and feet, alone or combined with dermatophytes [172].

Yeasts are true fungi that lack hyphae and therefore cannot be classified as molds. Yeasts typically affect fingernails rather than toenails.

Yeast infection, particularly *Candida* spp., is responsible for up to 30% of fingernail onychomycosis, whereas nondermatophyte molds are not commonly detected in diseased fingernails. *Candida albicans* is the yeast most commonly isolated (5.6%) [157].

Mixed infections of nondermatophyte molds with dermatophytes have been described in varying percentages of 3% to 11% [177,178]. In one epidemiologic study from Canada, *Scytalidium dimidiatum* accounted for less than 1% of cases of onychomycosis [179]. In France, *Scytalidium* spp. are the most frequent nondermatophyte fungi in onychomycosis (3.6%), and 9% are mixed infections. All of these patients were residents or had visited tropical or subtropical countries [180]. Disseminated infection from an onychomycosis due to *Fusarium* is exceptional but has been documented [181].

The most common pathogen identified in the pediatric population is *T. rubrum*, and the most prevalent site involved is the toenails. Family history of OM and concurrent tinea pedis infection are seen, but most children present with neither [158].

The appearance of the nail and accompanying lesions may provide clues to the likely identity of the infecting organism, although it is seldom possible to identify the species on clinical grounds alone. For instance, irrespective of right or left handedness, unilateral hand involvement is a common feature of dermatophytosis caused by *Trichophyton rubrum*; in such patients, both feet are commonly infected. Similarly, onychomycosis confined to the fingernails is more suggestive of a *Candida* infection, especially in paronychia and onycholysis, although infections caused by either *Scytalidium dimidiatum* (*Hendersonula toruloidea*) or *Scytalidium hyalinum* may cause the same nail changes.

Predisposing Factors

Some of the contributing factors that are associated with eliciting onychomycosis are humidity, occlusive footwear, repeated nail trauma, genetic predisposition, concurrent disease, poor peripheral vascular circulation, HIV infection, as well as other forms of topical or systemic immunosuppression [171, 173, 182, 183].

Other significant predisposing factors are a family history of onychomycosis, footwear, hyperhidrosis, local trauma psoriasis, peripheral circulatory alterations, and local factors, such as climate. The disease is more common in diabetic patients and hemodialysis patients. [168].

Onychomycosis is the second most common nail disorder in dialysis patients. Studies report that dialysis duration and diabetes mellitus are independent risk factors [171, 172, 184, 185].

Toenails are predominantly affected in onychomycosis and the major risk factor is occlusive footwear. Consequently, the prevalence of infection is often higher in urbanized populations. Fingernail infection, which is less common, is usually associated with occupational exposure to damp or wet conditions. Nail diseases such as psoriasis or damage to the nail plate also predispose to infection [172].

Clinical Presentation

The first clinical classification for onychomycosis was published in 1972 [186]. Modifications have been made since then and the most widely used classification was published in 1998 [187]. Fungal infections of the nail apparatus may be classified according to the invasion pattern of infection in the nail plate, including the site and mode of invasion. There are seven clinical presentations: 1. distal and lateral subungual onychomycosis, 2. superficial onychomycosis, 3. proximal subungual white onychomycosis, 4. endonyx onychomycosis, 5. mixed pattern onychomycosis, 6. secondary onychomycosis, and 7. total dystrophic onychomycosis. Some authors also include candidal paronychia as an infection pattern.

A recent revised classification by Hay et al. [188] has extended this to include mixed and secondary forms of onychomycotic infection and refined the definition of superficial and proximal subungual infection.

Distolateral Subungual Type (DLSO)

Distal subungual onychomycosis affects the nail bed, nail plate, and the hyponychium. Infection usually initiates with tinea pedis from the surrounding skin, the most common form is distolateral subungual onychomycosis (DLSO). DLSO remains the commonest form of fungal invasion of the nail plate, where the site of invasion is from the lateral or distal undersurface of the nail plate.

DLSO begins with invasion of the stratum corneum of the hyponychium and distal nail bed, most commonly forming a white or yellowish opacification at the distal edge of the nail but, on occasion, other color changes such as brown, black (Figure 15.1), and orange discoloration have been described as well (Figure 15.2).

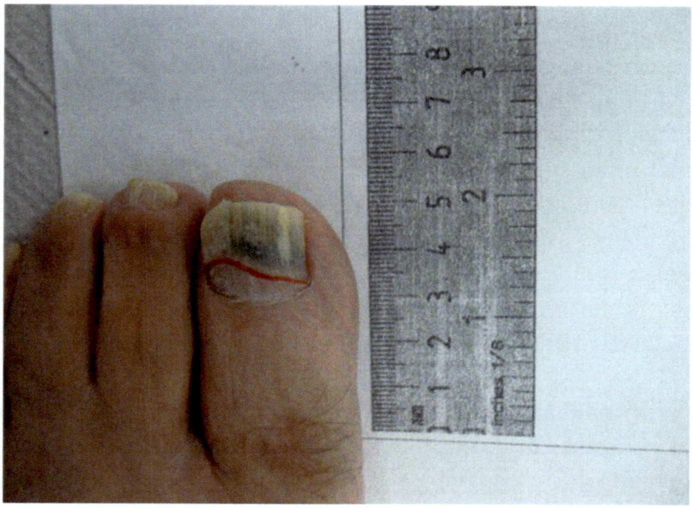

Figure 15.1. DLSO Distolateral Subungual Type.

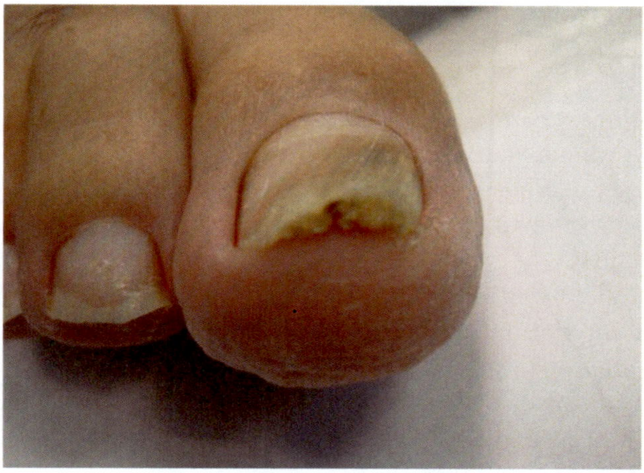

Figure 15.2. DLSO Distolateral Subungual Type.

The infection then spreads proximally up the nail bed to the ventral nail plate. Hyperproliferation or altered differentiation of the nail bed in response to the infection results in subungual hyperkeratosis, while progressive invasion of the nail plate results in an increasingly dystrophic nail [189]. DLSO may be complicated by other changes such as longitudinal streaking of the nail, sometimes called a dermatophytoma. Streaking or dermatophytoma can be seen in other patterns of onychomycosis but is commonest with DLSO [188] (Figure 15.3).

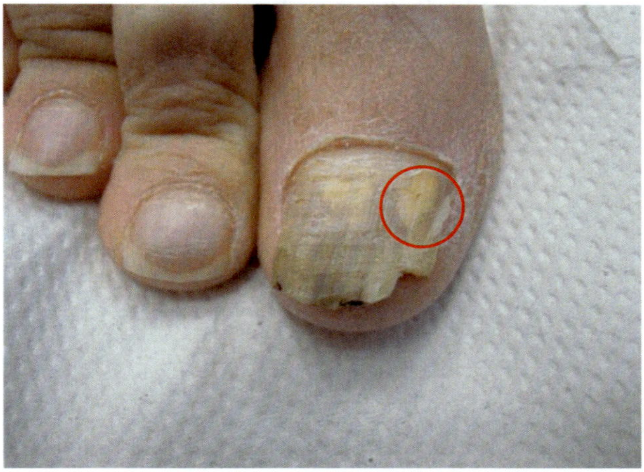

Figure 15.3. Dermatophytoma.

Onycholysis is occasionally the only physical abnormality associated with distolateral nail plate invasion [188]. If onycholysis is the only sign of nail abnormality it is important to verify fungal invasion of the nail either by direct microscopy or mycological culture.

DLSO is associated with a variety of different fungi with the most common being *T. rubrum*, *T. mentagrophytes*, *E. floccosum*, *C. albicans*, *Fusarium* spp., *Scytalidium* spp., and *Scopulariopsis brevicaulis* [188].

DLSO caused by *T. rubrum* may result in the fungus spreading from the plantar and palmar surfaces of the feet and hands, a pattern seen in the one hand-two foot tinea syndrome [189].

DLSO caused by *Scytalidium dimidiatum* or *Scytalidium hyalinum* present in a pattern similar to that of dermatophyte onychomycosis, but secondary paronychia appears to be a more common feature in fingernail infections, and extensive onycholysis may also be a prominent feature of these infections [189]. Paronychia associated with DLSO is also seen in some *Fusarium* infections.

Aspergillus spp., *Acremonium* spp., *Penicillium* spp., and *Pyrenochaeta unguis-hominis* most commonly present with hyperkeratosis and brown or green discoloration; the toenails are most commonly affected [189].

Microsporum spp. can also manifest with DLSO; this is the most common clinical presentation followed by TDO and SWO, and rarely PSO. *M. gypseum* is the most common pathogen isolated among the *Microsporum* species causing DLSO [172].

Proximal Subungual Onychomycosis (PSO)

PSO primarily originates from infection under the proximal nail and nail fold with the infection slowly extending distally, organized in diffuse patches or transverse striate patterns (Figure 15.4).

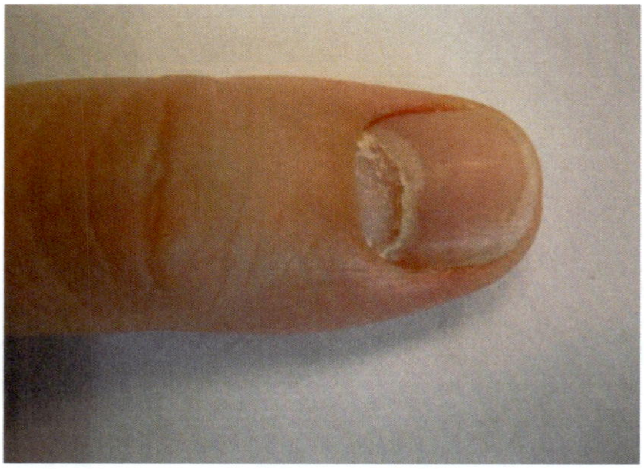

Figure 15.4. Proximal subungual onychomycosis.

Those forms presenting with transverse bands (striate pattern) are often associated with a concurrent superficial onychomycosis. This form of infection is difficult to treat and always requires oral therapy, although relapse is common [188].

Proximal White Subungual Onychomycosis (PWSO)

Proximal white subungual onychomycosis (PWSO) is considered to be rare and can affect both fingernails and toenails. PWSO is seen with a wide range of organisms including dermatophytes, usually *T. rubrum*, *T. megninii*, *T. schoenleinii*, and also *Fusarium* spp.; *C. albicans*, and *Aspergillus* spp. have been recorded as causes [188,189]. The causative organisms are thought to penetrate via the stratum corneum of the proximal nail fold, which is the primary site of the fungal invasion.

T. rubrum and *T. megnini* can clinically appear as a white to beige opacity on the proximal nail plate. This opacity gradually enlarges to affect the entire nail and eventuates in subungual hyperkeratosis, leukonychia, proximal onycholysis, and/or destruction of the entire nail (Figure 15.5).

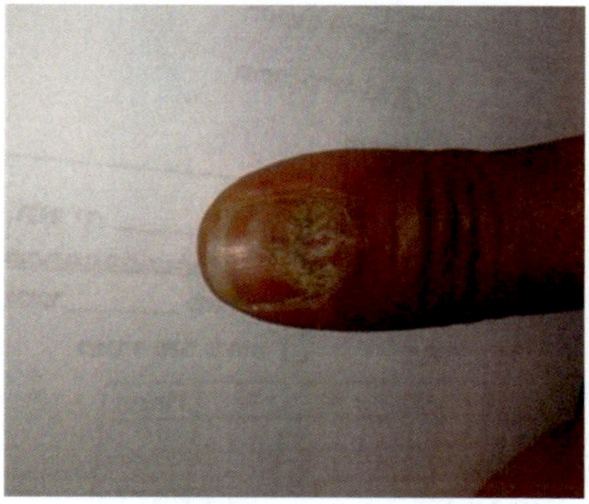

Figure 15.5. PWSO-Proximal White Subungual Onychomycosis.

PSO is associated with immunosuppression, particularly HIV/AIDS, and is considered a rapidly developing form. Patients with PSO should be screened for HIV, as PSO has been considered a marker for this disease (Figure 15.6).

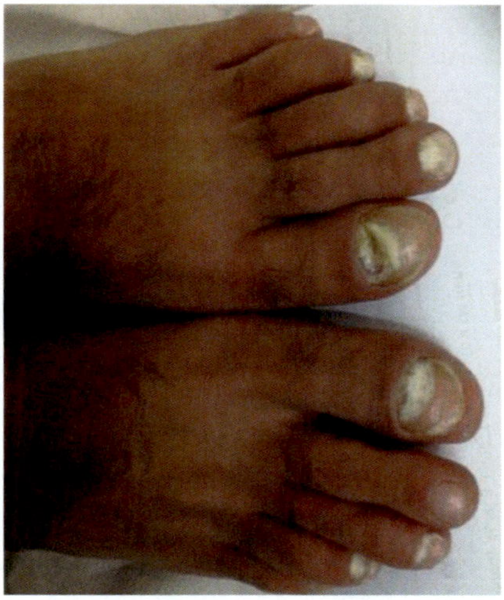

Figure 15.6. HIV patient with PSO proximal subungual onychomycosis.

Proximal Subungual Onychomycosis and Paronychia

Proximal nail plate invasion may also occur with paronychia; the most common fungi associated with this pattern are *Candida* spp. as well as *Fusarium* and other mold infections [172]. It should be borne in mind that other fungi can cause nail fold infection with or without nail plate invasion. The best known examples are *Scytalidium dimidiatum* and *Scytalidium hyalinum* and *Fusarium* spp. [188] (Figure 15.7).

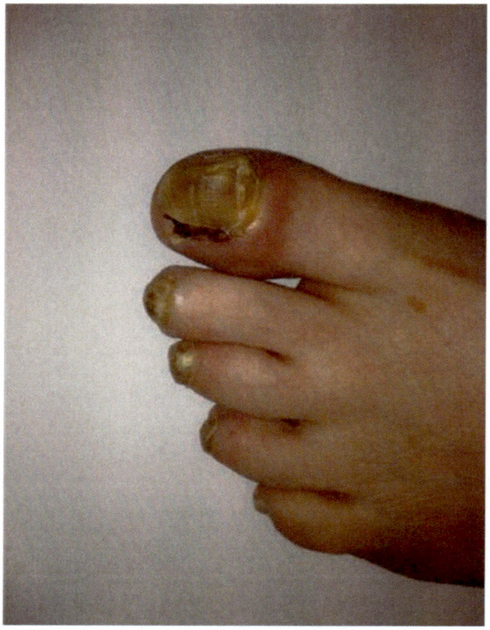

Figure 15.7. Onychomycosis and paronychia.

Nondermatophytic onychomycoses are becoming more frequent worldwide and represent a clinical challenge due to the fact that there is poor response to the converntional systemic antifungal treatment. In cases where PSO is combined with paronychia, the suspicion of mold or yeasts causing onychomycosis should be eboked. In case of severe superficial white onychomycosis, *T. mentagrophytes* or other types of molds should be considered.

Superficial Onychomycosis (SO)

Superficial onychomycosis may present with a wide range of dyschromias depending on the organism involved.

The pattern of nail plate invasion may present with superficial patches (patchy type) or be organized in transverse striae that may resemble different types of leukonychia [190,191]. Several nails may be involved at the same time or SO may appear de novo on the superficial nail plate or emerge from under the proximal nail fold; hence it is impractical to use topical therapy as it is seldom effective. In the classic forms that present with patchy infiltration of the upper aspect of the nail plate, topical therapy can be used as initial treatment but there are no large clinical therapeutic studies to support this advice.

White Superficial Type (WSO)

White superficial type is fairly rare. It results from direct invasion of the dorsal nail plate and may be seen as white to dull in color (Figure 15.8).

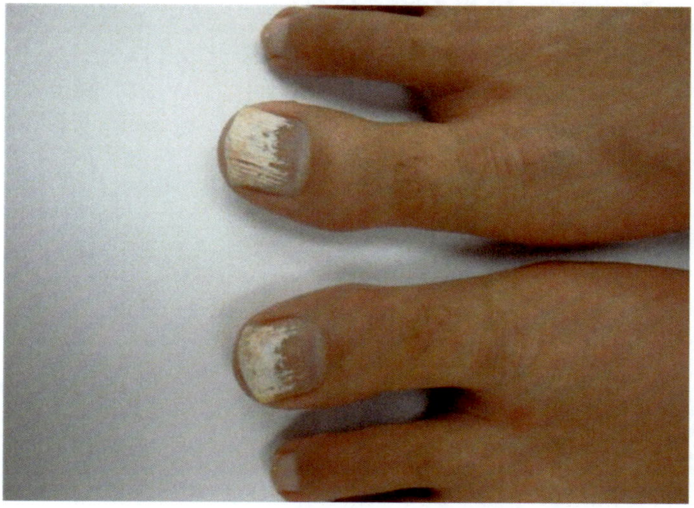

Figure 15.8. WSO-White Superficial Onychomycosis.

The causative organisms produce a clinical picture of small superficial white patches with distinct edges. These later coalesce and may gradually cover the whole nail, hence the term leukonychia trichophytica (mycotica). Older lesions tend to acquire a yellowish color. In other cases, the superficial infection is arranged in linear bands (striate leukonychia). It is usually caused by *Trichophyton interdigitale*, although nondermatophyte molds such as *Aspergillus*, *Scopulariopsis*, *Fusarium oxysporum*, and *Acremonium* spp. are also known pathogens. *Candida* spp. may invade the hyponychial epithelium to eventually affect the entire thickness of the nail plate and have occasionally been isolated.

In HIV positive patients or immunocompromised patients the superficial white onychomycosis or PSO may occur with a dermatophyte, e.g., *T. rubrum* or *Fusarium*. However, here the pattern of infection is usually different, as there is often proximal subungual infection as well [189].

Superficial Black Onychomycosis

Superficial black onychomycosis is rare and presents in a similar pattern of nail plate invasion and dystrophy that can be caused by dematiaceous or black fungi. *Scytalidium dimidiatum* and *T. rubrum* may both cause superficial black onycomycosis.

Endonyx Onychomycosis (EO)

In endonyx onychomycosis the nail plate invasion is distinguished by the combination of lamellar splitting of the nail, discoloration of the nail plate (e.g., milky patches), and the absence of nail bed invasion. The route of infection is thought to follow fungal hyphae penetrating the distal nail plate directly. It is distinguished pathologically by the absence of inflammation and fungi in the nail bed or subungual hyperatosis but many fungal hyphae in the interior of the nail plate [188].

Trichophyton soudanense in particular seems to be mainly associated with the infection that causes endothrix scalp infections. However, cases caused by other organisms, such as *T. violaceum*, have been seen [188,189] (Figure 15.9).

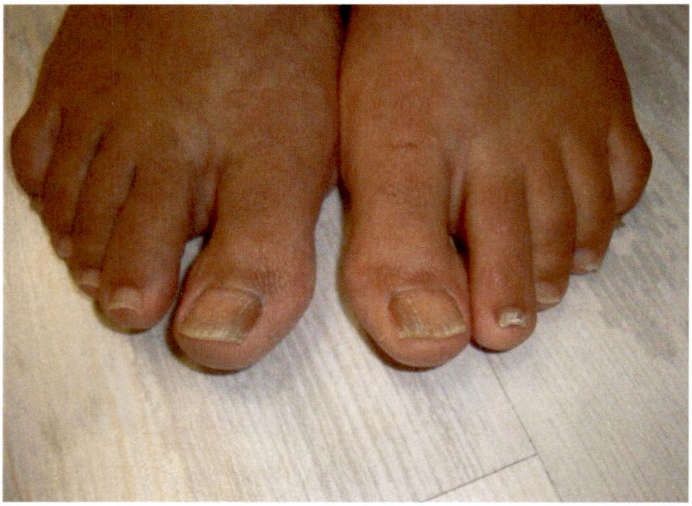

Figure 15.9. EO-Endonyx Onychomycosis.

Mixed Pattern Onychomycosis

Although the different patterns of onychomycosis have been described as distinct entities, they may also coexist both in the same individual and also in the same nail. For instance, a patient may show DLSO and subungual onychomycosis SO or PSO and SO on the same nail plate. Mixed pattern onychomycosis almost always requires oral therapy [189].

Total dystrophic onychomycosis (TDO)

Total dystrophic onychomycosis (TDO) represents the most advanced form of all previous types of onychomycosis. TDO is clinically classified as the end stage of a variety of different modes of nail plate invasion caused by different organisms [189]. The most common clinical type that follows is DLSO but other forms, particularly PSO, can result in this end stage (Figure 15.10).

In TDO the nail plate crumbles away and disappears leaving a nail bed that is thickened and ridged and usually covered with fragments of nail plate. End stage nail infection may be secondary to dermatophytes such as *T. rubrum* and all nails may be involved in chronic generalized dermatophytosis [189].

TDO is also observed in patients suffering from chronic mucocutaneous candidiasis (CMC) or other immunodeficiency states. Clinically the whole nail unit is thickened as a result of extensive hyperkeratosis that reflects the rapidity of nail plate invasion, and in nail disease secondary to immunosuppression [188]. *Candida* invasion rapidly involves all the tissues of the nail apparatus. The thickening of the soft tissues results in a swollen distal phalanx. The nail plate is thickened, opaque, and yellow-brown in color. Mucous membrane involvement such as oral candidiasis is generally present in these patients. This manifestation occurs more often in childhood or infancy and tends to recur despite treatment [189].

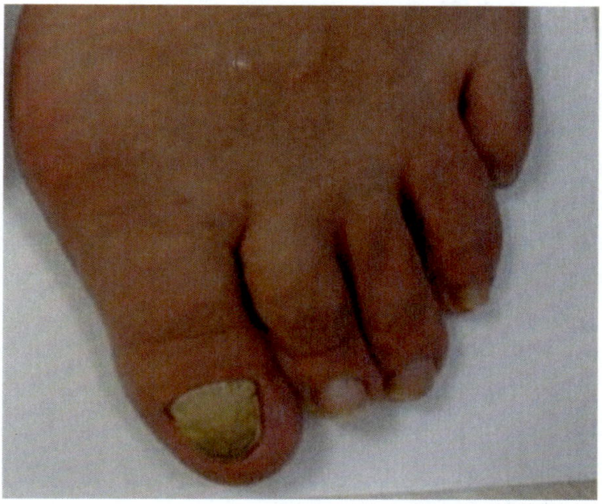

Figure 15.10. TDO-Total Dystrophic Onychomycosis.

Secondary Onychomycosis

Fungal infection of the nail plate may develop secondary to some other dermatological condition. Fungi can penetrate the nail plate and the surrounding tissues secondary to other nonfungal pathologies.

The best recognized causes of these are psoriasis [189] and traumatic nail dystrophy, but it can also occur in keratodermas or onychogryphosis (Figure 15.11).

The importance of recognizing this underlying pathology is that the appearances of the nail are usually more typical of the underlying condition (e.g., in psoriasis hyperkeratosis the nail plate is more clinically prominent). In these secondary forms of fungal nail dystrophy diagnosis can be particularly difficult based solely on clinical suspicion, and laboratory investigations are usually necessary to confirm the presence of fungi.

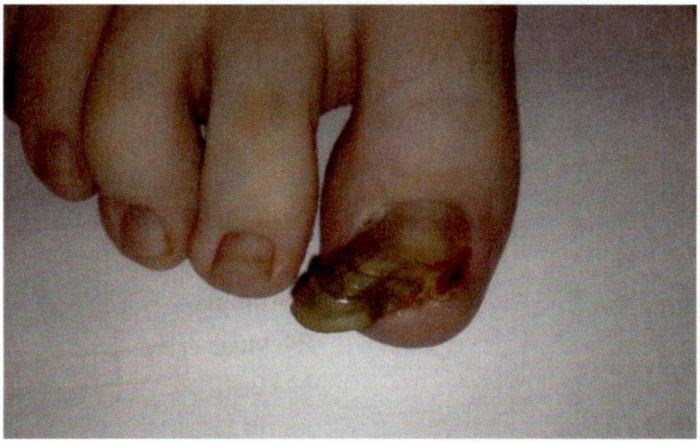

Figure 15.11. Onychogryphosis.

Differential Diagnosis

Pachionychia congenita

Pachonychia congentina is an autosomal dominant keratoderma disorder in skin pathology located in the palms and soles with oval plaques, skin blisters, and nail deformation. At the nail units there is hyperkeratosis of the nail beds and thickened elevated nails (from the proximal to the distal side of the nail plate). Since it is a congenital disorder, the nail pathology begins early in life.

In case mycological analysis will be positive, systemic antifungal treatment will not lead to total cure.

Onycholysis

Onycholysis is a common nail disorder and defined as a separation of the nail plate from its nail bed. The serration starts from the lower distal part of the nail plate close to the hyponychium and progresses proximally; the color of the separated nail plate becomes opaque and whitish (Figure 15.12). There are many reasons for onycholysis, among them repeated minor traumas, genetic disorders, psoriasis, and self-inflicted damage in the ventral part of the nail (Figure 15.13). Fungal infection may also play a role in causing onycholysis; mycological analysis should be done. If the only cause for the onycholysis is the fungal infection, this onycholysis (onychomycosis) will cure up to normal nail appearance if there is no irreversible damage to the nail bed. Non-dermatophyte molds may be found in the nail bed and on the ventral part of the distal nail plate, but very often these kinds of fungi are considered as saprophytes, unless a mycological sample was taken from the same nail and the same fungus was found and no systemic and/or topical antifungal medication is needed. It is needless to stress that antifungal treatment will not be useful.

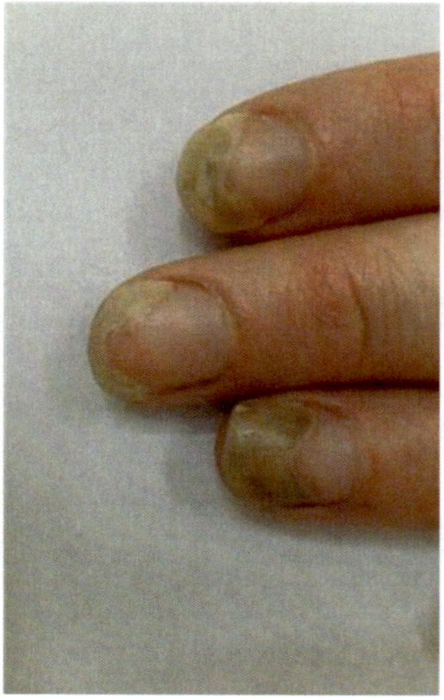

Figure 15.12. Onycholysis.

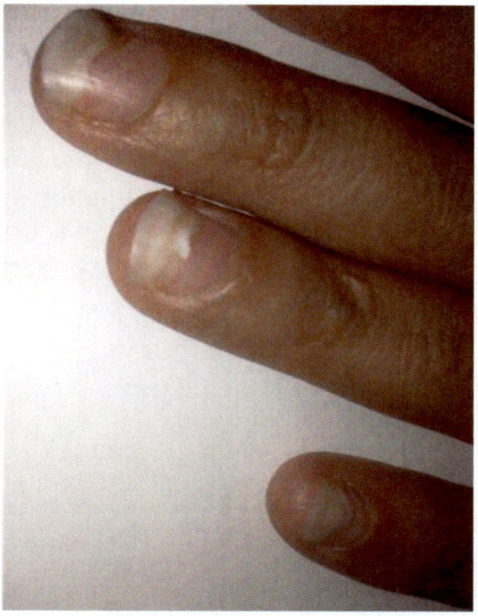

Figure 15.13. Onycholysis due to psoriasis, 'onycholysis psoriasis'.

In case dermatophyte infection was found in the onychomycosis nail, it is difficult to determine if the dermatophyte is responsible for the onycholysis. A relevant systemic antifungal is recommended because a dermatophyte is sometimes considered a pathogen. If there is no subungual debris in the ventral part of the nail plate, the onycholysis is most probably not related to the fungus.

Nail trauma

Having a normal appearing nail is due to normal nail bed and normal nail matrix. If the nail bed and/or the nail matrix are abnormal, a deformed nail appearance will be presented. The greater the abnormality of the nail bed and/or the nail matrix, the greater the deformation of the nail plate.

Nail trauma could be divided to acute major trauma (Figure 15.14) and chronic nail trauma such as repeated minor trauma from wearing tight shoes (Figure 15.23); as a result there is retrograde pressure from the shoes to the nail plate and via the nail plate to different locations on the nail matrix, resulting in nail deformation. Onychomycosis of the distal and lateral subungual subtypes usually present as a thick rough nail and the pressure of the shoes to the thickened nail may affect or injure the nail matrix; injury to the nail matrix is reversible or irreversible depending on the severity of the pressure and the period of time of this pressure. Different nail matrix traumas will show different nail plate deformations.

Traumatic nail that shows nail plate deformation, such as thickened nail, may be a point of entry for different fungi and as a result mycological onychomycosis. A patient with these combined disorders may be checked by his caregiver and may be sent for mycological analysis; the results will be positive for fungi. The caregiver may think – by mistake – that the fungus that was revealed by the mycological analysis is the only pathology in the nail plate deformation and will be considered as "pure" onychomycosis. Relevant systemic antifungal treatment may diminish or kill the fungus itself but not the deformation, which occurred due to nail matrix insult. In case of combined disorders (nail trauma and onychomycosis) not always seen or diagnosed by the caregiver – careful inspection should be made to try to diagnose the nail deformation that is not related to the onychomycosis itself. Once the caregiver will diagnose which of the deformations is related to trauma and not related only to the onychomycosis, the patient will not have an expectation for achieving complete cure.

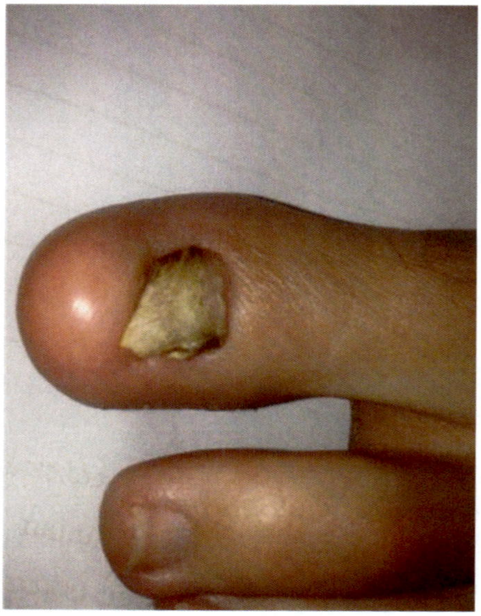

Figure 15.14. Nail trauma.

Nail psoriasis

The prevalence of nail psoriasis in psoriatic patients is very common, varying between 20% and 90% [168].

Nail psoriasis occurs more often in patients with severe disease. There is a positive association between nail psoriasis and duration of skin lesions, and between its severity and the severity of skin and joint involvement. Between one and five percent of patients have affected nails without skin lesions. There are several nail changes due to psoriasis and they depend on the location of psoriasis (Figure 15.5).

The precise location of the pathology of psoriasis of the nail unit (nail bed/nail matrix) will result in differential clinical presentations, namely nail matrix psoriasis usually presents as pitting, leukonychia, erythema of the lunula, and mild to severe nail deformation. On the other hand, psoriasis of the nail bed presents as "oil drop" ("salmon patch" (Figure 15.16)) splinter hemorrhages, subungual hyperkeratosis, and onycholysis or other combinations of the above. Each of the nail pathologies could appear separately or any combination could occur. In other words, the clinical presentation of nail psoriasis depends not only on the precise location but also the severity of the psoriasis itself at the specific location. Because of the huge variation of the clinical presentation of nail psoriasis, part of the clinical presentation will be included in the list of differential diagnoses due to its similarity to onychomycosis, while other clinical presentations such as nail pitting will not be included. Therefore every psoriatic patient with different nail involvements with clinical resemblance to onychomycosis should get a mycological test as there could be a combination of psoriasis and onychomycosis. There is a possibility that proper treatment of the fungi won't necessarily cure all infected nails, or even only some or none. There is no way to predict treatment success.

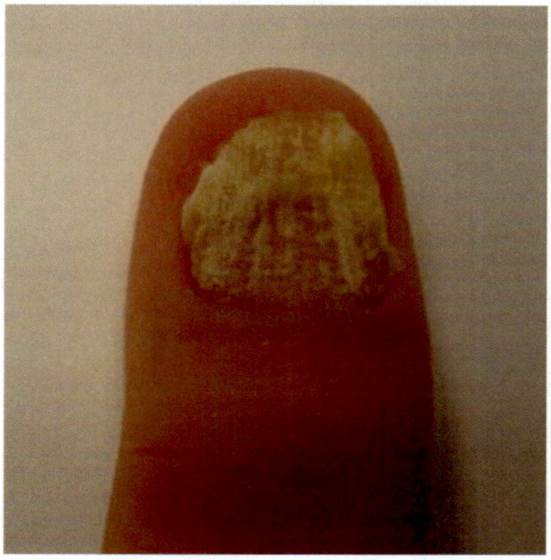

Figure 15.15. Nail psoriasis.

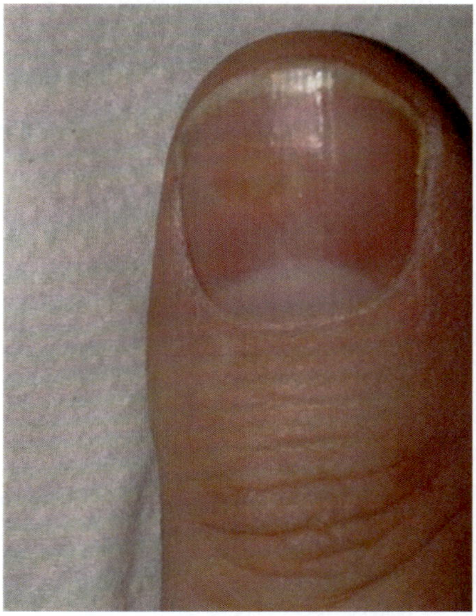

Figure 15.16. Salmon patch.

There are studies that suggest that a combination of onychomycosis and psoriasis in a patient causes the Koebner phenomenon, and treating the fungi will eliminate the psoriasis in the involved nails . The patient must be notified that the systemic treatment (especially terbinafine rather than itraconazole) may worsen the existing psoriasis. As a general rule systemic treatment with terbinafine should be avoided.

In the case of a mixed condition of psoriasis and onychomycosis, there is no way to determine the percentage of each disease, and the ratio between them could even differ per nail, which can cause different cure rates in different nails (Figure 15.17, Figure 15.18).

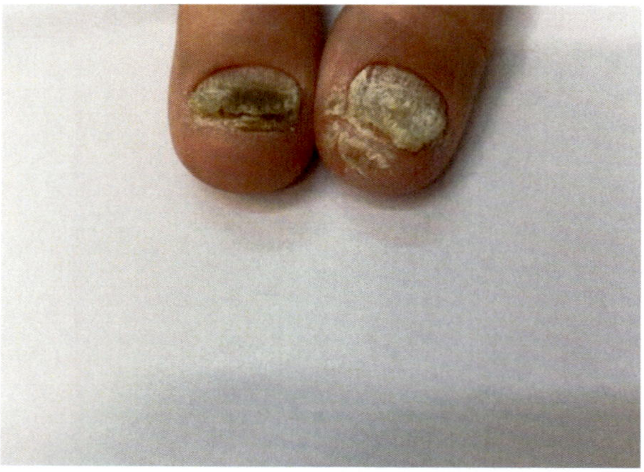

Figure 15.17. Psoriatic nails with onychomycosis.

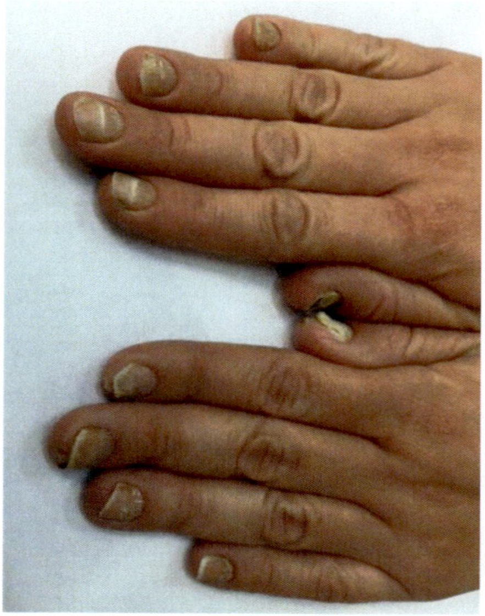

Figure 15.18. Psoriatic nails with leukonychia.

Lichen planus of the nails

Lichen planus of the nails is one of many skin manifestations of lichen planus. Lichen planus of the nail usually appears with the skin manifestation of lichen planus but also may manifest only on the nails. As much as 10% of lichen planus patients also have involvement of the nails. One or more nails may be involved; involvement of all 20 nails is called twenty-nail dystrophy.

The involvement of the nail/s in lichen planus has many clinical manifestations such as shallow or elevated ridges and/or superficial or deep grooves that may be parallel, creating triangular shapes; mild onycholysis may be seen at the distal end of the nail plate. The nails could be thin (usually) or thick, rough, and irregular (Figure 15.19). Shedding or disappearance of the nail plate may also occur. The nail bed may become hyperpigmented, especially in darker skin patients. Involvement of the cuticle is common and as a result pterygium beside the scar of the hyponychium may occur.

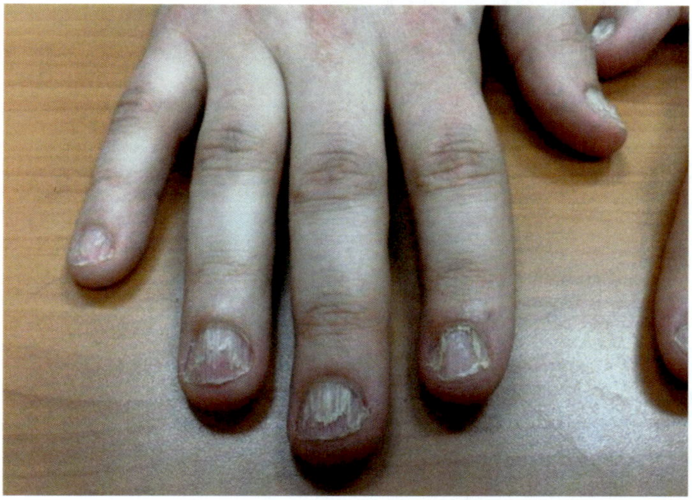

Figure 15.19. Nail Lichen Planus.

If the patient has twenty-nail dystrophy, it is most probably that even if fungus is revealed it is just a saprophyte rather than pathogenic one, especially due to the fact that the clinical presentation of twenty-nail dystrophy is different and not one of the other classical clinical presentations of onychomycosis (rough, deformed, etc.)

In case of involvement of one or several nails, especially if hyperkeratotic nail/s is observed, even when mycological analysis is positive the patient has to understand that relevant systemic antifungal treatment will not necessarily achieve complete cure. The amount of the nail/s improvement depends on the relationship between the fungus itself and the nail lichen planus.

Median nail dystrophy

Median nail dystrophy, synonym canaliform nail dystrophy, is a unique deformation of the nail plate usually at its central longitudinal axis. Its starts from beneath the proximal nail toward the distal nail plate creating a Christmas tree shape. One or more nails might be involved with a predilection to the thumb nail. This phenomenon is unknown but self-infliction of the cuticle toward the proximal nail fold may affect the nail matrix, which affects the nail plate with swelling of the proximal nail fold with or without the lateral nail folds, which in unique circumstances may be distinguished from chronic simple paronychia (Figure 15.20) [192].

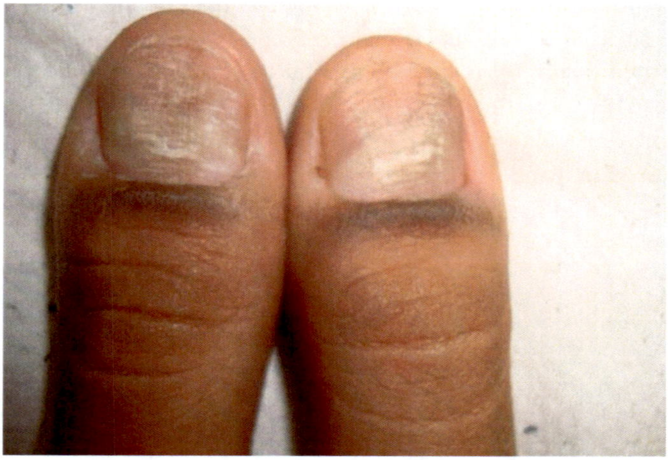

Figure 15.20. Median nail Dystrophy.

Usually the two big fingernails are affected, with or without other nails, and no subungual hyperkeratosis may be seen, suggesting there is no fungal infection. In case fungal infection will be observed – if it is a dermatophyte infection – relevant treatment will be given. In case of molds or yeasts the clinical presentation should be different from median 1 nail dystrophy.

Subungual wart

Subungual warts are caused by human papillomavirus and located just beneath the distal subungual nail plate, which is attached to the nail bed (Figure 15.21). Sometimes when the wart is wide – along the space beneath the distal nail plate – it may resemble distal and lateral subungual onychomycosis. Looking carefully at the wart, black/grey dots (due to proliferation of the small blood vessels in an upward direction toward the epidermis) may be seen and this indicates that this is a wart scraping for mycological analysis; this area will result in mild bleeding.

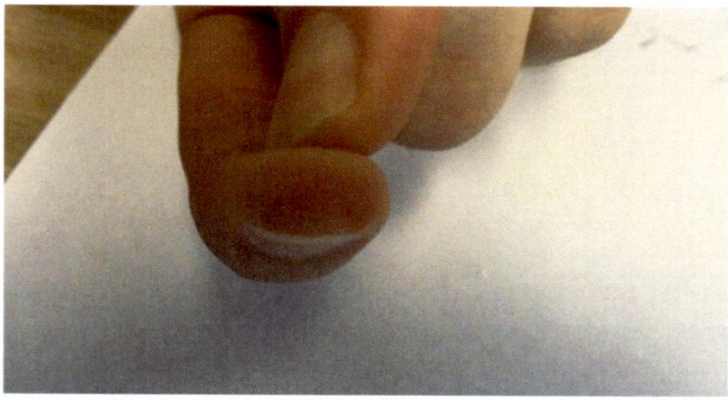

Figure 15.21. Subungual wart.

Subungual Exostosis

Subungual exostosis is a bone growth under the nail plate. Usually it is a solitary lesion but there may be more than one. In case the exostosis is located beneath the nail plate – subungual exostosis – no subungual debris will be seen. X-ray of the involved finger will reveal the diagnosis.

Hand Eczema

Hand eczema is a chronic dermatitis that could be also acute or subacute dermatitis. Once the inflammatory process is close to the nail matrix/nail bed there is the possibility of the involvement of the nail matrix and/or the nail bed, and as a result mild to severe deformation of the nail plate may be observed, depending on the severity and the proximity of the inflammatory process from the nail matrix/nail bed (Figure 15.22).

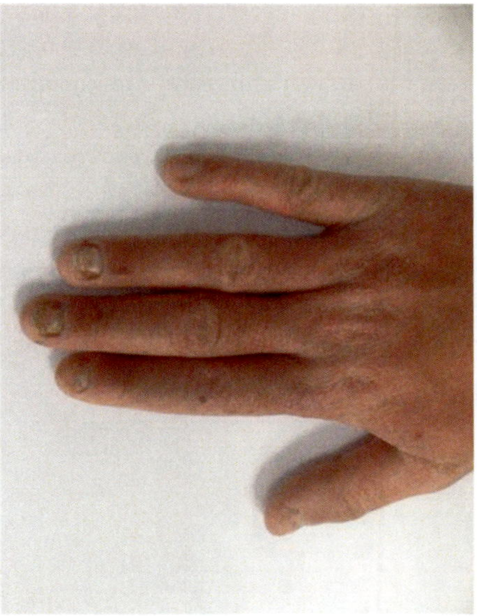

Figure 15.22. Hand eczema.

The clinical presentations of the nail deformation are variable and also depend on the precise location of the inflammation. Basically, the suspicion of onychomycosis will occur if the clinical presentation looks like one of the 7 subtypes of onychomycosis. Other changes will be excluded from the list of onychomycosis differential diagnosis.

In case of any suspicion for onychomycosis, mycological analysis should be taken, and in case of positive result, two questions should be asked. Is the onychomycosis pure onychomycosis? Or are there are two disorders – onychomycosis and hand eczema?

Looking carefully at the hands, basic anamnesis, clinical history, and if there is severe eczema close to the nail matrix/nail bed it is most probably a combined disease.

Pityriasis Rubra Pilaris (PRP)

PRP is one of the papulosquamous disorders, a relatively rare disease, and is divided schematically to 5 subtypes. In general there is a hyperkeratosis of the follicular papules covered by fine scales.

Nail involvement often occurs and may resemble onychomycosis. In case of a PRP patient with onychomycosis (mycologically) two questions need to be asked. Is the onychomycosis pure onychomycosis? Or are there are two disorders – onychomycosis and PRP? Hence there is no need to have the skin PRP be close to the nail matrix/nail bed for the involvement of the nails (not like in hand eczema). Mycological analysis should be taken followed by antifungal treatment.

Thick nails

There are many reasons for thick nails. In addition to the most common reason – fungal infection onychomycosis (the thickened nail changes the color of the nail and beneath or above the nail plate there is a deterioration of the nail plate), there are other reasons for thick nails. If one or several fingernails or toenails are thickened, trauma is one of the most common reasons. If all the nails become thickened systemic alteration is the reason to be suspected such as psoriasis, chronic eczema, pulmonary disorders, cardiovascular diseases, and different metabolic disorders such as hypothyroidism. Another factor causing thick nails is that with age the nail becomes thickened and harder. Usually thickened fingernails or toenails lose their transparency and develop a yellow/brown opaque shade.

Usually the 5th toenail suffers from deformation in patients who wear tight shoes (usually women) due to constant retrograde pressure from the sides of the shoes through the nail plate toward the nail matrix (Figure 15.23).

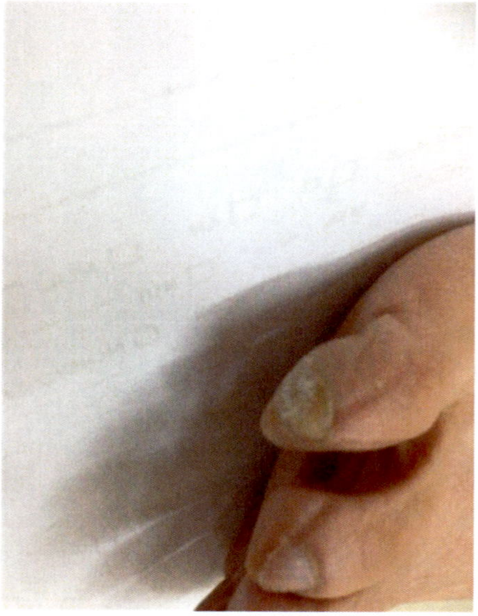

Figure 15.23. Repeated minor trauma from the lateral sides of the shoes- nail trauma.

Once the nail matrix becomes deformed – due to continual retrograde pressure – the deformed matrix creates a thick deformed nail plate [193]. One point to stress is that if the 5th toenails are the only deformed toenails, and mycological analysis was taken and the mycological results were positive, it should be noted that maybe that after suitable systemic antimycotic treatment those 5th toenails will not achieve a complete cure because another factor exists in addition to the fungus itself – the matrix deformation leading to nail deformation. The antifungal medication only treats the reversible deformation caused by the fungus itself.

In case of one thick nail due to trauma, for example, and this toenail was also contaminated with fungus, which was revealed by mycological analysis, it is almost impossible to predict the outcome of the relevant systemic antifungal treatment, because it is impossible to know the relative contribution of each disorder (Figure 15.24). Although complete cure or almost complete cure could be achieved in this combined disorder, it is recommended to treat the patient as a pure onychomycosis. It is needless to stress that the patient has to understand that although fungal infection was found treatment will not necessarily achieve compete cure.

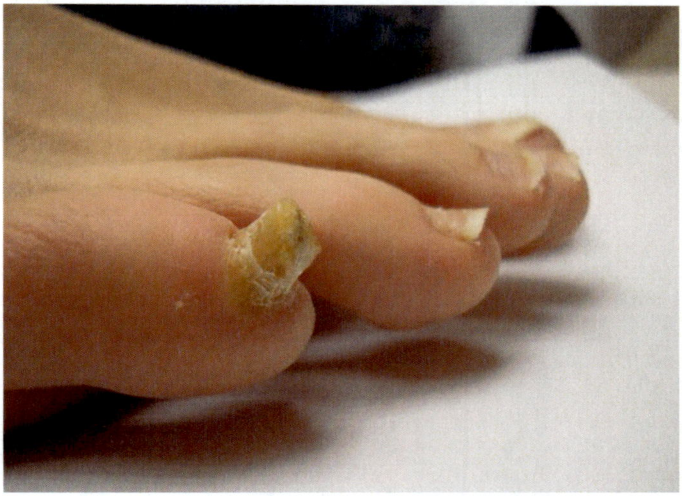

Figure 15.24. Trauma of the nail 5th toenail.

Distal nail splitting/brittle nails/onychorrhexis

Brittle nails is an alteration in the compactness of the nail plate and characterized by a fragility, weakness, flaking, and splitting of the distal part of the nail plate. Sometimes crumbling of the nail plate may occur. Women are affected twice as often as men.

Brittle nails can be divided to idiopathic brittle nails and secondary brittle nails. Idiopathic brittle nails refers to nail changes such as transverse splitting and lamellar separation, longitudinal ridging, and distal fissuring of the nail plate. The idiopathic brittle nails may be caused by intrinsic and/or extrinsic factors. The intrinsic factors include the level of the sulfur, lipids, and water in the nail plate – the relative amount of each component is very important for normal nail structure, and change in the relationship between these components may lead to different levels of brittle nail. Among the extrinsic factors the environmental and/or occupational factors (excessive use of water and/or different chemical detergents, etc.) play an important role in causing brittle nails.

Secondary brittle nails refers to dermatological (psoriasis, lichen planus, Darier disease, alopecia, areata, etc.) or systemic diseases such as avitaminosis, zinc or selenium deficiencies, which may affect directly or indirectly the nail plate compactness, which can lead to brittle nails. Drug intake such as penicillamine, retinoids, antimetabolic agents may also lead to brittle nails. With respect to onychomycosis, the fact that there is no thickening of the nail plate, no accumulation of subungual debris, supports that there is no pathogenic fungal infection. In case mycological analysis was taken it could be superimposed (dermatophytes) or non-dermatophyte mold saprophytes.

Rough nails/twenty rough nails/twenty-nails syndrome

Rough nails means that the superficial nail plate is rough and not smooth (Figure 15.25). It could be one nail, several, or all the nails (fingernails and/or toenails). The reason is unknown but it could be secondary to dermatological disorders such as lichen planus, psoriasis, alopecia areata, atopic dermatitis, vitiligo. Once all 20 nails get involved, the term used is twenty-nail dystrophy. The clinical presentation is variable and consists of longitudinal ridges, thinning of the nails, the distal free edges of the nail plate could be brittle and/or split, and the nail plate is not transparent as in normal nails.

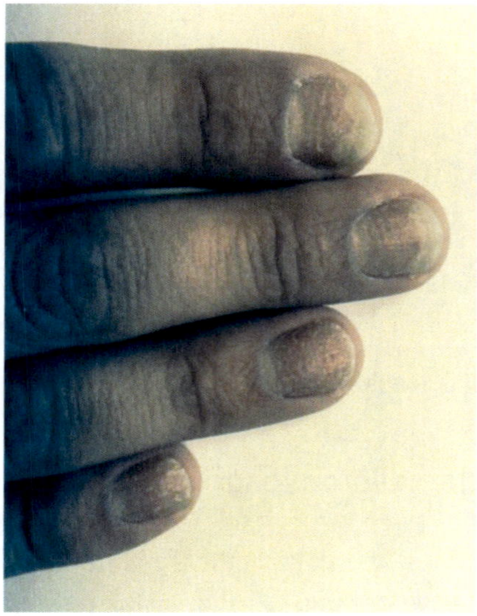

Figure 15.25. Rough nails.

Clinically, trachyonychia is not to be considered as a differential diagnosis for onychomycosis except in suitable circumstances; it might be differentiated from superficial white onychomycosis.

Looking carefully at the nail plates, concentrating on the pathological morphology of the nail plates, involvement of other nails, suitable clinical morphology of classical onychomycosis, and skin diseases (as mentioned above), combined with mycological analysis will provide the ability to differentiate between onychomycosis and trachyonychia. It is not impossible to have both disorders together.

Yellow nail syndrome

Yellow nail syndrome refers to secondary nail changes for internal disorders such as lymphedema, pleural effusion, chronic sinusitis, and bronchiectasis. The nail changes include thick yellow nails; the nails may sometimes be cloudy in color or yellow-green.

The fact that there is no subungual hyperkeratosis, no whitish scale on the superficial nail plate, and the nail surfaces all look about the same, supports that this is not onychomycosis.

Subungual onychopapilloma

Subungual onychopapilloma is a benign nail lesion that begins at the distal part of the matrix or the proximal part of the nail bed. During the nail growth there is a longitudinal erythronychia that sometimes ends in a notch at the distal part of the nail plate. Although the name of this disorder may cause the misperception that this is human papillomavirus in origin, there is not enough proof of the cause of HPV.

Clinically, there is distal subungual hyperkeratosis located under the free end of the nail plate. The erythronychia/subungual onychopapilloma is located in the central area of the nail plate. Subungual onychopapilloma is usually located on the big fingernail but several or other fingernails and/or toenails could be involved. It is very common to see the longitudinal line proximal to the distal subungual hyperkeratosis in lateral onychomycosis. The onychomycotic line usually has the same color all along the line; very often involvement of other nails with onychomycosis or even the same nail might have another clinical presentation of onychomycosis. Mycological analysis may help for final diagnosis (Figure 15.26).

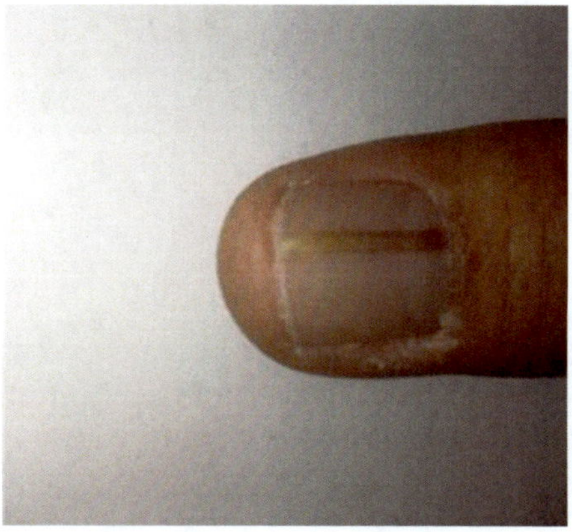

Figure 15.26. Subungual onychopapilloma.

Subungual SCC

Subungual SCC is a rare non-melanoma malignant tumor, originating from the squamous layer of the epidermis with various degrees of differentiation (Figure 15.27). It usually appears beneath or around the nail plate and mimics several different lesions such as infected verruca vulgaris, pyogenic granuloma, chronic paronychia, and subacute/chronic eczema. Subungual SCC may present as subacute dermatitis with mild serous discharge or even serous/hematogenic fluid, which does not react to systemic antibiotics. Sometimes bacterial smear and culture are taken and the relevant systemic antibiotic is given with no impressive improvement. Classical onychomycotic nail has no inflammatory process with expectation of onychomycosis combined with paronychia; therefore onychomycosis clinically and mycologically accompanied with chronic/sub-acute discharge inflammation and no response to relevant systemic and topical antibiotics should always be suspected as a neoplastic process until proven otherwise. Sometimes the first histopathology results will not reveal the tumor (this is because the biopsy was taken from an incorrect location); repeated biopsies should be taken until the correct diagnosis is achieved.

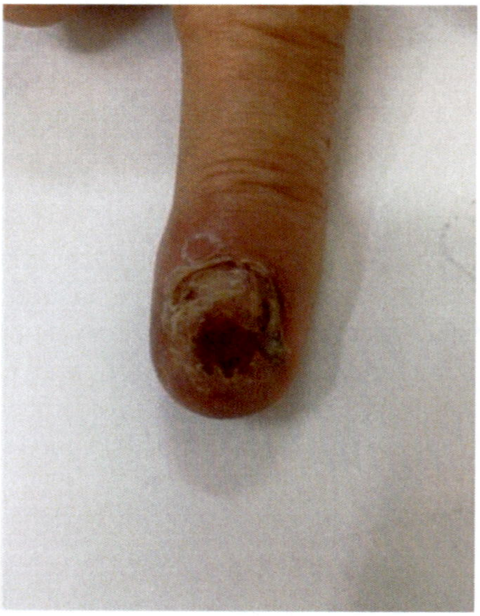

Figure 15.27. Subungual SCC.

Subungual melanoma

Subungual melanoma refers to melanoma that arises from the nail matrix or under the nail plate or around and beneath the nail plate (within or beneath the lateral or proximal nail folds (Figure 15.28). The thumb (or the big toenail) is the most common nail to be involved.

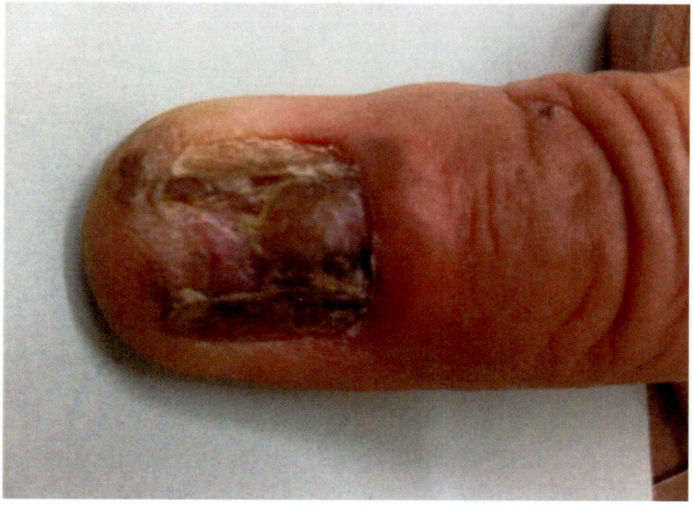

Figure 15.28. Nail Matrix Menaloma.

Subungual melanoma is irregular in shape, but generally an irregular longitudinal melanonychia may be noted. Ulceration and/or bleeding from the nail areas are very suspicious markers for melanoma. The width of the longitudinal melanonychia at its proximal area is larger compared to the distal area. Sometimes Hutchinson's sign may be seen – which is an important sign of melanoma.

It is very important to stress that it is possible to have onychomycosis together with melanoma of the nail unit; in another words, positive mycological analysis in a nail with clinical signs of melanoma. Biopsy of the suspicious areas should be done to rule out or confirm the suspicions of melanoma.

Longitudinal melanonychia

Longitudinal melanonychia refers to brown to black longitudinal pigmentation beneath the nail plate just within and along the nail bed (Figure 15.29). The cause could be endogenous or exogenous. The most common cause is benign nevus or lentigo, but malignant melanoma sometimes cannot be excluded until proven otherwise. In such cases nail biopsy should be taken to rule out or to confirm the final diagnosis. Sometimes an onychomycotic nail might have longitudinal melanonychia. Mycological analysis may reveal the fungus, e.g., *T. rubrum*, and the caregiver might think that the dark color of the nail is due to the fungus itself (hence the name rubrum – the dark red color as with dark red wine).

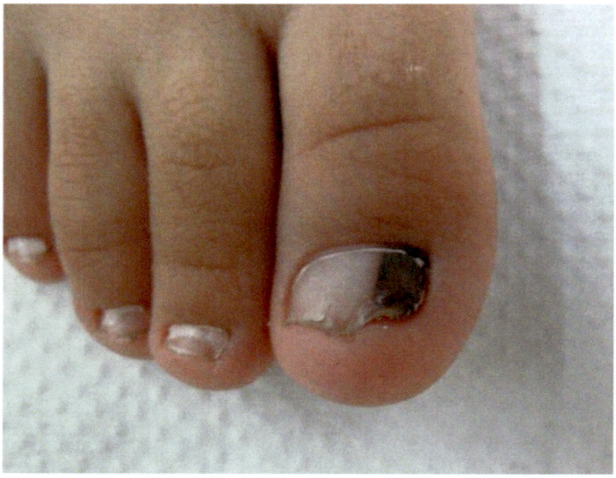

Figure 15.29. Longitudinal melanonychia.

Look carefully at the nail plate and if a longitudinal band is noticed – although positive mycological analysis was obtained and was positive for fungus – nail matrix biopsy should be taken, especially if dermoscopy supports the suspicion.

Leukonychia

Leukonychia is defined as white discoloration of the nails. It could be partial or total (Figure 15.30). The partial group can be divided to 3 subtypes depending on the clinical presentation (two or more subtypes could present in the same nail and rarely may proceed to total leukonychia): 1. leukonychia striata (transverse leukonychia, Mees' lines), 2. leukonychia punctata, 3. longitudinal leukonychia.

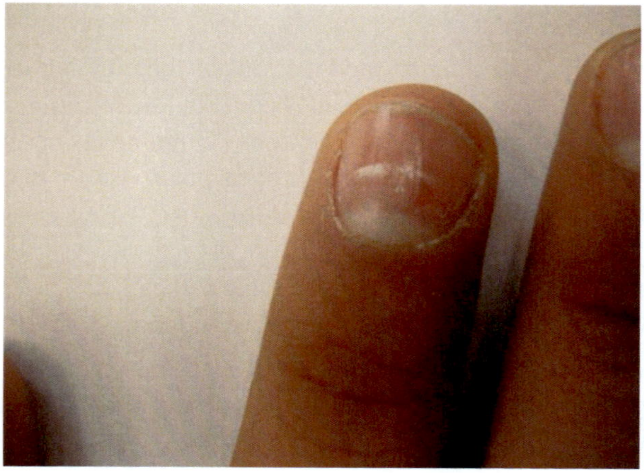

Figure 15.30. Leukonychia.

Total leukonychia is defined when the entire nail plate develops a white discoloration. In general, it is much more common having leukonychia in the fingernails compared to the toenails. The most common cause of partial leukonychia is repeated minor trauma to the distal nail plate. This kind of partial leukonychia progresses distally, and as the nail plate grows the leukonychia patches come out together with the nail plate and disappear gradually. Total leukonychia is usually caused by systemic disorders such as hypoalbulinemia as a part of nephrotic syndrome or drug reaction appearing as leukonychia. On the other hand, partial leukonychia occurs due to repeated minor trauma that the patient might not be aware of.

Regarding onychomycosis, the subtype superficial white onychomycosis may sometimes be confused with leukonychia (or vice versa). Superficial white onychomycosis can easily be differentiated from leukonychia by scraping the nail plate from its superficial (dorsal) part. In superficial white onychomycosis the whitish color will peel off while scraping the nail plate; in contrast, while scraping leukonychia patches, the whitish color remains about the same; this is because the whitish color in superficial white onychomycosis is located at the outmost layers (superficial/dorsal) of the nail plate, while in leukonychia the whitish color is located beneath and not on top of the nail plate.

Koilonychia

Koilonychia or spoon nails usually refers to iron deficiency anemia and Plummer–Vinson syndrome. Clinically the nail plate is thin and has a spoon shape; brittleness of the distal nail plate may be noted. There is no thickening or whitish scaly material on the superficial area of the nail plate; therefore regular koilonychia will not usually be considered as a differential diagnosis of onychomycosis.

Clubbing nails

Clubbing nails is defined as longitudinal and lateral curves located on the fingernails and/or toenails (Figure 15.31).

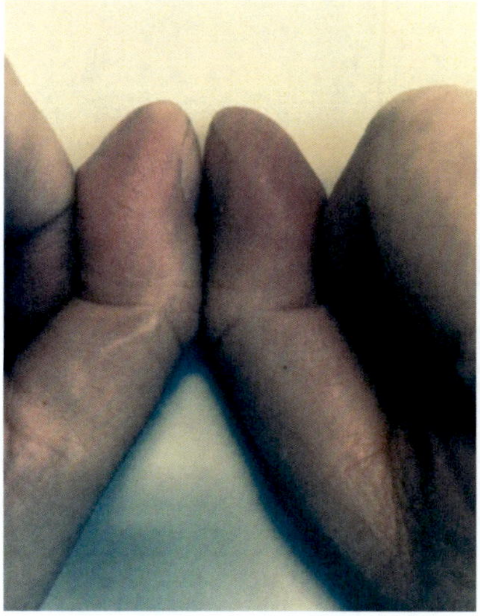

Figure 15.31. Clubbing.

Clubbing nails could appear from an unknown origin but are usually associated with several internal disorders such as lung disorders (lung cancers, tuberculosis, interstitial lung disease, bronchiectasis, long abscess, blood vessel malformations, etc.), cardiovascular diseases (congenital cyanotic heart disorders, Tetralogy of Fallot, SBE, etc.), and gastrointestinal disorders (cirrhosis, hepatopulmonary syndrome, Crohn's disease, ulcerative colitis), and other autoimmune and/or endocrine disorders. The pathogenesis is not clear but there is a type of swelling of the soft tissue just beneath and proximal to the nail bed. The swelling of this soft tissue causes the nail plate to lie on the nail bed with longitudinal and horizontal curves. The nail plate itself is not thick and/or crumbled/deformed and therefore clubbing could not really play a role in terms of differential diagnosis of onychomycosis. Sometimes the clubbed nails are thick or have a whitish/yellowish color, which in unique circumstances may resemble onychomycosis.

Mycological analysis should be done and suitable systemic antifungal treatment should be recommended in the case of positive mycology (dermatophye) results. In such a case it is important to clarify to the patient that the clubbing will not improve with the systemic treatment, only the deformation caused by the fungus itself.

Onychomatricoma

Onychomatricoma is defined as a benign nail matrix tumor. This rare tumor is located beneath the nail plate and clinically may easily be confused by non-experienced caregivers with distal and lateral onychomycosis (Figure 15.32). In onychomatricoma there is a thickened nail and slight over-curvature – horizontally, especially at its distal part.

Close inspection through the frontal aspect of the nail plate will reveal tiny holes, which is a huge clue for the diagnosis of onychomatricoma. These tiny holes are created by the fibroepithelial branches of the tumor that extend from the nail matrix. Onychomatricoma appears in one toenail or fingernail in contrast to onychomycosis, which usually appears in several nails.

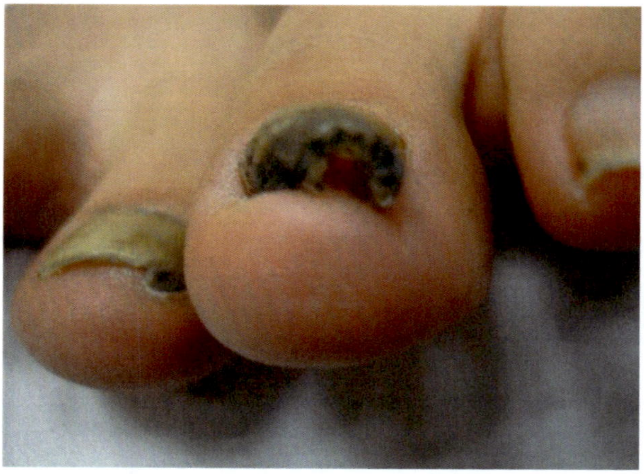

Figure 15.32. Onychomatricoma.

With suspicion of onychomatricoma (especially the existence of holes) nail matrix biopsy should be taken to confirm the diagnosis, and immunohistochemical analysis for cytokeratin should be obtained to establish the diagnosis. As mentioned in other differential diagnoses, it is possible that onychomatricoma and onychomycosis may occur together, and in this case mycological analysis might mislead that onychomycosis is the correct and the only diagnosis.

Onychomadesis

Onychomadesis is a nail disorder that presents as periodic growth and arrest of the nail plates; hence the nail growth begins from the nail matrix (Figure 15.33). The clinical presentation should be seen at the proximal part of the nail plate. The reason for the temporary dysfunction of the nail matrix is unknown, but some conditions have been described such as nail trauma, loss of blood supply, emotional stress, medications, and blister formation.

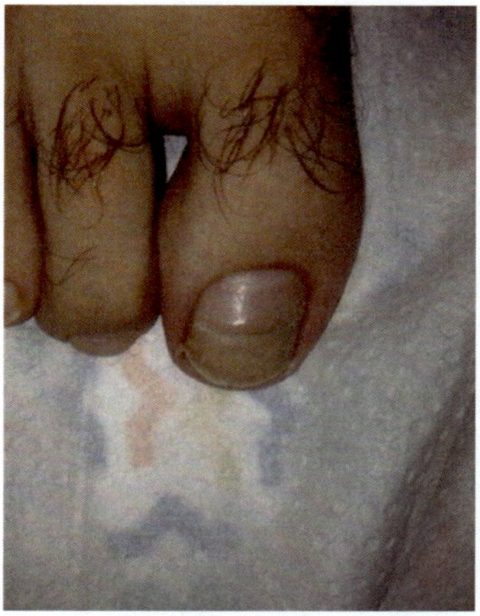

Figure 15.33. Onychomadesis.

Onychomadesis may be seen in fingernails, toenails, or both. Involvement of several or all the nails could occur. Onychomadesis is rare in young children.

Clinically there is the appearance of "new" growing nail just beneath the "old" nail, which pushes the "old" nail outward distally. A horizontal line that separates the "new" nail and the "old" nail is apparent. The deformation seen in onychomadesis may sometimes be confused with onychomycosis but the horizontal line appearance in one or several toenails and/or fingernails may lead to the correct diagnosis of onychomadesis. Having positive mycological results of dermatophyte infection, nondermatophyte molds will be considered as a secondary infection.

Diagnosis

Onychomycosis is responsible for the majority of dystrophic nails but it is essential to obtain diagnostic laboratory confirmation prior to initiation of treatment, especially when treatment is usually long-term with potentially toxic oral antifungal treatments.

The most frequent methods for establishing diagnosis are with direct microscopy (KOH examination of subungual debris) and fungal culture of the nail plate. But these diagnostic methods may yield false-negative results. On diagnostic uncertainty, histopathological examination with Periodic Acid Schiff (PAS) staining of the nail clipping and molecular testing can be used.

Direct microscopy (KOH examination)

In direct microscopy small pieces are taken from clinically infected areas of the nail and particularly of subungual hyperkeratosis. Samples are then embedded with 10–30% potassium hydroxide.

The slide may be warmed over a Bunsen flame. Sixty milliliters of a 20% KOH solution is mixed with 40 mL of pure dimethylsulfoxide (DMSO). This technique is useful for the preservation of specimens, but globular artifacts may sometimes be seen and these must be distinguished from yeasts.

The nail specimen is then examined for fungal hyphae or arthrospores.

In *Candida* infections, yeast forms can be present. In certain non-dermatophyte infections conidia may be formed in situ. This is characteristic of *Scopulariopsis* infections, although it may also occur in onychomycosis caused by *Aspergillus* spp. The hyphae of *Scytalidium dimidiatum* and *Scytalidium hyalinum* are very similar in appearance to those of dermatophytes and need to be examined by experts in order to establish diagnosis. (Baran)

Direct microscopic examination of KOH-prepared nail samples is the simplest, most inexpensive method used in the diagnosis of mycotic infections. However, KOH examination is often negative and nails with hyphae reported on KOH examination often yield negative cultures. KOH preparations have been reported to have a false-negative percentage of 5% to 15%, possibly because of the low visibility of scantily scattered fungal material in the nail sample [194]. The simplest way to minimize false-negatives caused by sampling error is to maximize sample size and repeat sample collection.

The following criteria are suggested to discern and distinguish contaminants, saprophytes, and pathogenic fungi.

1. When a dermatophyte is isolated, it will always be considered the causative agent of onychomycosis.
2. The diagnosis for NDM or yeasts is made when compatible elements such as mycelia, arthrospores, or yeast cells are seen on direct microscopy of the nail.
3. To diagnose an NDM infection, the fungus must be isolated on actidione-containing or actidione-free medium in at least 5 of 20 inocula.

Whereas culture is the most specific test for onychomycosis and PAS examination of nail clippings is the most sensitive, it requires waiting weeks for a result, making direct microscopy the most frequent method used for diagnosis.

Culture

Mycotic culture is considered the most specific test for the diagnosis of onychomycosis and can determine the exact pathogen involved. The different organisms can be recognized using morphological and/or biochemical criteria. Scrapings from subungual keratosis and nails should be planted into Sabouraud agar and incubated at 26°C.

The presence of chloramphenicol or streptomycin and penicillin in the medium prevents the growth of contaminant bacteria. However, wherever possible, nails should be plated on medium both with and without cycloheximide (actidione), as it inhibits some non-dermatophytes that may cause onychomycosis.

Sometimes it is difficult to isolate fungi, even from nails that are positive on direct microscopy. The problem lies in the fact that many patients have already received topical or systemic treatment. In order to improve the isolation rate, various methods have been devised such as the use of a grinder, a dental drill fitted with a suction nozzle that collects the nail dust for microscopy and culture.

The clinical appearances of the nails, the presence of "atypical" hyphal elements in nail clippings, and repeated isolations of a non-dermatophyte are all helpful clues to the possible involvement of an unusual organism.

Scopulariopsis brevicaulis forms filaments as well as spores of characteristic size and morphology in nails. According to Ornsberg, the demonstration of *S. brevicaulis* on direct microscopy and the presence of more than 10 colonies in culture are diagnostic of infections caused by this organism. If there are fewer than three colonies, and *S. brevicaulis* is not seen on direct microscopy, the organism is probably present as a commensal. *S. brevicaulis* is often found in toenails infected by dermatophytes, particularly *T. rubrum* or *T. interdigitale.* The dermatophyte responsible for the primary infection may eventually be isolated after repeated scrapings have been taken. *Aspergillus* spp. may also form conidia in nails *in vivo* [189].

In a single nail a count of 11 or more culture-positive inocula of 15 plates, in combination with positive potassium hydroxide (KOH), is associated with a greater than 70% probability that the mold is the etiologic agent, particularly with *Acremonium* spp [195].

Histopathology

Histopathology examination of the nail can demonstrate whether a fungus is invasive or merely colonizing subungual debris. Onychomycotic nail biopsy may show the location of the hyphae and may give some hints to the possibility of the port of entry.

Depending on the site of involvement, nail clippings should be taken from the edge or the lateral part of the nail plate together with a shallow portion of subungual tissue. Samples are then embedded directly into paraffin without prior fixation. The specimens are stained with hematoxylin and eosin, PAS, and toluidine blue; calcofluor and Grocott's stain can also be used. Nail biopsy of a nail clipping with subungual hyperkeratosis may show fungal elements while the culture might be negative.

PAS stain is usually sufficient to demonstrate fungi but they cannot be further identified, since both dermatophytes and molds may produce hyphae and large, thick-walled arthrospores.

Fungal invasion leads to orthokeratosis of the nail bed epithelium. Hyperkeratosis accompanying onycholysis is a common feature of dermatophyte infections, which are the most common causes of DLSO, whereas in *Candida* onychomycosis, gross hyperkeratosis is mainly seen in total nail plate involvement in patients with chronic mucocutaneous candidiasis; in other cases of true *Candida* onychomycosis, thickening of the nail plate may be minimal [189].

However, some fungi do produce distinctive morphological features in nails that aid identification; for example yeasts plus hyphae and pseudo hyphae with *Candida albicans* or rough-surfaced conidiospores with *S. brevicaulis*.

Hyphae are seen between the nail laminae parallel to the surface and have a predilection for the ventral nail and stratum corneum of the nail bed. The epidermis may show spongiosis and focal parakeratosis, and there is a minimal dermal inflammatory response.

Nail clippings often show abundant Munro-like abscesses in onychomycosis; since fungi may be sparse, one cannot make the diagnosis of nail psoriasis from the presence of intracorneal abscesses in the absence of fungi alone. However, if fungi can be demonstrated histologically in the hyponychium of a nail from which fungi have not been isolated, the culture result is clearly false negative.

Distal and lateral subungual onychomycosis develops from an infection of the hyponychium and almost invariably shows fungi in the hyperkeratosis of the distal nail bed. The progression of the fungus proximally may reach the distal matrix area and include a different degree of inflammation at the proximal nail fold.

In PSO, histopathology shows that the entire nail plate is infiltrated with fungi, which are lying in a longitudinal parallel arrangement. However, the picture is complicated in that other surfaces such as the superior aspect of the plate and the distal or lateral margins may also be involved. Possibly because of the rapid spread, these patients do not show much nail thickening [189].

In WSO, the organisms are present superficially on the dorsal nail and display unique "perforating organs" and "eroding fronds". Onychomycosis may be caused by the pseudo-hyphae of different types of *Candida* spp. (especially *C. albicans*) penetrating the nail plate, cuticle, and even the stratum spinosum of the nail bed.

Histological examination of the nail plate, with the underlying tissue, will not only demonstrate the fungal elements but also reveal the depth of their penetration into the nail plate. This may provide further evidence of the pathogenic role of fungi isolated in culture, particularly if they can be identified in situ on morphological grounds, or by immunofluorescent labeling using specific antisera.

Histology of the primary distal and lateral subungual onychomycosis: Fungal invasion leads to orthokeratosis of the nail bed epithelium. In advanced nail disease, a more severe inflammatory reaction affects the nail bed with penetration of mononuclear cells and polymorphonuclear leukocytes into the subungual keratin, sometimes mimicking Munro's microabscesses. Parakeratosis may present. Ultimately, though, diagnosis still depends on the laboratory identification of the fungus. Invasive onychomycosis can also be proved convincingly by use of histology and appropriate stains such as Periodic Acid Schiff reagent (PAS) [189].

Onychomycosis caused by different types of molds is primarily considered as laboratory contaminates or super imposed fungus. Not like dermatophytes which almost always considered as real pathogen for onychomycosis. Revealing any dermatophyte in suspecting an onychomycotic nail will be sufficient for dermatophytic onychomycosis. The primary finding in suspicion of onychomycotic nail will not be considered primarily as pathogenic one unless taken 3 times, 2 weeks apart from the same deformed nail and the same mold will be revealed [129, 196].

Molecular Diagnosis

The use of molecular methods to detect fungal DNA or RNA in nail fragments is gaining ground although at present there are only a few commercially available systems for diagnosis.

Generally these either use one or more probes that are specific to common organisms such as *T. rubrum,* or panfungal probes that detect a wider range of organisms. At present, there is some difficulty in determining specificity versus carriage/true infection. Some authors advise using an algorithm that utilizes direct microscopy as the first measure followed where necessary by molecular testing using a polymerase chain reaction (PCR) technique. This method is likely to become more common in the future as microbiology laboratories adopt molecular diagnostic tools [189].

Treatment

The management of onychomycosis depends on several factors including the severity of nail involvement, associated tinea pedis, efficacy and potential adverse effects of any treatment regimen, and people who simultaneously take contraindicated drugs. While it seems reasonable not to treat minimal nail involvement, concurrent tinea pedis should always be treated, particularly in the setting of diabetes mellitus to prevent cellulitis, or in those patients who already had erysipelas or cellulitis and also have onychomycosis/tinea pedis. Those patients have to be treated correctly for their onychomycosis/tinea pedis. This is because onychomycosis and tinea pedis are well known contributors to erysipelas and cellulitis.

Topical Therapy

In those patients with distal nail involvement and/or contraindication for systemic treatment, topical therapy should be considered. Ciclopirox 8% lacquer applied daily for 48 weeks achieved mycologic cure in 29–36% of cases and clear nails (clinical cure) in 7% of mild to moderate cases of onychomycosis caused by dermatophytes. 77 Despite its much lower efficacy compared with oral antifungal agents, use of topical ciclopirox avoids the risk of drug interactions.

Amorolfine 5% applied twice weekly is another agent specifically prepared for use as a nail lacquer. It is the first member of a new class of antifungal drugs, the morpholine derivatives, which show activity against yeasts, dermatophytes, and molds that cause onychomycosis. Amorolfine may have higher mycologic cure rates (38–54% after 6 months of treatment) compared to ciclopirox lacquer; however, prospective controlled trials validating a significant difference are needed.

Topical treatment for onychomycosis is usually not effective enough and it is due to the fact that the different antimycotic properties have some difficulties in penetrating the nail plate downwards to the nail bed. A novel method (not yet published) of treatment has been developed to improve drug penetration through the nail plate to the nail bed. This method is based on drilling two horizontal lines of holes in the nail plate up to the nail bed. These two lines have to be drilled just proximal to the border between the diseased and healthy portions of the nail plate, 1.8–2 mm apart. (Figure 15.34)

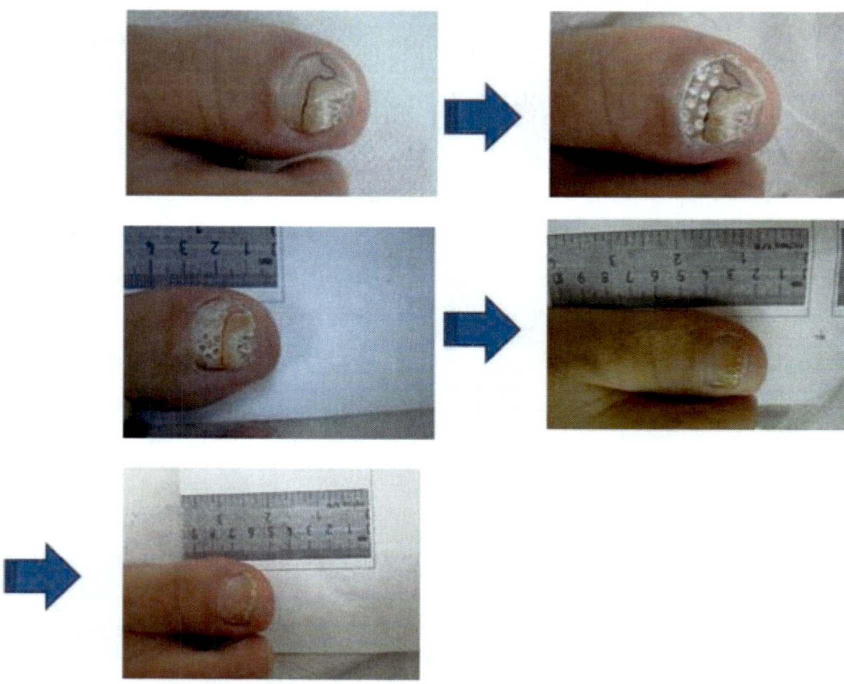

Figure 15.34. Drilling.

The automatic device drills rapidly until a pre-defined humidity level is reached and stops short of penetrating the nail bed, thus preventing any pain or discomfort for the patient. Once the two lines of holes are ready a solution of antifungal agent is to be applied twice daily. Once a week the holes have to be renewed (this is because while the nail grows out, the holes are usually filled by keratin debris and may prevent the antifungal solution from reaching the nail bed).

Systemic Therapy

An oral antifungal is required for onychomycosis involving the matrix area, or when a shorter treatment regimen or greater chance for clearance or cure is desired. Selection of the antifungal agent should be based primarily on the causative organism, the potential adverse effects, and the risk of drug interactions in any particular patient. Terbinafine is fungistatic and fungicidal against dermatophytes and *Aspergillus*, and less so against *Scopulariopsis*. Terbinafine is not recommended for *Candida* onychomycosis since it demonstrates variable efficacy against *Candida* spp. A course of terbinafine 250 mg daily for 6 weeks is effective for most fingernail infections, while a minimum 12-week course 12–16 is required for toenail infections. Most adverse effects are gastrointestinal such as diarrhea, nausea, taste disturbance, and elevation of liver enzymes. Evidence suggests that a 3-month continuous regimen of terbinafine is the most effective oral treatment available today for onychomycosis of the toenails. Clinical cure rates among different studies are approximately 50%, although the success rate is lower in patients over 65 years.

Itraconazole is fungistatic against dermatophytes, nondermatophyte molds, and yeasts. Safe and effective schedules include pulse dosing with itraconazole 400 mg daily for 1 week per month or a continuous dose of 200 mg daily, both of which require 2 months or 2 pulses of treatment for fingernails and at least 3 months or 3 pulses for toenails. Itraconazole is dosed by weight in children at 5 mg/kg/day. 81 Elevated liver enzymes occur in 0.3–5% of patients during therapy and return to normal within 12 weeks of discontinuation. Although itraconazole has a broader spectrum of activity than terbinafine, studies have shown a significantly lower rate of cure (about 25% vs. 50%) and higher relapse rate (about 50% vs. 20%) with itraconazole compared with terbinafine. Fluconazole is fungistatic against dermatophytes, some nondermatophyte molds, and *Candida*. The usual regimen for fluconazole is 150–300 mg once weekly for 3–12 months.

Griseofulvin is no longer considered standard treatment for onychomycosis (yet still the gold standard for tinea capitis) because of its prolonged treatment course, potential for adverse effects and drug interactions, and its relatively low cure rates. Combination therapy regimens may have a higher clearance rate than either oral or topical treatments alone. Oral terbinafine combined with amorolfine nail lacquer was shown to result in clinical cure and negative mycology in 59% of patients compared to 45% of patients treated with oral terbinafine alone. However, another study failed to show any additional benefit of combining oral terbinafine with ciclopirox 8% solution. *In vitro* fungicidal activity demonstrated by thymol, camphor, menthol, and oil of *Eucalyptus citriodora* offers the potential for additional therapeutic strategies to treat onychomycosis. Thymol 4% prepared in ethanol may be used as drops applied to the nail plate and hyponychium. The application to nails of commercially available topical preparations with thymol, such as Vicks VapoRub™, has anecdotally led to success. Final options for refractory cases include surgical avulsion or chemical removal of the nail with 40% urea compounds in combination with topical or oral antifungals.

Photodynamic Therapy for onychomycosis

Photodynamic therapy (PDT) is one of several modalities for the treatment of onychomycosis. This type of treatment is based on the activation of visible light by different photosensitizing agents. This combination produces reactive oxygen species, which leads to cell death. Because photosensitizing agents may be absorbed (differently – depending on the fungus type) by fungi, this type of treatment has been promoted. The effects *in vitro* of PDT have already been proven.

In a study published in the *Journal of Advanced Drug Delivery* [197], 5-aminolevulinic acid (mALA) was applied above the nail plate and was occluded for 3 hours; then the nail was radiated by red fluorescence 630 nm at 37 j/cm^2 for 7 minutes and 24 seconds. This regimen was applied twice more at 15-day intervals. After 3 consecutive treatments the direct smear and fungal culture were negative. After 3 months, and up to 24 months, the direct smears and cultures remained negative.

In another study published by Sotiriou and his colleagues in *ActaDermato-Venereologica* [198], 30 patients were treated with a unique regimen: urea 40% was applied under occlusion for 10 days, then PDT (red light 570-670 nm light source $40J/cm^2$) with 20% mALA was applied for 3 hours. There was a total of three treatments every 2 weeks; no systemic medication was allowed. Complete cure was defined as up to 10% of subungual hyperkeratosis combined with negative mycology (direct microscopy and culture). The results of this small study were encouraging due to the fact that 43.3% were cured after 12 months and 36.6% remained with complete cure after 18 months.

Multicenter studies on large series of patients are needed to prove the efficacy and safety of different methods of PDT on onychomycosis patients.

Laser Treatment for Onychomycosis

The laser treatment regimens are variable. Different laser machines are available for onychomycosis and the promotion of laser treatment for onychomycosis has been fruitful compared to the clinical results worldwide.

Review of the relevant literature revealed that there are not more than a dozen publications on laser treatment of onychomycosis. The biggest study contained 131 patients [199] while the smallest study contained 8! Patients [200]; the rest of the studies had around 20 patients or less [200-204]; only one study had a control group [205]. Each of these studies had different criteria for enrolling the patients and effectiveness of the different laser machines, which led to a huge variability (see the section "Onychomycosis in clinical studies" in this chapter).

The exact mechanism of action of the different lasers is not yet fully understood. But, infrared wavelengths of 780–3000 nm (this is the wavelength range usually used in treatment of onychomycotic nails) exert their energy effect by heating the nail plate in order to heat the fungus itself [206]. The principle method of the upgraded laser machines is having a pulsed beam and not the continuous beam; this pulsed beam may lead to selective photothermolysis [207]. In addition to the effect of selective photothermolysis, there is some breaking of the uninvolved tissue (between the pulsed beams) and it has the ability to become cold, preventing the so-called collateral damage. This idea was established due to the fact that *in vitro* studies show that there is impressive efficacy of the pulsed beam lasers for clipped onychomycotic nails. Those studies shown that 50°C is sufficient to kill the fungus (*T. rubrum*) [208].

The clinical studies that were done in the last few years have shown variable results. The levels of the majority of these studies were low due to the fact that they included small numbers of patients and low level of evidence was noted. Only two small clinical studies were randomized controlled studies. Some of the studies have shown some efficacy by measuring 5 mm of healthy nail with no relation to outcome or relapse rate.

There is not enough clinical–laboratory correlation, and there are no comparative studies of traditional onychomycosis treatment and the different laser regimens. Each study was done with its own criteria; there was no uniformity in these studies. Serious clinical studies that include the following parameters need to be done: large series of patients, placebo control, traditional treatment control, longer period of time for follow up, and using the onychomycosis severity index (OSI) factor (the more severe the onychomycosis the less the chance to achieve complete cure). Using these strict criteria will lead to determination of the effectiveness of the laser itself and prevent misinterpretation of the clinical and mycological results.

In recent years, laser machines have been strongly promoted for the treatment of onychomycosis by being advertised as promising, safe, and very effective, while trying to mislabel the systemic antifungal agents as unsafe and dangerous.

The advantage of the laser for onychomycosis is that there are no adverse drug events and/or drug interactions.

The disadvantages of the laser treatments are that there is not enough data regarding the efficacy of the different lasers; hence the clinical studies are not big and impressive enough to base a decision on. There is not enough knowledge regarding the matching of the sub-type of onychomycosis to the type of the laser that is suitable to treat it. The cost of laser treatment is higher or much higher compared to conventional medical treatment.

To establish the assumption that laser therapy for onychomycosis is sufficient/successful, more information from large double blind-clinical studies is needed.

Onychomycosis in Clinical Studies

Many clinical studies regarding onychomycosis show the efficacy of different systemic antimycotic drugs with a huge gap and range from 14% to 90%. Searching the relevant literature reveals that there are several different criteria such as in the definition of clinical cure; in different studies this may range between 80% and 100%, relating only to the mycological culture with no importance given to the direct microscopy, while other studies relate to both direct microscopy and culture. All onychomycosis clinical studies ignore the age of patients, yet it is well known that the older the patient, the lower the cure rate achieved. If in one onychomycosis clinical study the average age is 20 years and in another onychomycosis study the average age is 70 years, it is very clear that there will be a difference between the two groups. In addition, the follow-up time is a factor that may influence the final results as well.

Another very important factor is the onychomycosis severity index (OSI). Almost all the onychomycosis clinical studies related to the big toenail as the target nail, and the final result also relates to the same big toenail. It is very convenient to measure the progression of the healthy nail during the treatment, but on the other hand the big toenail is prone to different traumas especially minor ones, which even the patient may not be aware of; this may prevent the nail's ability to heal totally. Not all the onychomycotic toenails achieve the same cure rate. Although one does not expect all studies to achieve the same results, variations in study designs might also cause some disparities in the cure rate; while variations in results are plausible, such a great variation is implausible.

A prospective study was done to compare the clinical and mycological cure rate of the big toenail to each of the involved toenails and the difference between the results according to different criteria. The results of this study show that the potential cure rate of the big toenail was lower compared to the second, third, and fourth toenails. The fifth toenail was not taken into account because this toenail is prone to pressure from tight shoes and this not a marker of successful treatment for onychomycosis. The final result shows that although the mycological results were about the same in all the involved toenails, the clinical cure rates were much better in the second, third, and fourth toenails compared to the big toenail on the same foot. The low cure rate of the hallux (the big toenail) can be explained by the fact that the big toenail is more prone to external traumas.

In order to prevent different results regarding clinical studies and onychomycosis in particular, consistency regarding the inclusion and exclusion criteria are needed, such as definition of clinical and mycological cure rate, calculation of onychomycosis severity index, uniformity regarding age, length of the treatment, and follow-up period of time. All the above are needed otherwise different results and conclusions will be achieved.

In addition, efficacy of drugs should be based on all of the involved toenails, excluding the fifth, rather than the big toenail alone. In clinical trials, when we take all the infected toenails into account, we ignore the possibility that the hallux might have been traumatized and was not completely cured, while other toenails of the same patient were cured. Examining the effectiveness of an antifungal drug should be based on its ability to eradicate fungi and not other conditions, let alone irreversible deformation ones. An antifungal drug is not necessarily an antideformation drug.

Follow-up

Although onychomycosis is not a fatal infection it can be associated with discomfort and negative self-image 3 and can predispose to soft tissue infection, particularly cellulitis [209].

Of 100 onychomycosis patients were treated for their onychomycosis, 37 developed mild, moderate or severe paronychia. Out of these patients with paronychia, 19 patients required surgical involvement. Consequently, it should be noted that ingrowing toenails may be a sign of effective treatment for onychomycosis. It is also important to be aware of the potential for drug–drug interactions before starting patients on oral antifungals and to consider the combination of physical and chemotherapeutic approaches [189].

Chapter 16

Pityriasis Versicolor

Synonym: Pityriasis versicolor is sometimes called "tinea versicolor", although the term tinea should be reserved for infection by a dermatophytic fungus.

Definition

Pityriasis versicolor is a chronic superficial mycosis that is caused by saprophytes of the genus *Malassezia*. Pityriasis versicolor gets its name from the delicate scales similar to bran (pityriasis, from the Greek pituron, bran) and the change in color of effected skin, ranging from pink or tan to dark brown, where it becomes lighter or darker than the surrounding skin (versicolor, from the Latin vertere turn on change – changeable in color).

Epidemiology

One of the most common fungal skin infections affecting young adults and adolescents worldwide in whom sebaceous gland activity is pronounced is pityriasis versicolor (PV). Although the disease is most prevalent in young and persons in their twenties and thirties, some cases of pityriasis versicolor have been reported in children [210, 211] and infants [212, 213].

An interesting study regarding a fishing community in Venezuela reported a total prevalence of 15.52%. 3 Although few studies on the subject exist, a review conducted in the United States between 1971 and 1974 showed a figure of 0.8% in a population of 28,000 people [214]. Another study in Sweden in 1979 found a 1.1% prevalence of PV in a total of 20,296 patients [215]. A subsequent study conducted in the same country in 1983 included 3302 people and found PV in 0.5% of men and 0.3% of women [216]. PV is most common in tropical and subtropical areas, due to the hot and humid climate. Pityriasis versicolor tends to be more prevalent in the summer months, without a distinction of sex or race [217,218].

Pathogens

The causative organisms of pityriasis versicolor are ubiquitous lipophilic yeasts of the *Malassezia* spp., which infectthe stratum corneum of the skin where sebaceous glands are abundant.

Pityriasis versicolor is a frequent superficial mycosis by *Malassezia* yeast, found in normal skin flora of 90-98% of adults [217,218].

The genus *Malassezia* includes a group of lipophilic yeasts whose natural habitat is the skin of humans and other warm-blooded animals. *Malessezia* was formerly called *Pityrosporum,* with only 3 species recognized for a long time (*Pityrosporum orbiculare*, *Pityrosporum ovale*, and *Pityrosporum pachydermatis*). In 1995, 7 species were included in *Malassezia* genus based on molecular analysis (*M. furfur*, *M. obtusa*, *M. globosa*, *M. slooffiae*, M. sympodialis, *M. pachydermatis*, and *M. restricta*). Currently, on the basis of common DNA sequences and molecular methods, the *Malassezia* genus has been expanded to 14 species *M. globosa*, *M. restricta*, *M. sympodialis*, *M. furfur*, *M. obtusa*, *M. slooffiae*, *M. pachydermatis*, *M. dermatis*, *M. japonica*, and *M. yamatoensis* were found to be related to human diseases [219,220]; other species such as *M. equine*, *M. caprae*, and *M. cunculi*, were also defined.

Malassezia are members of the fungal skin microflora; in healthy humans they colonize lipid-rich areas such as the scalp, face, back, and chest because they require a lipid source for growth. The presence of lipids in the skin favors *Malassezia* during postpuberty due to the apex of sebaceous glands development stimulated by sex hormones during this time of life. *Malassezia* in the skin microflora is generally permitted to grow asymptomatically because of the leniency of the immune system. The yeasts become pathogenic when the immune balance is disturbed. When this occurs they can convert from round yeast forms (saprophytic form) to pathogenic mycelial forms (opportunistic phase) that invade the stratum corneum causing mycosis. Keratinase is also produced and causes loosening of the stratum corneum and subsequent scale formation.

Pityriasis versicolor is considered an opportunistic infection related to host susceptibility rather than to exposure. This transformation has been linked to a series of factors, including genetic factors, age, climate, local environmental factors (heat, humidity, hyperhidrosis), diabetes mellitus, hepatic or renal diseases, malnutrition, pregnancy, oral contraceptives, immunodepression, and immunosuppressant therapy [221].

The *Malessezia* spp. are implicated in the pathogenesis of several human diseases, including pityriasis versicolor, seborrheic dermatitis, Malassezia folliculitis, atopic dermatitis and psoriasis. Additionally, the species *M. pachydermatis* and *M. furfur* can cause systemic infections. The most common *Malassezia* spp. cultured from lesions of pityriasis versicolor are *M. globose, M. sympodialis* and *M. furfur* [222]. *M. sympodialis* has a predilection for the back and chest and *M. furfur* has a predilection for the back and abdomen. Other species such as *M. slooffiae* and *M. furfur* are relatively less common but not completely absent. Differences between the studies may be a result of geographic variation in species prevalence, although further investigation is required to confirm this hypothesis. However, there is evidence that these species are also common on both nonlesional skin area in both nonlesional skin area of patients with or without pityriasis versicolor. It was shown that there is endogenous factors, promoting the development of pityriasis versicolor in those patients.

Different malassezia spp. Are located in the vast majority of clinically healthy patients without having pityriasis versicolor [222].

Clinical Presentation

Pityriasis versicolor is a common, chronic, superficial fungal disease characterized by the appearance of round to oval macular lesions with delicate scaling primarily found on the upper trunk, neck, and upper aspects of the arms (Figure 16.1), Figure 16.2).

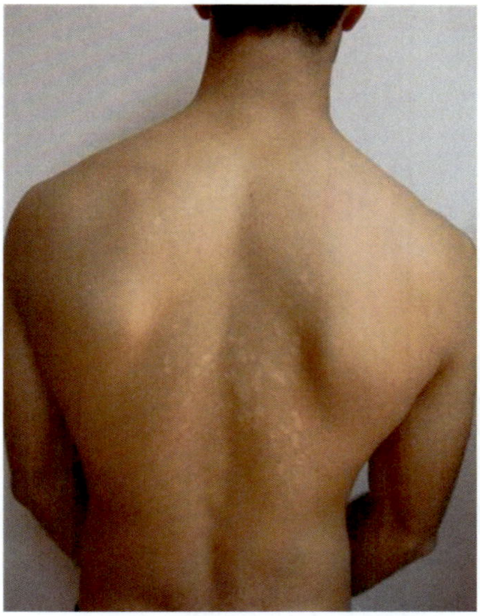

Figure 16.1. Pityriasis versicolor.

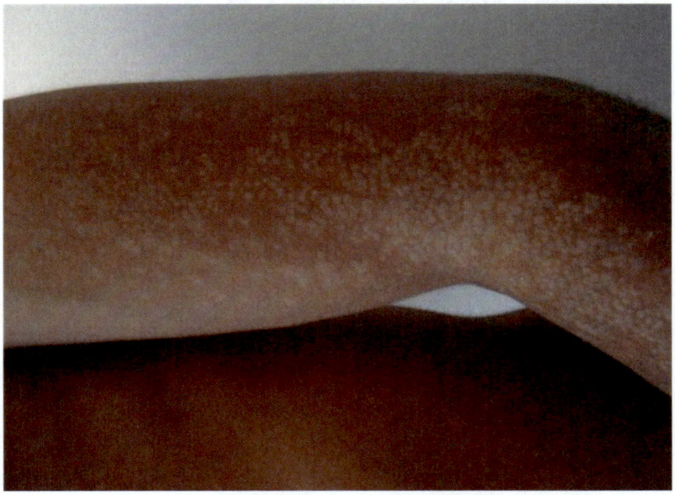

Figure 16.2. Pityriasis versicolor.

Clinically, pityriasis versicolor results in well demarcated, finely scaling thin plaques with variable pigmentation, occurring most frequently on the upper trunk and extremities. These lesions vary in color, and can be hypopigmented (white) or hyperpigmented (pink, tan, brown, or black).

Flaking is evident, although in larger lesions this may occur only at the border [222]. The furfuraceous scales can be observed better by stretching the skin distally and tension placed on skin lesions; a wrinkling of the skin with visible scale may be evident; this is known as Zileri's Sign. Scraping the area with a sharp blade or glass slide may reveal a powder or scale attributable to the effect of keratinase (Figure 16.3, Figure 16.4). This observation can be especially useful in austere environments without the ability to perform more definitive testing.

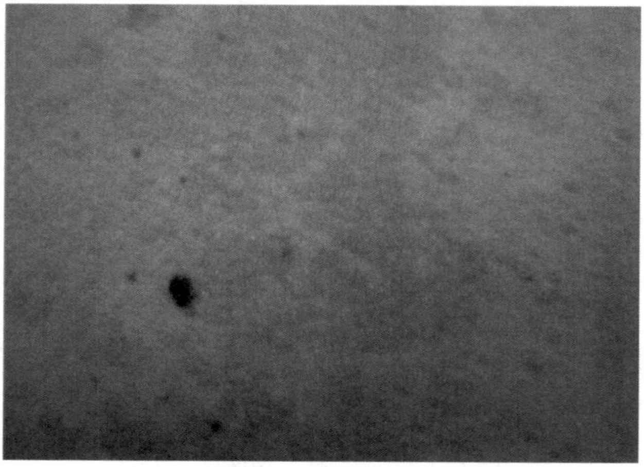

Figure 16.3. Before scarping.

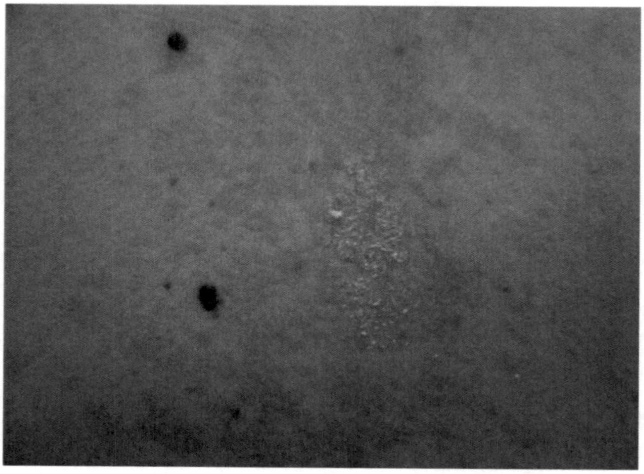

Figure 16.4. After scraping.

Generally, pityriasis versicolor isregarded as an asymptomatic cosmetic disorder; however, some patients report moderate-to-severe pruritus [222], which often arises due to sun exposure or sweating due to sport activity, usually appearing in healthy individuals.

Although pityriasis versicolor's most usual sites of involvement are the trunk, neck, and arms, it may also occur on the face, scalp, and other areas of the body either in addition to the more common distribution of lesions or as the sole area of involvement [222]. Involvement of the palpebra, areolae, and penile shaft are less frequent. Other uncommon locations have also been described, such as the eyelids, armpits, and perineum. The disease, in certain circumstances, may be difficult to distinguish from erythrasma (erythrasmoid PV) when erythrasma occurs in the groin areas, it may show a clinical representation of PV. Finding of PV only in the groin area occurs rarely.

The most common clinical forms of the disease are hypopigmented (PV alba or achromians variant) and hyperpigmented PV. Although most patients present macules of the same color, being either hypo-or hyper-pigmented, lesions are sometimes of 2 colors: a pink or brown may be seen in covered area and whitish color in the exposed areas. Recently, a red variant (PV rubra) was described, and another blackish (PV nigra) macule, as well as the possible transformation from one type [223]. Another less common form is inverse tinea versicolor, where lesions of pityriasis versicolor are confined to the flexural areas. Hypo- or hyper-pigmentation may persist for months after active infection is treated.

Malassezia (pityrosporum) folliculitis is a type of folliculitis filled with *Malassezia* yeasts within the hair follicles. The predicted locations are on the chest, face, and upper arms. Clinically it has dome-shaped red-pink papules and/or pustules, often itching (Figure 16.5). Malassezia folliculitis is often confused with acne, as both diseases appear in similar locations and both prefer oily skins.

Figure 16.5. Pityrosporum folliculitis.

There are several risk factors to having malassezia folliculitis. The external factors are heat, humidity, and oily sunscreens/creams; the internal factors are oily skin, tendency to sweat, pregnancy, diabetes mellitus, and immune deficiency. Systemic treatment that disturbs the balance between the normal bacterial flora and the large quantity of the *Malassezia* yeast causes the *Malassezia* yeast to proliferate. The diagnosis of malassezia folliculitis is done by direct smear/biopsy. The treatment is the same as for pityriasis versicolor.

Azelaic acid is an organic molecule that is found in several plants such as wheat and barley, and also created by different *Malassezia* spp. such as *M. furfur*. Azelaic acid is well known as a tyrosinase inhibitor, which leads to decreasing melanin synthesis and prevents the hyperpigmentation.

Predisposing Factors

Pityriasis versicolor is a frequent mycosis. The triggering of mycosis is due to a set of predisposing factors: use of skin moisturisers, high humidity and temperature of the climate, hyperhidrosis, use of systemic corticosteroids, previous outbreaks of PV, oral anticoagulants, and in principle genetic predisposition, among others. Systemic corticosteroids would increase the frequency of mycosis by changing the lipid composition of the cutaneous surface or by immunocompromising the individual [219,224,226-228]. The disease is more common among first-degree family members, suggesting genetic factors may play a role [229].

Patients with varying degrees of immunosuppression such as due to Cushing's disease or steroid intake have been found to be predisposed to development of widespread pityriasis versicolor [222]. It is also seen frequently in patients with uncontrolled diabetes (5.2%) [230].

Hot and humid weather is an important triggering factor. A history of recurrences during the summer months and/or heavy sweating is typical, as increased sebaceous gland involvement provides the humid environment necessary for the growth of the hyphal form [231].

Although pityriasis versicolor tends to be more prevalent in the summer months and in tropical locations than in temperate regions, evidence points to the importance of endogenous host factors in the development of the disease. These may include malnutrition, use of oral contraceptives, use of systemic corticosteroids or immunosuppressants, hyperhidrosis may be considered. Although many contributing or aggravating factors have been described, regarding the transformation of the saprophytic yeast to the parasitic mycelial form remains subject for debate [218].

Differential Diagnosis

Clinically, pityriasis versicolor can resemble other dermatologic disorders, and differential diagnosis should include:

Vitiligo

Vitiligo is a skin condition that expresses depigmentation of the skin in various locations. Practically, the cells that create the melanin (the melanocytes) stop the discharge of melanin just because the melanocytic cells are no longer active. The mechanism of vitiligo is not fully understood but several suggestions exist, such as immunological reasons, oxidative stress, or viral infections. Clinically, vitiligo may appear at any place on the body but it is common to see vitiligo around the eyes and at the distal parts of the extremities, in contrast to pityriasis versicolor, which often occurs on the upper back, chest, and upper shoulders. The main difference between the disorders is that the pityriasis versicolor always has scales, which can be noted by gentle scratching with the fingernail, while in vitiligo there is no scale at all (Figure 16.6). The color of the vitiligo patches is bright white while in pityriasis versicolor the color is variable, ranging from whitish/yellow to dark brown; hence the name versicolor.

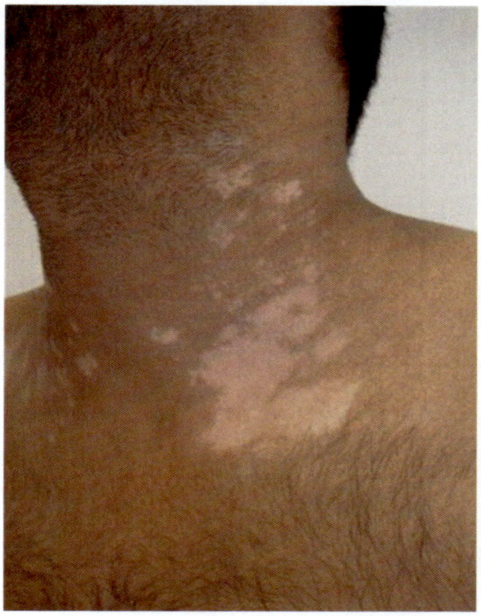

Figure 16.6. Vitiligo.

Tinea corporis –

See more on Chapter 11

Seborrheic Dermatitis

See more on page 47

Pityriasis rosea

Pityriasis rosea is one of the papulosquamous disorders characterized by a mild inflammatory skin disease that is expressed by pale red-pink-colored papules and plaques covered with unique scale arising from the center of the lesion that pulls off centrifugally (like the rose flower – hence the name rosea) (Figure 16.7).

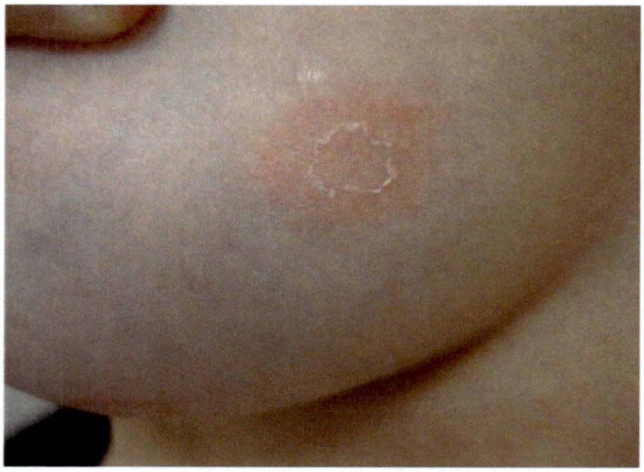

Figure 16.7. Pityriasis Rosea.

The rash usually begins with the appearance of a first relatively big lesion – the so-called herald patch (or "mother patch"); after a few days or weeks there is a widespread eruption (smaller than the "mother patch") usually located at the torso and the proximal areas of the lower and upper extremities, with an approximate duration of 6–8 weeks. The rash disappears spontaneously, without any residuals. This kind of rash is usually asymptomatic, but sometimes itching or tingling sensation could occur.

The disease is said to be caused by a viral agent, but some investigators have suggested a fungal cause to be involved, yet so far no definite fungal agent was found.

Pityriasis rosea usually disappears by itself without treatment.

Pityriasis alba

Pityriasis alba is a one of the minor examples of atopic dermatitis in children and young adults, which is usually located on the face with predeliction to the cheeks and the upper external part of the arms, but could occur at any location of the upper torso. The lesions are oval or elliptic in shape, mild or very mild erythematous patches of 1–5 cm, covered by tiny scales. It is usually several lesions but could be one or more than 15 lesions. In relation to pityriasis versicolor, pityriasis alba occurs much more often in young children while pityriasis versicolor occurs more often in young adults (rarely in young children). The locations in pityriasis versicolor are much more commonly at the upper back and chest while in pityriasis alba is usually located on the cheeks. The scales in pityriasis versicolor pull off easily and are a little bit greasy/slightly damp, while in pityriasis alba the fine scales are dry and do not pull off easily. Lastly, the lesion borders in pityriasis versicolor are well circumscribed while in pityriasis alba the lesions are gradually confluent with the normal skin.

Chloasma/melasma

Melasma (chloasma) is hyperpigmented irregular macules ranging from a few millimeters to the whole face – from the confluence of the patches (Figure 16.8). But usually the melasma is seen on the cheeks, forehead, and below the nose (upper part of the upper lip). Melasma occurs up to 10-fold more often in women than in men. There is a high correlation with women taking contraceptive pills and pregnant women. The borders of melasma lesions depend on the depth of the hyperpigmentation process itself. Practically, the melasma lesion can be divided to 3 types regarding the depth of the hyperpigmentation: epidermal, dermal, and mixed pattern.

The epidermal type shows well-circumscribed borders, the color is darker than the dermal subtype, and responds better to conventional treatment. This subtype of melasma may be diagnosed using a Wood's lamp, which shows the well-circumscribed lesion and the uniformity of the color in the patch.

The dermal subtype is the most common, has no well-demarcated borders, does not react well with Wood's lamp, and does not react to treatment well.

The mixed type is a combination of the two above subtypes that can be seen by the Wood's lamp but there is no uniformity in the whole lesion. Regarding treatment, there is a partial improvement because the superficial part reacts well to the treatment while the dermal subtype does not.

Although pityriasis versicolor could be dark in color, the location and the lack of scales support the diagnosis of melasma.

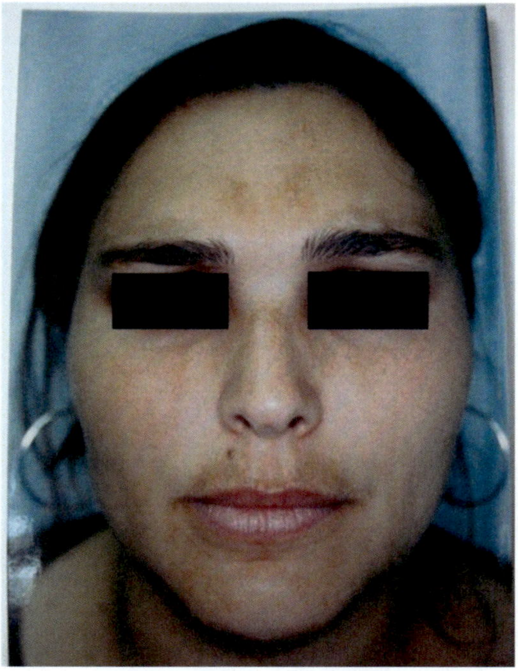

Figure 16.8. Melasma.

Nevus anemicus - Nevus anemicus is a congenital vascular anomaly, presented as hypopigmentation macules, as a result of vasoconstriction (Figure 16.9).

Erythrasma - in cases involving the groin - see in erythrasma.

Confluent and reticulated papillomatosis of Gougerot and Carteaud

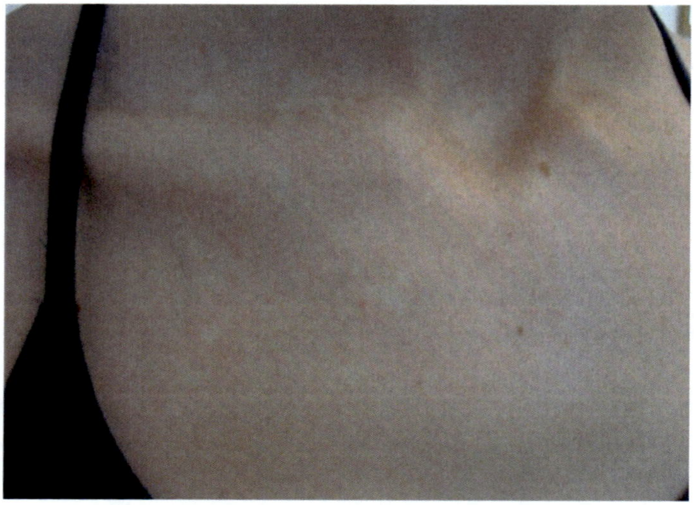

Figure 16.9. Nevus Anemicus.

Confluent and reticulated papillomatosis of Gougerot and Carteaud is a tiny flat papule of 2–5 mm, brown grey in color, covered by fine scales. The lesions are often crowded and the appearance of a network may be seen. The cause is unknown but several suggestions are mentioned in the literature such as hormonal, *Malassezia* (due to the fact that some cases react well to antifungal treatment), and hereditary causes. The lesions are located first at the middle of the chest and the back, and then spread gradually to the sides of the torso; sometimes itching sensation may occur.

Confluent and reticulated papillomatosis of Gougerot and Carteaud is much more common in women than in men and has exacerbations and remissions.

Although there is good reaction to systemic minocycline, no bacteria were found in the lesions.

Compared to pityriasis versicolor, the chronicity, the configuration of the lesions, and the characteristic nature of the scales may distinguish between the diseases.

Secondary syphilis

Syphilis is a bacterial venereal disease caused by the spirochete *Treponema pallidum*. This is a usually sexually transmitted disease, but may also be transferred from mother to fetus in utero, or through infected blood product transfusion. If untreated, syphilis progresses through primary, secondary, latent, and tertiary stages. Syphilis has a many clinical presentations and can mimic many other infections mediated processes in advanced stages. For this reason, the other entity for secondary syphilis is "the great impostor". It is not so well known that there is a form of cutaneous syphilis, the so-called annular syphilid, which is also strikingly characteristic of the skin color, particularly those of African ethnicity. This is an early manifestation of the disease and a modification of the flat papular or discoid syphilid. The lesions apparently begin as flat papules that enlarge peripherally and clear up in the center, forming circular elevated rings. By the coalescence of several rings, various gyrate and festooned patches are produced. The eruption is seen most often on the face, but may also occur on the trunk and extremities, especially the back.

There is a huge variability regarding the clinical presentation of secondary syphilis. Even the same secondary syphilis rash in different people may range from mild cases to very severe cases.

The extremely variable manifestations of tertiary syphilis produce an extremely broad differential diagnosis. Care must be taken to consider syphilis in cardiac, dermatologic, and neurologic disorders. Syphilitic patients should be checked for other sexually transmitted diseases, including chlamydia, gonorrhea, trichomoniasis, bacterial vaginosis, and HIV infection. When making a primary diagnosis of a generalized rash or an STD, syphilis must be included in the differential diagnoses because of its varying manifestations, and prophylactic treatment or serologic studies considered.

Diagnosis

The diagnosis of pityriasis versicolor is most commonly based on clinical signs and symptoms and confirmed by direct microscopy.

The diagnosis is clinical and relatively easy. The very fine plaques that are covered by fine scale should be scratched gently and collected for direct microscopy. It can be confirmed either by using a 10–15% potassium hydroxide solution or by applying scotch tape on previously scratched lesions (scotch-skin test) and viewing the hyphae and spores of the yeast under a light microscope. A specimen for microscopy should be taken from the scaling edge of a lesion, as these areas are most likely to contain viable organisms. The keratin and debris in the specimen should be dissolved using either 10–15% potassium hydroxide or Albert's solution. Staining of the fungal elements will present as a characteristic "spaghetti-and-meatballs" pattern, reflecting the presence of both hyphae and spores, and is considered the gold standard for diagnosis. Some authors report that the number of yeast and hyphae in the lesions of pityriasis versicolor is greater than in normal skin, while others have shown that the difference is not statistically significant [222].

Wood's light examination (filtered UV light with a peak of 365 nm), in addition to microscopic examination, is also a useful diagnostic tool but is only positive in one-third of cases [2]. Lesions may fluoresce a characteristic bright yellow or gold color. The color of the fluorescence may also aid in differential diagnosis and can be used to detect subclinical lesions, as it is unique to the mycelial form of *Malassezia*. Recent evidence has suggested that only *M. furfur* produces the indole compounds that fluoresce under Wood's light, indicating that this species is implicated in at least some cases of pityriasis versicolor [222].

Neither skin biopsy nor culture is normally required for diagnosis but may be essential when diagnostic uncertainty occurs in a cutaneous biopsy specimen characterized by the presence of a mild dermal infiltrate of mononuclear cells and polymorphous leucocytes. Although few of these inflammatory cells reach the superficial skin layers, the skin-invading fungi are normally confined to the stratum corneum. The *Malassezia* yeasts stain well with Periodic Acid Schiff and methenamine silver.

Fungal cultures are usually unnecessary for routine diagnosis as well, as they will often lead to negative results because the fungus does not contain the lipids required for growth in culture media. Culture can be essential to identify the species present in the lesions or those forming part of the normal flora. The *Malassezia* yeasts, with the single exception of *Malassezia pachydermatis*, do not grow in standard mycological media, such as Sabouraud agar, and need a specific oily surrounding which may help the malasezzia yeast to grow in culture [218].

The development of molecular methods made it possible to identify yeasts directly from skin scales and there us no need for culture. The performance of such methods is mostly dependent on the sensitivity of the nucleic acid extraction procedure.

Polymerase chain reaction (PCR) method can be applied for the identification of 11 *Malassezia* strains. The phenetic analyses, however, are usually a time-consuming, multistep process, necessitating several experimental techniques.

To overcome this limitation, studies have used a variety of molecular methods such as nested PCR, real-time PCR, pulsed-field gel electrophoresis (PFGE), amplified fragment length polymorphism (AFLP), denaturing gradient gel electrophoresis (DGGE), random amplification of polymorphic DNA (RAPD), single-strand conformation polymorphism, terminal fragment length polymorphism, restriction fragment length polymorphism (RFLP), and sequence analysis.

Despite the usefulness of these molecular techniques, potentially serious drawbacks are associated with each, such as inefficiency in differentiating all the species, challenging technical requirements, high cost of analysis, and questionable reproducibility.

Treatment

Treatment of pityriasis versicolor infection with most topical and systemic agents is usually easy and effective. However, the treatment of PV is becoming increasingly challenging with the emergence of resistant *Malassezia* species. Once diagnosed, PV is usually treated as it may lead to emotional distress because of its appearance, and it will persist for many years if left untreated.

Malassezia yeasts are susceptible to a wide range of nonspecific and specific antifungal topical treatments, and several effective oral agents. Older topical treatments tend to lack antifungal activity and generally possess keratolytic properties. These agents include selenium sulfide, propylene glycol, sulfur, and tar-containing compounds. The mechanism of this agent is through the antimicrobial effect. Traditionally, the most frequently used topical treatment has been a 2.5% selenium sulfide shampoo applied once a day for 7–14 days. It acts by physically or chemically removing the infected stratum corneum. Of the non-imidazole topical agents, zinc pyrithione shampoo appears most effective compared with placebo. Sulfur salicylic acid shampoo is also effective.

Specific antifungal agents used for the topical treatment for pityriasis versicolor include the azoles (ketoconazole, bifonazole, clotrimazole, itraconazole, fluconazole, miconazole, econazole, fenticonazole, metronidazole, sulconazole, tioconazole, imidazole, hydroxylpyridones (ciclopirox olamine), allylamines (terbinafine), benzylamines (butenafine), tacrolimus, and pimecrolimus [222].

Rilopirox, a new synthetic pyridine derivative initially designed as an intravaginal antifungal treatment against *Candida albicans*, seems to also be effective against tinea versicolor. Topical lanoconazole, a racemic imidazole antimycotic agent, was also found effective against superficial infections of *Candida albicans* and *Malassezia* spp. 9 NND-502 might be beneficial in the treatment of *Malassezia*-associated skin diseases [232]. Also, adapalene gel, though commonly used for acne treatment and overall more expensive, has been shown to eliminate disease, likely through decreasing sebaceous gland activity, removing abnormal keratin-producing cells, and acting as an anti-inflammatory agent.

Other even less frequently used topical compounds such as tea tree oil (*Melaleuca alternifolia*), honey, and cinnamic acid have demonstrated activity both *in vitro* and *in vivo* against *Malassezia* spp., simultaneously displaying anti-inflammatory properties [233].

Honey applied for 3 weeks every 8 hours was also found to be effective, resulting in a 79% cure rate [231].

Generally, patients are instructed to apply shampoos daily for several weeks, leaving on the skin for 5 to 10 minutes before washing, while creams are routinely used once to twice daily for 1 month. After total cure is achieved, it is recommended to use the shampoo once or twice weekly as prophylactic treatment.

Patients should have a fair trial with topical antimycotic shampoos or creams before considering initiating oral treatment. Stubborn conditions of pityriasis versicolor that do not react enough to the conventional topical treatment should be treated properly with systemic fluconazole or itraconazole, etc.

Systemic therapies used to treat PV include oral itraconazole, ketoconazole, fluconazole, and pramiconazole [234]. They are all effective against PV when compared to placebo; no significant difference exists between them. Different dosing regimens such as 200 mg/d for 5 or 7 days of itraconazole, 300 mg/wk for 2 weeks of fluconazole, 200 mg oral ketoconazole daily for 10 days, and 200 mg/d for 2 days of pramiconazole are effective for the treatment of pityriasis versicolor. Fluconazole is considered among the safest [231]. Of note, single doses of 300 mg oral fluconazole or 400 mg oral ketoconazole followed by a workout to sweat the medication into the skin have been commonly used in the military; however, single doses are less efficacious than longer oral treatment options [231].

Ketoconazole was the first effective oral azole and has been used to treat pityriasis versicolor. Itraconazole, particularly recommended when there is resistance to topical preparations, and fluconazole [222] have been reported to be effective treatments of pityriasis versicolor. Oral terbinafine is not effective for pityriasis versicolor. The reason why there is high efficacy of topical in treating pityriasis versicolor, compared with the systemic terbinafine, is not completely understood. One possible reason might be that although topical treatment may be sufficient to kill all superficially located *Malassezia* yeasts, such treatment might result in an uneven distribution of the drug in the dermis, epidermis, sebum, stratum corneum, and deeper layers of skin such as pilosebaceous follicles [222]. If the concentrations were marginal the effectiveness would be borderline, and only the susceptible *Malassezia* strains will react to the treatment. Gupta et al. [235] have already shown that the *Malassezia* species vary in their *in vitro* susceptibility to various antifungal agents, including terbinafine. Moreover, orally administered terbinafine may not be circulated effectively to body regions with a greater number of sebaceous glands. Because these sites often have higher *Malassezia* counts, the effectiveness of the drug may be reduced [222].

Drug resistance is another recently increasing problem that affects all antifungal agents. It concerns many types of infections including PV. No sufficient data concerning resistant PV and its management is available in the literature. Detection of resistant strains is facilitated by accurate identification of the species in question.

Hypopigmentation may last weeks to months after effective treatment. This hypopigmentation may lead the patient to think treatment was ineffective; however, disappearance of the scale is evidence that the hyphal yeast has likely been eradicated. Thus, sun exposure and time are necessary for correction of pigmentation changes. Although not readily available, in those with persistent hyperpigmentation despite therapy, a 5-day twice daily application of cycloserine (an inhibitor of TAM 1 enzyme thought to be a key cause of hyperpigmentation) may be beneficial [231].

Follow-up

Pityriasis versicolor is regarded as a cosmetic disorder, as most patients are asymptomatic. The disease in often treated based on the psychosocial impact that it may have on the individual and the non-self-limiting nature of the disease.

Even though *Malassezia* yeasts causing pityriasis versicolor are susceptible to a wide variety of antifungal agents the disease often has a relapsing nature and needs to be treated frequently.

Recurrence is very common, often with a seasonal pattern. In the first year, the recurrence rate can be as high as 60%, increasing to 80% in the second year [232]. Oral itraconazole may be effective in the prophylaxis of pityriasis versicolor. Faergemann et al. [236] reported that in a 6-month study, itraconazole (400 mg) administered once monthly was effective against the recurrence of pityriasis versicolor, in comparison to placebo. Ketoconazole has also been used effectively in prophylactic regimens for pityriasis versicolor, with single monthly doses of 400 mg or 200 mg once daily for the first 3 days of each month.

It is essential that patients are educated that hypo- or hyper-pigmentation may persist for months after active infection is treated because this may lead the patient to think treatment was ineffective; however, disappearance of the scale is evidence that the hyphal yeast has likely been eradicated.

Follow-up – it is very important to inform the patient that the recurrence rate is very high. Topical and systemic treatment should be suggested to the patient as a preventive or prophylactic measure.

Things to be checked:

1. The immune system and the tendency to have PV.
2. The recurrence of PV and the importance of prophylactic treatment.

Chapter 17

Tinea Nigra Palmaris

Tinea nigra is caused by *Hortaea werneckii*, which is classified in the family Dematiaceae, class Hyphomycetes, phylum Deuteromycota, but may also be caused by other species of dematiaceous fungi such as *Stenella araguata*. The dermatomycosis tends to occur in areas with an increased concentration of eccrine sweat glands. Hyperhidrosis appears to be a risk factor for this disease. *Cladophialophora saturnica*, a new species, has been described to cause tinea nigra in an immunosuppressed patient with HIV. Overall, it is uncommon and appears as hyperpigmented macules, usually on the palms, rarely on soles, and more rarely on the body. The pigment arises from accumulation of a melanin-like substance in the fungus. It was first described in 1891 and named keratomycosis nigricans palmaris.

Tinea nigra has lipophilic adhesion to human skin. It is a superficial mycosis exclusively of the stratum corneum. It is thought that infection occurs following trauma to the affected area from a contaminated source, soil, dirt, wood, or compost, and inoculation with the pathogen. Incubation lasts 2–7 weeks. The lesion grows slowly over months and can reach a few centimeters in diameter depending on the duration. It receives nourishment from using decayed lipids and has mechanisms of adaptation to high salinity and high acidity environments. It is not uncommon in tropical regions of Central America, South America, Africa, and Asia.

It appears to be less common in the Black population, but this may reflect impaired recognition of the disease. Three times more females are affected than males. It usually infects the pediatric and adolescent populations. Patients are asymptomatic and rarely itch. The lesion is usually solitary and typically located on the palmar surface of the hands and may extend to the fingers or from the planter surface to the toes. Although tinea nigra is often easily diagnosed on clinical grounds alone, the use of dermoscopy for palmar or plantar pigmentation may enhance the recognition of tinea nigra.

A culture of skin scrapings on Sabouraud agar at 25°C yields the growth of yeast-like, shiny black mucoid colonies in approximately 1 week. In 2–3 weeks, the colonies become olivaceous brown and develop airborne mycelia.

Topical application of antifungal agents usually resolves tinea nigra within 2–4 weeks. Prolonged therapy may be necessary to prevent relapse. Repeated vigorous scrubbing or topical application of keratolytic agents can reduce pigmentation.

Differential Diagnosis of Tinea Nigra Palmaris

A. Yaws

Yaws is a tropical disease. Infection of the skin is caused by the *Treponema pallidum pertenue*; after contamination there is a subcutaneous swelling of 1–5 cm, but it could be bigger. This is followed by a rupture of the covering skin and appearance of an ulcer. The contamination is from infected person to healthy person by direct contact with the lesional area. After several months there is healing of the ulcers, which remain scars, and after several weeks, months, or even years, there is a recurrence of the disease in the joints and/or bones followed by painful sensation and new skin lesions may appear. Hyperpigmentation of the palms may be noted at the primary stage, but usually not only the palms are involved. Three stages of yaws disease are known: primary, secondary, and tertiary. Mycological analysis should be made in case of suspicion of tinea nigra palmaris.

B. Addison's Disease

Addison's disease is a rare endocrine system disorder; namely, the adrenal glands fail to produce the steroid hormones. There are several degrees of this adrenal failure, and the clinical symptoms are related to the severity of this adrenal failure. The symptoms include abdominal pain, fatigue, weakness, up to very low blood pressure and coma. There is hyperpigmentation of the sun-exposed and friction areas, around the mouth and/or oral mucosa. Regarding to tinea nigra palmaris, the pigmentation may occur also at the palms especially at the palmar areas. The pigmentation is not limited to the palms, but is also seen on other locations of the body. Clinically, the borders of the hyperpigmentation in Addison's disease in the palms are not well circumscribed as may be noted with tinea nigra palmaris. Mycological analysis will determine the diagnosis of tinea nigra palmaris.

Chapter 18

White Piedra and Black Piedra

Piedra (from Spanish, stone) is a superficial asymptomatic fungal infection of the hair shaft. It was classified in 1911 by Horta [237] into two types: black piedra, caused by *Piedraia hortae,* and white piedra. The fungi causing white piedra were originally called *Pleurococcus beigeli,* they were later referred to as *Trichosporon beigelii,* and are currently known as *Trichosporon asahii*. These include five species: *T. ovoides, T. inkin, T. mucoides,* and *T. cutaneum.* Of these, *Trichosporon asahii* has been mostly associated with white piedra, although there is some evidence to suggest T. *ovoides* is the main fungi of white piedra of the scalp.

The two types of piedra arise in diverse climatic conditions: black piedra is most common in the tropical regions, including many Central and South American countries, as well as in Southeast Asia. White piedra is more common in temperate and semitropical climates.

Furthermore, both black and white piedra affect hair in different anatomical regions. Black piedra typically infects scalp hair, while white piedra often affects pubic, axillary, and facial hair, including eyebrows and eyelashes. However, white piedra is also associated with scalp hair and in Brazil, is reported most commonly with scalp hair. White piedra, has also been observed in horses, monkeys, and dogs; while black piedra, occurs only in monkeys and humans.

Both the white and black types of piedra cause hair breakage due to the weakening of the shaft the cuticular penetration. In immunocompromised patients, dissemination of *T. asahii* may ensue, typically presenting with purpuric or necrotic cutaneous papules and nodules. Identifying the causative organism may require cultures or biopsy samples from skin lesions. . The environment (animal hair, soil, or stagnant water) and typical skin flora are the two leading sources of infectious agents causing piedra. In black piedra, *Piedraia hortae* is found in the soil; infection, however, has also been found in stagnant water and crops. In white piedra, typically *T. asahii* has been demonstrated to be present in soil, air, water, vegetable matter, or sputum. However, the kind of infection in humans is unclear. *Trichosporon* spp. has also been associated with causing of onychomycosis. In addition, *T. asahii* fungemia may be diagnosed in debilitating patients irrespective of a malignancy. This is seen primarily in neutropenic patients and, rarely, in patients with AIDS. Cutaneous disseminated papulae or purpural nodules are the mainstay of clinical presentation in these patients.

A unique and probably underreported variation of a mixed black and white piedra has been reported. It is typically restricted to the scalp hair of young Muslim women who cover their hair with a scarf (hijab).

In many patients Piedra may be asymptomatic. The minute nodules in hair shaft may go undetected by many patients. . White piedra is marked by irregular, white, cream-colored, or brown soft nodules or gelatinous sheaths whicb are easily detached from the hair shaft. White piedra may accompany a synergistic coryneform bacterial infection. Rarely, *Trichosporon* spp. may be accompanied by *Candida parapsilosis* along hair shafts, although it is unclear if this is truly a co-infection.

Black piedra may present as firmly attached, hard, dark nodules of a few millimeters in diameter. The fungus grows into the hair shaft, possibly leading to hair breakage as a result of the structural instability.

Hair breakage occurs in both forms of piedra; the surrounding skin is healthy.

Differential Diagnosis of White and Black Piedra

A. Trichomycosis Axillaris

Trichomycosis axillaris is a bacterial disease, although the name trichomycosis is "mycologic". Trichomycosis axillaris is a superficial bacterial disease caused by *Corynebacterium* spp. – mostly *Corynebacterium tenuis*. Large numbers of these bacteria are located around the hair shafts that are located at rich sweat gland areas such as the axillary areas.

Clinically, there is a small mass of sticky material (the *Corynebacterium* bacteria and the debris of hair keratin) that covers the circumference of the hair shaft. The location of trichomycosis axillaris differs from that of white and black piedra. The clinical appearance is also different; while in white and black piedra alike, the hair shaft is covered segmentally by an appearance of a dense and well-circumscribed mass around the hair shaft, in Trichomycosis axillaris, the bacteria cover almost the whole length of the hair shaft and no clinical well-circumscribed borders may be noted.

B. Monilethrix

Monilethrix is an abnormality in the hair shaft, having a periodic narrowing along the hair shaft. Besides this unique abnormality of the hair shafts, there is appearance of hypotrichosis in the scalp (sparse hair growth).

Monilethrix is caused by several gene mutations and there are many patterns of inheritance.

Under certain circumstances it may resemble white/black piedra. In white piedra there is no change in the morphology of the hair shaft itself, but there is addition of mass that periodically covers the hair shaft (may look like a pediculosis capitis).

Close inspection will show that there is no change in the hair shaft itself. Mycological analysis will diagnose the white/black piedra.

C. Trichorrhexis Nodosa

Trichorrhexis nodosa is a deformation of the hair shaft that presents as a thickening of one or several points along the hair shaft. These thickened areas are weak and tend to break easily, which leads to hair loss and damages the appearance of the hair. This unique hair defect is caused by a combination of a genetic tendency combined with environmental factors, such as warm drying and massive brushing, and overuse of different chemicals/creams/solutions on the scalp hairs. Close inspection using a microscope will show the broken hairs, while in white and black piedra there is mass of material that covers the hair shafts segmentally.

Mycological analysis will help to distinguish between Trichorexis nodosa and white and black piedra.

Culturing

Place hair in 10–15% potassium hydroxide preparation on a glass slide. If the nodule is from black piedra, tightly packed and pigmented hyphae and ascospores are seen attached to the hair shaft. If the nodule is from white piedra, darkly stained and lightly arranged hyphae, blastoconidia, and arthroconidia are seen attached to the hair shaft.

Piedraia hortae, the cause of black piedra, grows slowly on Sabouraud dextrose agar and is not inhibited by cycloheximide. Microscopic examination reveals septate hyphae, chlamydospores, and irregularly shaped hyphal elements. These cultures are of the asexual phase of the fungus. Organisms in the sexual phase are difficult to grow in culture. *Trichosporon asahii,* the typical cause of white piedra, rarely grows on Sabouraud dextrose agar because of inhibition by cycloheximide, which is present in dermatophyte test medium and in Mycosel and mycobiotic agars. In addition, *Trichosporon* spp. grow best at 28–30°C.

Mycological culture on Mycosel plus molecular identification may be used to confirm the diagnosis.

Treatment

Spontaneous remissions occurs often. However, in the absence of such a remission, treatment is necessary in the form of shaving or cutting the hair. This is curative and usually no follow-up is required as recurrences are rare. Black piedra is treated by using oral terbinafine. White piedra can be treated with topical antifungals, including imidazoles, ciclopirox olamine, 2% selenium sulfide, 6% precipitated sulfur in petroleum, chlorhexidine solution, Castellani Paint, zinc pyrithione, and amphotericin B lotion.

Treatment of white piedra may pose a therapeutic challenge. The agent may withstand several topical and systemic antifungal treatments. However, a combination of oral azole antifungals and shampoos have been shown to be effective in certain cases, and should therefore be tried in an attempt to obviate the need for shaving the scalp . Should these topical remedies fail, oral itraconazole may serve as a good choice for the treatment of uncomplicated white piedra affecting the scalp hair. Disseminated trichosporosis may prove difficult to treat, yet itraconazole is often tried. Itraconazole with caspofungin provides enhanced antifungal activity against *T. asahii*.

Chapter 19

Cutaneous Candidiasis

Candida spp. are universal fungi representing the most prevalent fungal pathogens affecting man. Candidiasis is contracted by contamination with a certain species of the genus *Candida.* The occurance of local and systemic disease caused by *Candida* spp. is increasing, and the expression is primarily dependant on the immune condition of the host. *Candida* spp. produce a broad spectrum of diseases, ranging from superficial mucocutaneous disease to invasive illnesses. *Candida* spp. are true opportunistic pathogens that achieve penetrate the circulation and deep tissues as a result of newly developed technological advances in chemotherapy, organ transplantation, and by means of contamination of instruments. Critically ill patients in medical and surgical ICUs, neonatal, and pediatric patients are at higher risk for opportunistic nosocomial fungal infections, primarily with *Candida* spp.

Candida spp. are yeast-like fungi forming true hyphae and pseudohyphae. They are usually confined to human and animal reservoirs but are not found in the hospital environment, including foods, countertops, air-conditioning vents, floors, respirators, and on medical personnel. *Candida* spp. are the leading cause of fungal infection in immunocompromised individuals, with oropharyngeal colonization found in 30–55% of healthy young adults and in 40–65% of normal fecal flora.

Well-recognized but poorly characterized virulence factors that contribute to the infectious capability of *Candida* spp. include predominantly surface molecules promoting adherence to other structures, acid proteases and phospholipases that facilitate penetration of and damage to cell envelopes, and the ability to convert to a hyphal form. The host defense systems also play an important role in the development of *Candida* infections. Host defense mechanisms include intact mucocutaneous barriers, satisfactory number of polymorphonuclear cells, adequate complement level, immunoglobulins, cell-mediated immunity, and mucocutaneous protective bacterial flora.

Over 200 species of *Candida* exist; to date, only a few have been associated with human disease. Clinically significant *Candida* species include the following:

C. albicans–the most common species identified (50–60%)
C. glabrata (15–20%)
C. parapsilosis (10–20%)
C. tropicalis (6–12%)
C. krusei (1–3%)

C. kefyr (<5%)
C. guillermondi (<5%)
C. lusitaniae (<5%)
Candida dubliniensis was first found in patients with HIV infections.

Cutaneous Candidiasis Syndromes

Oral candidiasis

Many systemic diseases and treatment for numerous conditions can predispose the individual to *Candida* infections. Oral candidiasis is the most common mucocutaneous mycosis of the oral cavity. *Candida* spp. are a common commensal organism, found in the oral cavity of 53% of the general population. One hundred and fifty species of this genus have been isolated in the oral cavity, and 80% of these correspond to *Candida albicans*, which may colonize the cavity alone or in combination with other species, particularly *Candida glabrata* or *Candida tropicalis* (observed in 7% of all healthy people and in 80% of all patients with candidiasis). Recently, *Candida dubliniensis* was isolated in patients infected with HIV. This species is also significant since it is associated with very severe mucositis candidiasis of the oral cavity, esophagus, and other locations, and because it is resistant to antifungal treatment.

The pathogenesis of candidiasis involves three factors: host, fungus, and oral microenvironment-modifying factors. Host predisposing factors include endocrine defects (e.g., diabetes mellitus, pregnancy, renal failure, and hyperthyroidism), immune depression (normally associated with antineoplastic treatments or immunosuppression in transplant patients, as well as agammaglobulinemia or cellular immune defects), HIV-AIDS, or hematological and immune disorders such as agranulocytosis (neutropenia). Additional predisposing conditions are malignant diseases including leukemias or lymphomas, aplastic anemia, drug treatments (long-term administration of broad spectrum antibiotics, antineoplastic drugs, corticosteroids, immunosuppressants and antidepressants), hyposialie (occuring in disorders such as Sjögren's disease, drugs, or radiotherapy), and terminal or end-stage systemic diseases. Oral microenvironment-modifying factors include dental erosion/loss of teeth, poorly fitting dentures, chronic antiseptic use, prolonged use of pacifiers by children, poor oral hygiene,smoking and alcoholism.

In addition, neonates are colonized during passage through the birth canal. Hence, the risk for thrush increases when the mother has an active vaginal yeast infection. Other sources of transmission to neonates include colonized mammary glands (for breastfed infants), improperly cleaned hands, nipples, and bottles. Kissing has also been implicated. Overgrowth of yeast on the oral mucosa leads to epithelial desquamation and accumulation of bacteria, keratin, and necrotic tissue. This necrotic tissue becomes a pseudomembranous-like tissue that attaches to the mucosa. This membrane is typically spared involvement of extensive areas of edema, ulceration, and necrosis of the underlying mucosa.

C. albicans frequently and asymptomatically inhabits the GI tract of many children and adults, and has been implicated as a reservoir for yeast contamination of the perineum. Therefore, thrush usually occurs simultaneously with candidiasis. Thrush is usually a mild and self-limiting illness, although it may cause discomfort sufficient to disrupt feeding in a newborn. When thrush occurs after early infancy or without a reasonable explanation the possibility of an underlying immunodeficiency must be considered. More than 90% of people infected with HIV who are not receiving highly active anti-retroviral therapy (HAART) eventually develop oropharyngeal candidiasis (OPC), while 10% eventually develop at least one episode of esophageal candidiasis.

Candidal infection may range from mild superficial mucosal involvement to severe disseminated forms. Axéll classification (1997) [238] divides oral candidiasis into two major categories:1) primary oral candidiasis and 2) secondary oral candidiasis. The primary oral candidiasis includes acute forms (pseudomembranous or erythematous) and chronic forms (hyperplastic nodular and plaque-like or pseudomembranous or erythematous). Secondary candidiasis includes all the oral manifestations of systemic mucocutaneous candidiasis as a result of the diseases mentioned above.

Primary Oral Candidiasis – The Acute Forms

Pseudomembranous candidiasis

One of the most common forms, it may occur at any age but especially in chronically ill patients or infants. The oral lesions are characterized by the appearance of soft, white, slightly elevated plaques most frequently on the buccal mucosa and tongue but can also be seen on palate, gingiva, and floor of the mouth. The white plaque can usually be wiped away with gauze, leaving a rather normal or erythematous mucosa (Figure 19.1).

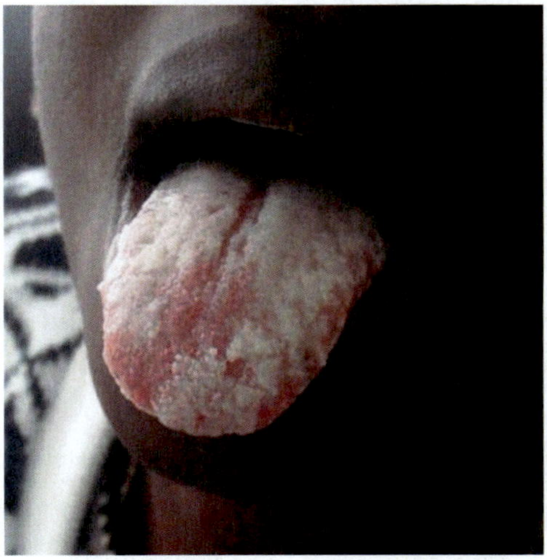

Figure 19.1. Pseudomembranous Candidiasis.

Erythematous candidiasis (also known as antibiotic sore mouth)

It usually occurs as a sequela of a course of broad spectrum antibiotics, steroids, or disease that suppresses immunity, commonly HIV. The lesion appears erythematous with diffuse borders due to increased vascularity. This is the only form of oral candidiasis that is painful. At the dorsal aspect of the tongue, central papillary atrophy may be seen that presents as asymptomatic symmetric erythematous lesions. It is erythematous due to loss of filiform papillae and related to smoking and candida (Figure 19.2).

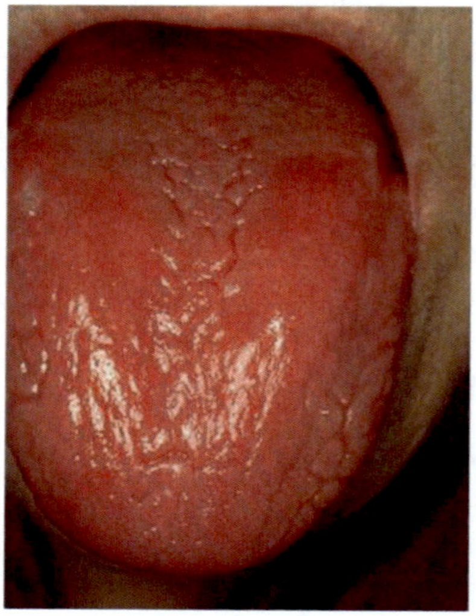

Figure 19.2. Erythematous Candidasis.

Primary Oral Candidiasis – The Chronic Forms

Chronic hyperplastic candidiasis – (also known as leukoplakia type of candidiasis)

The lesions are firm, white persistent plaques usually on lips, tongue, and cheeks. The lesions may be homogenous or nodular and persist for years. There is a correlation between the presence of *Candida* in the lesions and premalignant potential with epithelial atypia, as in leukoplakia. Some cases are correlated with iron and folate deficiency and defective cell-mediated immunity (Figure 19.3).

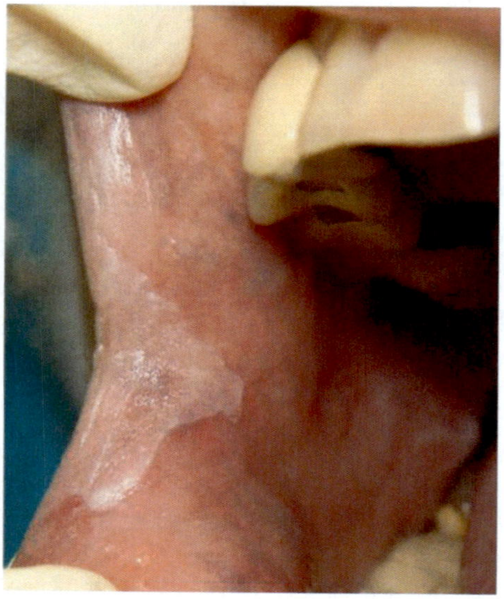

Figure 19.3. Chronic Hyperplastic Candidiasis.

Candida-Associated Lesions

Denture stomatitis – (chronic atrophic candidiasis)

This is a diffuse erythema and edema of the denture-bearing area often occurring with angular cheilitis. It is usually asymptomatic except for soreness. Mandibular mucosa is rarely affected. Some studies have found that women are more affected than men. Usually dentures are the situation predisposing to the *Candida* infection (Figure 19.4).

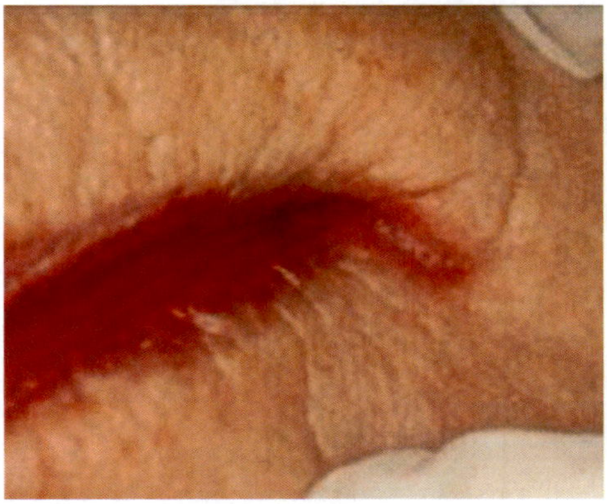

Figure 19.4. Denture Stomatitis.

Leukoplakia, lichen planus, and lupus are keratotic lesions that may be superimposed by *Candida* and appear similar to chronic hyperplastic candidiasis clinically, but they will not regress after antifungal treatment.

Secondary oral candidiasis

This is a group of different forms of infection that have many things in common. In general, there is chronic *Candida* involvement of the skin, scalp, nails, and mucous membranes. As a group, the patients have an impairment of the immune system.

Id reaction as a hypersensitivity reaction to the Candida antigen can manifest as a vesicular and papular rash on the skin of patients with chronic candidiasis.

Any form of oral candidiasis is diagnosed based on the clinical recognition of the lesions. These can be confirmed by the identification of *Candida* from oral samples by microscopy and/or isolation in culture, among other methods. In the case of *Candida*, its detection in the oral cavity is not pathognomonic of infection since it is a common commensal organism in this location. A definitive diagnosis of candidiasis requires the confirmation of tissue invasion by *Candida*. For this reason, a negative culture result is of greater use in discarding candidiasis a putative diagnosis of infection than a positive culture result is in confirming one. Thus, in the absence of clinical manifestations of oral candidiasis, a positive culture result for *Candida* is not sufficient to conclude that the patient has oral candidiasis. The most frequently used methods for diagnosing primary candidiasis include stains (i.e., 10% KOH), smears, and cultures (Sabouraud dextrose agar). In determining the species of *Candida*, CHROMagar Candida® and Candida ID® offer both sensitivity and specificity, in addition to being accessible and simple to use for identifying *Candida* spp. When diagnosing invasive candidiasis, and in cases where *C. albicans* must be distinguished from *C. dubliniensis*, ELISA or PCR have been preferred. A new method known as CHROMagar-PAL® has recently been proposed, combining CHROMagar Candida® and Pal agar. It provides simple and rapid differentiation of *C. albicans* and *C. dubliniensis*, even in mixed cultures. Multiplex PCR is also popular because it directly identifies yeasts in samples without the need for nucleic acid extraction – thereby eliminating time lost culturing the samples and (somewhat) reducing the costs.

Generalized cutaneous candidiasis

This is an unusual form of cutaneous candidiasis that manifests as a diffuse eruption over the trunk, thorax, and extremities, but mainly at skin folds found in the groin and peri-anal areas. Physical examination reveals a widespread rash that begins as individual vesicles and than spreads into large confluent areas.

Intertrigo

This affects skin surfaces that are in close proximity, providing a moist, warm environment that comes to be marked by a pruritic red rash. Physical examination reveals a rash that begins with vesiculopustules, then spreading and eventually rupturing, causing maceration and fissuring. The area involved has a characteristic scalloped border with a white rim consisting of necrotic epidermis surrounding the erythematous macerated base. Often, satellite lesions appear and may coalesce and extend into larger lesions. Erosio interdigitalis blastomycetica is essentially *Candida* that has infected the finger or toe webs that are subject to constant friction and occlusion that promotes sweating. On the hands, the third web space is the most common area affected, and on the feet, the fourth webspace is most common. Patients most commonly affected are those with diabetes and those whose hands and feet that are frequently immersed in wet environments (Figure 19.5).

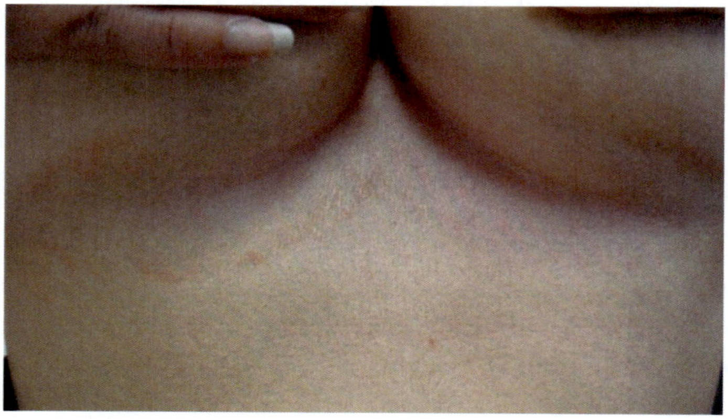

Figure 19.5. Intertrigo mechanic.

Candida folliculitis

Is an infection predominantly found in facial hair follicles of the beard and moustache of men which can (albeit rarely) become extensive. The reported causes of Candida folliculitis in immunocompetent individuals include the use of antibiotics and steroids, IV drug abuse, obesity, hypothyroidism, diabetes, and oral contraceptive use. *C. albicans* has also been reported to cause folliculitis barbae. In general, in addition to the above mentioned predisposing factors for *Candida* infections, *Candida* colonization of the mouth, or the mouth of the partner, and an infected razor have been suggested for the development of Candida folliculitis. There are reports of Candida folliculitis occurring in patients with hypothyroidism, agranulocytosis, malignant tumors, and immunodeficiency syndromes.

Candida species are thought to be a rare cause of a folliculitis outbreak. Elucidating pathogenesis of cutaneous candidiasis in immunocompetent patients is essential due to its role as a normal commensal organism in the human body. It is thought that *C. albicans'* pathogenic effect is directly related to cell adherence. *In vitro*, the organism is found to actively adhere to stratum corneum corneocytes. It has also been found that cell populations of patients treated with antibiotics and/or steroids exhibited twice the ability to bind *Candida* in comparison to healthy control populations. High temperatures, particularly 37°C, favor rapid pseudohyphal growth, especially in intrafollicular areas. The differential diagnosis for these cases includes malassezia folliculitis, steroid-induced acne, acne vulgaris, bacterial folliculitis, Majocchi's granuloma (dermatophyte infection of follicles), and tinea corporis, most of which can be ruled out after KOH wet preparation examination and skin biopsy.

Paronychia and onychomycosis

Paronychia and onychomycosis are associated with frequent immersion of the hands in water and with diabetes mellitus. The patient will have a history of a painful and erythematous area around and beneath the nail and nail bed. Physical examination reveals inflammation that becomes warm, glistening, tense, and erythematous, and may extend under the nail. This is associated with secondary nail thickening, ridging, discoloration, and, occasionally, with nail loss. Further details are found in Chapter 15. Long standing paronychia leads to chronic paronychia (Figure 19.6).

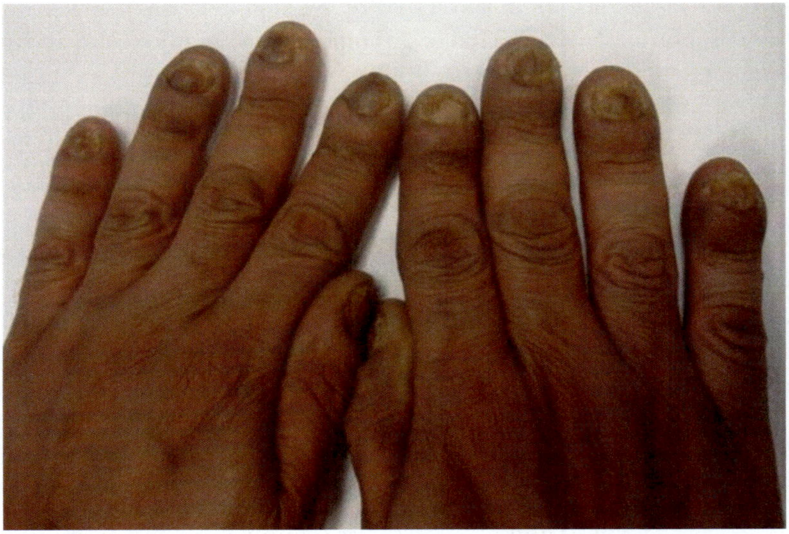

Figure 19.6. Chronic Paronychia.

Chronic mucocutaneous candidiasis

Is a *Candida* infection of different locations on the skin including the hair, nails, and mucous membranes, which tends to persist for a long period of time. History: Most infections begin in infancy or during the first two decades of life with rare onset in people older than 30 years. Patients typically survive for prolonged periods and rarely experience disseminated fungal infections. The most common cause of death is bacterial sepsis. This type of candidiasis is frequently associated with endocrinopathies, e.g., hypoparathyroidism; Addison's disease; hypothyroidism; diabetes mellitus; autoimmune antibodies to thyroid, adrenal, gastric tissues (approximately 50%) and melanin-producing cells; thymomas; dental dysplasia and polyglandular autoimmune disease. Physical examination reveals disfiguring lesions of the scalp, face, hands, and nails. It is also occasionally associated with oral thrush and vitiligo.

Gastrointestinal tract candidiasis

Oropharyngeal candidiasis

These patients often present with a history of HIV infection, diabetes mellitus, exposure to broad-spectrum antibiotics or inhaled steroids. They typically wear dentures. Some may complain of sores and painful, burning mouth or tongue, dysphagia, and have whitish thick patches on the oral mucosa. The clinical presentation of the oropharynx will show diffuse erythrasma covered by whitish-yellowish fine plaques around the oropharynx such as the tongue, gums, and oral mucosa. There are five types of oropharyngeal candidiasis (OPC): Membranous candidiasis: Among the most common types, characterized by creamy-white curd like patches on the mucosal surfaces. Erythematous candidiasis: This is associated with an erythematous patch on both hard and soft palates. Chronic atrophic candidiasis (denture stomatitis): This is also thought to be among the most common forms of the disease. Presenting signs and symptoms include chronic erythema, and edema of the portion of the palate in contact with dentures. Angular cheilitis: An inflammatory reaction, this type is characterized by soreness, erythema, and fissuring at the corners of the mouth. Angular cheilitis is usually due to *Candida* infection that is located at the lateral sides of the mouth. Clinically there are erythematous cracks covered by thin whitish plaques. Soreness and uncomfortable sensation may occur. Mixed: A combination of any of the above mentioned types is possible. Esophageal candidiasis: The patient's medical history usually includes chemotherapy, use of broad-spectrum antibiotics or inhaled steroids, HIV infection, hematologic or solid-organ malignancy. Patients may be asymptomatic or may display one or more of the following symptoms: normal oral mucosa (>50% of patients), dysphagia, odynophagia, retrosternal pain, epigastric pain, nausea, and vomiting. Physical examination almost always reveals oral candidiasis. Non-esophageal gastrointestinal candidiasis: The patient usually has a history of neoplastic disease of the GI tract, particularly of the esophagus or the stomach. Less commonly, chronic gastric ulcerations, gastric perforations, or malignant gastric ulcers occur with concomitant candidal infection. The small and large bowel are the third most common sites of infection (20%). Approximately 15% of patients develop systemic candidiasis. Findings on physical examination differ according to the site of infection. However, because approximately 20–25% of the total population is colonized with *Candida,* the diagnosis must rely on more than just positive culture results. Typical symptoms may include: epigastric pain, nausea and vomiting, abdominal pain, fever and chills, and abdominal mass (in some cases). Endoscopy with or without biopsy is necessary to confirm the diagnosis.

Candida keratitis

Fungal infections of the cornea (mycotic or fungal keratitis, keratomycosis) present as suppurative, usually ulcerative lesions. Mycotic keratitis has been reported in many different parts of the world, particularly tropical areas. In keratitis due to *Candida albicans* and related fungi, there is usually some pre-existing ocular (e.g., insufficient tear secretion, defective eyelid closure) or systemic (e.g., diabetes mellitus, immunosuppression) condition; this type of keratitis may also supervene on a pre-existing epithelial defect because of herpes keratitis or abrasions caused by contaminated contact lenses.

Genitourinary tract candidiasis

Vulvovaginal candidiasis (VVC)

Is the second most common cause of vaginitis. Three of every four women experience at least one bout of vulvovaginal candidiasis during their lifetime. A typical patient's history includes vulvar pruritus, vaginal discharge, dysuria, and dyspareunia. About 10% of women without precipitating risk factors experience repeated episodes of VVC. Physical examination typically reveals a vagina and labia that are erythematous with a thick curd-like discharge, and a normal cervix upon speculum examination.

Candida balanitis

Male patients report pruritus along with whitish patches on the penis. Candida balanitis is acquired through direct sexual contact with a partner with VVC. Physical examination reveals vesicles on the surface of the penis that later develop into patches with a whitish exudate. The rash occasionally spreads to the thighs, gluteal folds, buttocks, and scrotum. Dry, red, superficially scaly, pruritic macules and patches on the penis are seen.

Diagnosis

Species identification – *C. albicans*, *C. dubliniensis*, and *Candida stellatoidea* can be identified morphologically via germ-tube formation (hyphae are produced from yeast cells after 2–3 h of incubation) or biochemical assays.

CHROMagar Candida allows for the presumptive identification of several *Candida* spp. using color reactions in specialized media that identifies colonies based on colors typical for various species of *Candida*. Biochemical essays using API20C and API32C may identify the *Candida* spp. with much greater accuracy. These assays evaluate the assimilation of numerous carbon substrates and generate profiles used in the identification of different fungal species.

A newer version of this test now allows for the simultaneous identification of either *C. albicans* or *C. glabrata*. Nonculture *Candida* detection assays – The Candida mannan assay has a sensitivity of 31–90% (less for non-albicans *Candida* spp.). The Candida heat labile antigen assay has a sensitivity of 10–71%. The D-arabinitol assay has a sensitivity of 50%, but is not useful for infection with *C. krusei* or *C. glabrata*. The enolase assay has a sensitivity of 55–75%, which improves with serial testing. The (1,3) β-D-glucan assay is an amebocytelysate assay with a sensitivity of 75–100% and a specificity of 88–100%. It is a broad-spectrum assay that detects *Aspergillus*, *Candida*, *Fusarium*, *Acremonium*, and *Saccharomyces*. β-D-glucan is a cell wall component in a wide variety of fungi and can be detected based on its ability to activate factor G of the horseshoe crab coagulation cascade. The Fungitell assay may be used in the evaluation of invasive fungal infections caused by the fungi mentioned above. *Cryptococcus neoformans* and Zygomycetes cannot be detected using this method. Novel, molecular assays are still in the early investigational phases, but appear promising. A new, rapid test for *Candida* infections of the bloodstream may reduce patient mortality from 40% to 11% by reducing the time for accurate identification and diagnosis of candidemia by 25 times compared to blood cultures. Called T2Candida, the new test employs PCR on blood samples, and then hybridizing the amplified *Candida* DNA to superparamagnetic nanoparticles coated with complementary DNA. The nanoparticles aggregate into "microclusters" that significantly alter the T2 magnetic resonance (T2MR) signal.

Ultrasonography may be useful for diagnosing *Candida*-related hepatosplenic abscesses. The classic bull's eye or target lesions are readily observed in the liver and spleen using this approach. CT scanning with contrast enhancement may prove efficacious for diagnosing hepatosplenic candidiasis, intra-abdominal abscess or peritonitis, renal abscess, and pyelonephritis. Echocardiography may be beneficial in confirming or excluding diagnosis of Candida endocarditis. This would be highly significant because fungal endocarditis is frequently associated with large vegetations that are readily observed on standard echocardiograms. Tissue biopsy of the involved areas is frequently helpful in establishing the presence of *Candida* infection. In this regard, bronchoscopy with bronchoalveolar lavage and transbronchial biopsy provides sufficient tissue for analysis and diagnosis of pulmonary candidiasis. For suspected infections of the esophagus and stomach, endoscopy provides direct examination.

Tissues "fixed" with chemical preservatives can be stained with hematoxylin and eosin. In addition, fungal hyphae may be demonstrated with Grocott methenamine silver, methylene blue, or periodic acid-Schiff reagent. *Candida* spp. may differ morphologically such that their yeast may be ovoid or round in shape, with hyphae or pseudohyphae.

Treatments for *Candida* infections may vary substantially based on the anatomic location of the infection, the underlying disease, and the immune status of the patients, risk factors for infection, the specific species of *Candida* involved, and, in some cases, the susceptibility of the *Candida* species to specific antifungal drugs. In the last few years, several significant chmodifications in the treatment of candidiasis have occurred. For example, use of the echinocandins caspofungin, micafungin, and anidulafungin, along with voriconazole and posaconazole expanded-spectrum azoles, as well as lipid formulations of amphotericin B in various forms of invasive candidiasis, and mucosal candidiasis.

Most localized cutaneous candidiasis infections are well treated with any topical antifungal agent (e.g., clotrimazole, econazole, ciclopirox, miconazole, ketoconazole, and nystatin). If the infective agent is a paronychia, drainage of the abscess is critical, followed by oral antifungal therapy with either fluconazole or itraconazole. Systemic antifungal therapy is prescribed for extensive cutaneous infections, infections in immunocompromised patients, folliculitis, or onychomycosis,. Infections in HIV-positive patients are generally slower to respond, and in approximately 60% of patients, recur within six months of the initial episode.

In such situations, in addition to correcting the immune dysfunction with HAART, higher doses of fluconazole (up to 800 mg/d) or itraconazole (up to 600 mg/d) may be useful. Posaconazole suspension at 400 mg orally, twice per day, has also been demonstrated to yield excellent results in these patients. Caspofungin 50 mg/d IV and anidulafungin 100 mg/d IV have also proved effective. Treatment with amphotericin B is rarely necessary, but, when used, low doses (0.3–0.7 mg/kg) have proven effective.

Chapter 20

Erythrasma

Erythrasma is a chronic superficial infection of the skin caused by *Corynebacterium minutissimum*, a Gram-positive, non-spore-forming bacillus that usually presents as normal human skin flora. *Corynebacteria* invade the upper third of the stratum corneum. These organisms proliferate under conditions such as heat and humidity. The organisms are seen in the intercellular spaces as well as within cells, dissolving keratin fibrils. The coral-red fluorescence of scales seen under Wood's lamp is secondary to the production of porphyrin by these diphtheroids.

Epidemiology

This infection is observed all over the world. The incidence of erythrasma is reported to be around 4% and is higher in darker phenotype individuals. Both sexes are equally affected; however, the crural form of erythrasma is more common in men. The incidence increases with age, but no age group is immune to the disease. Infection commonly involves the interdigital areas of the toe webs, followed by the groin and axilla. The submammary area, periumbilical region, and intergluteal folds are less commonly involved in erythrasma. Toe web lesions appear as maceration, with the fourth interdigital space most frequently affected.

Predisposing factors

For erythrasma include: excessive sweating/hyperhidrosis, gentle cutaneous barrier, obesity, diabetes mellitus, warm environment, poor hygiene, advanced age, and immunocompromised states. The widespread form is most commonly found in immunocompromised individuals. In such individuals, *C. minutissimum* has caused infections other than erythrasma, including abscess, intravascular catheter-related infections, primary bacteremia, peritoneal catheter-related infections, endocarditis, pyelonephritis, cellulitis, endophthalmitis, arteriovenous fistula infection, cutaneous granuloma, and meningitis.

Clinical picture

The typical appearance of erythrasma is well-demarcated, brown-red macular patches. The skin has a wrinkled appearance with fine scales. Dark discoloration associated with erythrasma is usually limited to body folds that are naturally moist and occluded. Infection commonly is asymptomatic, but it can be pruritic. Widespread involvement of trunk and limbs is possible. The duration of erythrasma ranges from months to years. Diabetes should be suspected in recurrent erythrasma. Due to the association of erythrasma with other corynebacterial skin infections such as pitted keratolysis and trichomycosis axillaris, all body folds and feet should be thoroughly examined.

Interdigital

Erythrasma is the most common cause of interdigital bacterial infections on the feet. This variant of erythrasma commonly presents as scaling and chronic maceration of the web spaces. The web space between the fourth and fifth toes is frequently affected. Interdigital erythrasma may be asymptomatic or pruritic.

Interdigital erythrasma may occur with concomitant dermatophyte or candidal infection.

Intertriginous

Intertriginous erythrasma presents with well-defined, erythematous patches or thin plaques in the axillae, inframammary region, umbilicus, or groin. With time, lesion color often changes to brown. Involved areas often have easily visible fine scales and wrinkling that may give the skin a "cigarette paper" appearance. Affected areas are asymptomatic or mildly pruritic.

Disciform

A rare disciform variant of erythrasma has been reported, consisting of generalized, round plaques not confined to intertriginous areas. Disciform erythrasma has been reported to occur more frequently in black females living in tropical climates.

Genital/perianal

Erythrasma has been implicated as an often overlooked cause of chronic pruritus ani. Rarely, erythrasma may also affect the vulva, causing chronic pruritus that may be misdiagnosed as a candidal infection.

Differential Diagnosis

- Intertrigo
- ACD
- ICD
- Psoriasis
- Seborrheic dermatitis
- Tinea cruris
- Tinea pedis
- Pityriasis versicolor
- Melasma

Diagnostic procedures

Wood's lamp examination of erythrasma lesions reveals characteristic coral-red fluorescence of lesions attributed to excess coproporphyrin III synthesis by these organisms, which accumulates in cutaneous tissue and emits the coral-red fluorescence. Results may be negative if the patient bathed prior to presentation. On diagnosis uncertainty, cutaneous biopsy can reveal the *Corynebacterium* in the horny layers of the skin.

Gram staining discloses Gram-positive filamentous rods in culture media.

Treatment

Erythrasma responds to a variety of topical and oral therapies, although recurrences are common. A number of topical and oral antimicrobial agents are recommended but evidence supporting or comparing treatment efficacy is limited. Thus, factors considered during selection of therapy include the extent of disease, the patient's ability to use and tolerate a specific therapy, and drug cost or availability. Because culture and antibiogram are not performed routinely in daily clinical practice, the recommended initial topical treatment is fusidic acid cream. If this drug is not available, then topical erythromycin solution may be an alternative. *C. minutissimum* is generally susceptible to penicillins, first-generation cephalosporins, erythromycin, clindamycin, ciprofloxacin, tetracycline, and vancomycin. However, multiresistant strains have been isolated.

In general, for patients with widespread disease, a systemic therapy with an oral antibiotic such as clarithromycin or erythromycin is warranted. For patients with localized disease, topical therapy with clindamycin, an azole antifungal, or benzoyl peroxide is usually satisfactory. Because topical azole antifungals can be effective for the treatment of both erythrasma and tinea, these drugs are considered an initial therapeutic choice in cases in which it is not possible to distinguish between the two conditions.

Photodynamic therapy (PDT) has been reported as a potential treatment for erythrasma. This technique takes advantage of the natural porphyrins produced by *C. minutissimum*. Using a red light emitting PDT device with a peak of 635 nm, patients were reported to have a reduction in size of their erythrasma lesions, but less than 25% of the treated patients had complete clearance.

In cases of topical treatment failure, erythromycin, single-dose clarithromycin, or amoxicillin–clavulanate should be chosen for the systemic treatment.

Follow up

The prognosis for erythrasma is excellent, but the condition tends to recur if the predisposing factors are not eradicated.

Complications are rare and include fatal septicemia in immunocompromised patients, infective endocarditis in valvular heart disease patients, and postsurgical wound infection.

Chapter 21

Conclusion

The authors wrote this comprehensive book with respect to the relevant differential diagnosis of each subtype in each chapter and broadly discussed the clinical presentations of mycotic disease compared to its relevant differential diagnosis. Concentrating on the specific differential diagnosis combined with the correct interpretation of the mycological analysis results provides insight for distinguishing other skin diseases from mycotic disease and, as a result, the precise treatment. This book clearly explains the common antimycotic drugs worldwide and their combinations with many other drugs and the alternative possibilities of these drugs' interactions. This book presents many high quality clinical pictures that clearly demonstrate the difference between mycotic disease and its relevant/resembling other skin diseases. This book is suitable not only for dermatologists but also for general physicians, medical students, mycological laboratory staff, and interested others.

Appendix: Drug Interactions

	griseofulvin	ketoconazole	terbinafine	itraconazole	fluconazole	voriconazole	posaconazole	amphothericin B-Fungizone	caspofungin
Neurodegenerative diseases									
interferon beta -1a	no	no	no	no	no	no	no	no	no
rasagiline	no	no	no	no	no	no	no	no	no
cabergolin	no	no	no	no	no	no	no	no	no
entacapone	no	no	no	no	no	no	no	no	no
glatiramer acetate	no	no	no	no	no	no	no	no	no
propranolol HCl	no	no	no	no	no	no	no	no	no
carbidopa & levodopa	no	no	no	no	no	no	no	no	no
fingolimod HCl	no	f+++	no	no	no	no	no	no	no
trihexyphenidyl HCl	no	no	no	no	no	no	no	no	no
riluzole	no	no	no	no	no	no	no	no	no
CNS stimulants									
adrenalin (as acid tartrate)	no	C/I (QT inc)	no	C/I (QT inc)	C/I (QT inc)	partial C/I (QT inc)	partial C/I (QT inc)	no	no
rasagiline	no	no	no	no	no	no	no	no	no
methylphenidate HCl	no	no	no	no	no	no	no	no	no
modafinil HCl	no	k--	no	It--	no	v+	no	no	no
Anti-vertigo preparations									
Cinnarizine	no	no	no	no	no	no	no	no	no
Alzheimer's disease									
doepezil HCl	don-	don++	no	don++	don+	don+	don+	no	no
memantine HCl	no	no	no	no	no	no	no	no	no
Anti-emetics; Anti-naeuseants									
aprepitant	a--	a++/k+	no	a++/it+	a++	a++	a++	no	no
granisetron	no	no	no	no	no	no	no	no	no
haloperidol	no	C/I (QT Incre)	no	C/I (QT Incre)	C/I (QT Incre)	C/I (QT Incre)	C/I (QT Incre)	no	no
palonosetron HCl	no	no	no	no	no	no	no	no	no
dimenhydrinate	no	no	no	no	no	no	no	no	no
Glaucoma									
Cinnarizine	no	no	no	no	no	no	no	no	no

	griseofulvin	ketoconazole	terbinafine	itraconazole	fluconazole	voriconazole	posaconazole	amphothericin B-Fungizone	caspofungin
Anti-depressants									
clomipramine HCl	c-	C/I (QT inc) clo+	no	C/I (QT inc) clo++	C/I (QT inc) clo+ itr +	QT inc clo+	QT inc	no	no
Mianserin	no	C/I (QT inc)	no		C/I (QT inc)	QT inc	QT inc	no	no
Escitalopram	no	no	no	C/I (QT inc)	esc++	esc++	no	no	no
citalopram hydrobrom	no	cit ++	no	cit ++	cit ++	cit ++	cit ++	no	no
duloxetine HCl	no	no	no	no	no	no	no	no	no
desipramine HCl	des -	C/I (QT inc) des+	no	C/I (QT inc) des+	C/I (QT inc) des++	QT inc des+	QT inc des+	no	no
venlafaxine	no	QT inc	no	QT inc	QT inc	QT inc	QT inc	no	no
amitriptyline	am-	C/I (QT inc) ami++	no	C/I (QT inc) ami++	QT inc ami++	C/I (QT inc) ami++	C/I (QT inc) ami+	no	no
fluvoxamine	no	QT inc ket+	no	QT inc itr+	QT inc	QT inc V++	QT inc	no	no
doxepin (as HCl)	no	C/I (QT inc)	no	C/I (QT inc)	QT inc	C/I (QT inc)	QT inc	no	no
milnacipran	no	no	no	no	no	C/I (QT inc)	no	no	no
lamotrigine	no	no	no	no	no	no	no	no	no
sertaline HCl-Zoloft	no	no	no	no	no	no	no	no	no
Maprotiline HCl	no	C/I (QT inc)	no	C/I (QT inc)	C/I (QT inc)	C/I (QT inc)	QT inc	no	no
mirtazapine	no	no	no	no	no	no	no	no	no
nortryptylin HCl- Aventyl	no	C/I (QT inc) nor++	no	C/I (QT inc) nor++	C/I (QT inc)	C/I (QT inc)	QT inc	no	no
paroxetine	no	QT inc	no	QT inc	QT inc	QT inc	QT inc	no	no
fluoxetine (as HCl)	no	QT inc	no	QT inc	QT inc	QT inc	QT inc	no	no
mirtazapine	no	no	no	no	no	no	no	no	no
trimiprane-trimipramine	no	C/I (QT inc)	no	C/I (QT inc)	C/I (QT inc)	C/I (QT inc)	QT inc	no	no
imipramine	im-	C/I (QT inc) imi+	no	C/I (QT inc) imi++	C/I (QT inc) imi+	C/I (QT inc) imi++	QT inc + imi+	no	no
trazodone	tr--	C/I (QT inc) tra++	no	C/I (QT inc) tra++ גם	C/I (QT inc) tra++	C/I (QT inc) ıtra++ גם itr--	tra++ & pos-- & QT inc partial C/I	no	no
venlafaxine HCl	no	(QT inc)	no	(QT inc)	(QT inc)	(QT inc)	(QT inc)	no	no
bupropion HCl	no	no	no	no	no	no	no	no	no

	griseofulvin	ketoconazole	terbinafine	itraconazole	fluconazole	voriconazole	posaconazole	amphothericin B- Fungizone	caspofungin
Anti-inflammatory agents (nsaid's)									
diclofenac sod.	no	di++	no	di+	di++	di++	no	no	no
celecoxib	no	cel+	no	cel+	cel+	cel+	no	no	no
etodolac (micronized)	no	no	no	no	no	no	no	no	no
nabumetone	no	no	no	no	no	no	no	no	no
naproxen sod.	no	no	no	no	no	no	no	no	no
ketoprofen	no	no	no	no	no	no	no	no	no
cyclosporin	Cy--	Cy++Keto+	no	Itra++	Cy++	no	Cy++Posa++	nephrotoxicity and ototoxicity C/I	Casp+++C/I
Methotrexate	no	no	no	no	no	no	no	no	no
Corticosteroid									
methylprednisolone acetate	met--	met++	no	met++& itr-	met++	met++	met++	hypokalemia	no
Immunosuppressants									
mycophenolate mofetil	no	m++	no	m++	no	no	no	no	no
azathioprine	no	no	no	no	no	no	no	no	no
muromonab -CD3	no	no	no	no	no	no	no	no	no
Muscle relaxants									
baclofen	no	no	no	no	no	no	no	no	no
purified botulinum toxin type A	no	no	no	no	no	no	no	partial C/I bo++	no
dantrolene	no	no	no	no	no	no	no	no	no
orphenadrine citrate	no	no	no	no	no	no	no	no	no

	griseofulvin	ketoconazole	terbinafine	itraconazole	fluconazole	voriconazole	posaconazole	amphothericin B-Fungizone	caspofungin
Growth hormones and growth disorders									
octreotide acetate	no	C/I QT inc	no	C/I QT inc	C/I QT inc	QT inc	QT inc	no	no
goserolin acetate eq.-Zoladex	no	no	no	no	no	no	no	no	no
Thyroid and antithroid and preparations									
levothyroxine sod.	no	no	no	no	no	no	no	no	no
methimazol	no	no	no	no	no	no	no	no	no
Diabetes insipidus									
desmopressin	no	no	no	no	no	no	no	no	no
Osteoporosis									
zoledronic acid anhydrous	no	no	no	no	no	no	no	no	no
risedronate sod.	no	no	no	no	no	no	no	no	no
raloxifene HCl	no	no	no	no	no	no	no	no	no
alendronate	no	no	no	no	no	no	no	no	no
Insulins									
Actrapid-novolin	no	no	no	no	no	no	no	no	no
Hyperglycemia									
acarbose	no	no	no	no	no	no	no	no	no
rosiglitazone maleate/metformin HCl	no	no	no	no	no	no	no	no	no
rosiglitazone	no	no	no	no	no	no	no	no	no
exenatide	no	no	no	no	no	no	no	no	no
glibenclamide-glyburide	no	gly++	no	gly++	gly++	gly++	gly++	no	no
metformin HCl	no	no	no	no	no	no	no	no	no
glipizide	no	gli++	no	gli++	gli++	gli++	gli++	no	no
sitagliptin	no	no	no	no	no	no	no	no	no
liraglutide	no	no	no	no	no	no	no	no	no
Hypoglycemia									
Glucagon HCl	no	no	no	no	no	no	no	no	no
Anti-obesity agents									
phentermin (as resinate)	no	no	no	no	no	no	no	no	no

	griseofulvin	ketoconazole	terbinafine	itraconazole	fluconazole	voriconazole	posaconazole	amphothericin B-Fungizone	caspofungin
Preparations acting on the prostate									
dutasteride	dut-	dut++	no	dut++	dut+	dut+	dut+	no	no
alfuzosin HCl	al-	C/I al++	no	C/I al++	al+	al+	al+	no	no
doxazosin	no	no	no	no	no	no	no	no	no
lipido sterolic extract serenoa repens	no	no	no	no	no	no	no	no	no
Urolitholytics									
pot. sod. Hydrogen && meas-potassium citrate	no	no	no	no	no	no	no	pot-	no
Male sexual disorders									
cyproterone acetate- Ethinylestradiol	partial C/I eth--	ethi++	no	ethi++	ethi++	ethi++	no	no	no
tadalafil	tad--	partial C/I tad++	no	tad++	tad++	tad++	tad++	no	no
clomiphene citrate	no	no	no	no	no	no	no	no	no
vardenafil	var--	partial C/I ver++	no	partial C/I ver++	var++	var++	var++	no	no
testosterone undecanoate- Aveed	no	no	no	no	no	no	no	no	no
sildenafil	sil--	sil++	no	sil++	sil++	sil++	sil++	no	no
Renal and bladder disorders									
tolterodine tart.	tol--	tol++	no	tol++	tol++	tol++	tol++	no	no

	griseofulvin	ketoconazole	terbinafine	itraconazole	fluconazole	voriconazole	posaconazole	amphothericin B- Fungizone	caspofungin
Disease modifying anti-rheumatic drugs									
methotrexate	no	no	no	no	no	no	no	no	no
tocilizumab	no	no	no	no	no	no	no	no	no
leflunomide	no	no	no	no	no	vor+	no	no	no
etanercept	no	no	no	no	no	no	no	no	no
adalimumab	no	no	no	no	no	no	no	no	no
canakinumab	no	no	no	no	no	no	no	no	no
anakira- Kineret	no	no	no	no	no	no	no	no	no
rituximab VIALS	no	no	no	no	no	no	no	partial C/I both nephrotoxicity and/or ototoxicity	no
hydroxychloroquine	no	no	no	no	no	no	no	no	no
infliximab	no	no	no	no	no	no	no	no	no
sulphasalazine- Azulfidine	sul--	no	no	no	no	no	no	no	no

	griseofulvin	ketoconazole	terbinafine	itraconazole	fluconazole	voriconazole	posaconazole	amphothericin B-Fungizone	caspofungin
Endometriosis									
danazol	no	no	no	no	no	no	no	no	no
triptorelin acetate	no	no	no	no	no	no	no	no	no
Breast disorders									
cabergoline	no	no	no	no	no	no	no	no	no
Menopausal disorders									
risedronate sod.	no	no	no	no	no	no	no	no	no
alendronate sod. Monohyd	no	no	no	no	no	no	no	no	no
estradiol & norethisterone acetate	es--	es++	no	es++	es++	es++	es++	no	no
Infertility									
clomiphene	no	no	no	no	no	no	no	no	no
Obstetrics									

Antibiotics	griseofulvin	ketoconazole	terbinafine	itraconazole	fluconazole	voriconazole	posaconazole	amphothericin B-Fungizone	caspofungin
amikacin sulph.	no	am++/am-	no	no	ami-	ami-	ami-	C/I nephrotoxicity and/or ototoxicity	no
amoxicillin trihydrate & clavulanicacid (as potassium clavulanate- amoxicillin / clavulanate	no	no	no	no	no	no	no	no	no
minocycline	no	no	no	no	no	no	no	no	no
azithromycin	no	azi++ & QT inc	no	no	QT inc	QT inc	QT inc	no	no
cefadroxil	no	no	no	no	no	no	no	no	no
cephalexin	no	no	no	no	no	no	no	no	no
ciprofloxacin	no	no	no	no	no	no	no	no	no
clarithromycin	cla-	partial C/I QT in &ket ++	no	no	partial C/I QT in &cla+	QT inc & cla+	QT inc & cla+ & p++	no	no
clindamycin	no	no	no	no	no	no	no	no	no
colistimetate sod.-colistin	no	no	no	no	no	no	no	partial C/I nephrotoxicity and/or ototoxicity.	no
doxycycline hyclate	no	no	no	no	no	no	no	no	no
benzanthine penicillin G	no	no	no	no	no	no	no	no	no
erythromycin	C/I ery--	partial C/I QT in &ket ++& ery+++	no	no	C/I ery++ & QT inc	C/I ery++ & QT inc	partial C/I ery++ & p++& QT inc	no	no
ceftazidime	no	no	no	no	no	no	no	no	no
gentamicin sulph.	no	gen++/gen-	no	no	gen-	gen-	gen-	partial C/I nephrotoxicity and/or ototoxicity	no
ertapenem	no	no	no	no	no	no	no	no	no
levofloxacin	no	QT inc	no	no	QT inc	QT inc	QT inc	no	no
moxifloxacin HCl	no	partial C/I QT inc	no	no	partial C/I QT inc	QT inc	QT inc	no	no
meropenem	no	no	no	no	no	no	no	no	no
metronidazole	no	ket+	no	no	no	v+	no	no	no
minocycline HCl	no	no	no	no	no	no	no	no	no
neomycin sulph.	no	no	no	no	no	no	no	no	no
ofloxacin	no	QT inc	no	no	QT inc	QT inc	QT inc	no	no
trimethoprim & sulphamethoxazole-trimethoprim/sulfamethoxazole	no	QT inc & sul+	no	no	QT inc & sul+	QT inc & sul+ & V+	QT inc	no	no
roxithromycin	no	no	no	no	no	no	no	no	no
imipenem & cilastatin sod.-imipenem/cilastatin	no	no	no	no	no	no	no	no	no
ciprofloxacin lactate	no	no	no	no	no	no	no	no	no
vancomycin HCl	no	no	no	no	no	no	no	nephrotoxicity and/or ototoxicity	no
cefuroxime sod.	no	no	no	no	no	no	no	no	no
linezolid	no	no	no	no	no	no	no	no	no

	griseofulvin	ketoconazole	terbinafine	itraconazole	fluconazole	voriconazole	posaconazole	amphothericin B-Fungizone	caspofungin
Sulfonamids									
trimethoprim	no	QT inc	no	QT inc	QT inc	QT inc	QT inc	no	no
trimethoprim & sulphamethoxazole	no	QT inc & sul+	no	QT inc & sul+	QT inc & sul+	QT inc & sul+ & v +	QT inc	no	no
Antituberculosis and antileprotic preparations									
isoniazid	no	C/I ket--	no	C/I itr--	no	vor++	no	no	no
rifabutin	no	k-- & r+	no	it -- & r+	fl-	C/I vor--	po-- & r+	no	no
rifamycin 3 & rifamycin SV (rifampicin)- rifampin	no	k-- & r-	t-	i-- & r-	f-- & r-	C/I vor-- & r-	p-- & r-	no	cas --
Antimalarials, tropical diseases									
mefloquine	no	partial C/I QT inc & me++	no	partial C/I QT inc & me++	me++	partial C/I me++	partial C/I QT inc & me++	no	no
atovaquone & proguanil HCl	no	no	no	no	no	no	no	no	no
hydroxychloroquine	no	no	no	no	no	no	no	no	no
Antitrichomonal agents									
tinidazole	no	no	no	no	no	no	no	no	no
metronidazole	no	ket+	no	no	no	v+	no	no	no
Antivirals									
acyclovir	no	no	no	no	no	no	no	partial C/I nephrotoxicity and/or ototoxicity	no
foscarnet trisod hexahydrate	no	QT inc	no	QT inc	QT inc	QT inc	QT inc	nephrotoxicity and/or ototoxicity	no
iopinavir & ritonavir- lopinavir/ritonavir	lo--& ri--	partial C/I lo++ & ri++	no	partial C/I lo++ & ri++	lo++ & ri ++	C/I ri+++& l++ & v--	lo++ & ri ++& p++	no	no
interferon- interferon alfa 2b	no	no	no	no	no	no	no	no	no
ribavirin	no	no	no	no	no	no	no	no	no
valaciclovir-valacyclovir	no	no	no	no	no	no	no	no	no
AIDS									
maraviroc	mar--	mar++	no	mar++	mar++	mar++	mar++	no	no
zidovudine & lamivudine	no	zi++	no	no	zi+	no	no	am+	no
indinavir	in--	partial C/I in++ & k+	no	partial C/I in++ & it++	in++	partial C/I in++	in++ & p++	no	no
ganciclovir	no	no	no	no	no	no	no	am+	no
lamivudine	no	no	no	no	no	no	no	no	no
etravirine	et--	et++ & k-	no	partial C/I et++	et++	partial C/I et++ & v+	et++	no	no
zidovudine	no	zi++	no	no			zi+	am+	no
atazanavir sulfate	at-	at++&k+	no	at++& i+	at+	partial C/I at++	at+	no	no
abacavir &lamivudine & zidovudine-lamivudine/zidovudine/abacavir	no	zi++	no	no	zi+	no	no	am+	no

x

	griseofulvin	ketoconazole	terbinafine	itraconazole	fluconazole	voriconazole	posaconazole	amphothericin B-Fungizone	caspofungin
Neoplastic disorders									
doxorubicin	no	do++	no	do++	do++	do++	no	no	no
everolimus	partial C/I ev--	partial C/I ev++	no	partial C/I ev++	partial C/I ev++	partial C/I ev++	partial C/I ev++	no	no
cystosine-Cytarabine	no	no	no	no	no	no	no	no	no
melphalan	no	no	no	no	no	no	no	no	no
anastrozole	no	no	no	no	no	no	no	no	no
nelarabine	no	no	no	no	no	no	no	no	no
bevacizumab	no	no	no	no	no	no	no	no	no
bicalutamide	no	no	no	no	no	no	no	no	no
vinblastine sulph	vi-	vi++	no	vi++	vi+	vi++	vi+	no	no
bleomycin sulphate	no	no	no	no	no	no	no	no	no
irinotecan HCl	no	C/I ir++	no	ir++	no	no	no	no	no
dexrazoxane	no	no	no	no	no	no	no	no	no
dacarbazine	no	no	no	no	no	no	no	no	no
triptorelincetuximab- triptorelin	no	no	no	no	no	no	no	no	no
estramustine phos	no	no	no	no	no	no	no	no	no
etoposide	no	et++	no	et++	et++	et++	et++	no	no
fludarabine phos.	no	no	no	no	no	no	no	no	no
gemcitabine	no	no	no	no	no	no	no	no	no
sorafenib (as tosylate)	so--	no	no	no	QT inc	QT inc	QT inc	no	no
BCG- bcg vaccine live	no	no	no	no	no	no	no	no	no
paclitaxel	pa++ /pa-	pa++	no	pa++	pa+	pa+	pa+	no	no
tamoxifen	no	ta--	no	ta--	ta--	ta--	ta--	no	no
nilotinib HCl monohydrate	ni--	partial C/I QT inc ni++ & k+	no	partial C/I QT inc ni++ & it+	partial C/I QT inc& ni--	partial C/I QT & ni++ & v+	QT inc & ni++ & po++	no	no
docetaxel	do-	do++	no	do++	do+	do+	do+	no	no

	griseofulvin	ketoconazole	terbinafine	itraconazole	fluconazole	voriconazole	posaconazole	amphothericin B-Fungizone	caspofungin
Anti-allergic and cold preparations									
desloratadine	no	d+	no	no	no	no	no	no	no
loratadine	lo--	C/I lo++	no	C/I lo++/it++	lo++	lo++	lo++/po++	no	no
chlorpheniramine	no	no	no	no	no	no	no	no	no
paracetamol & diphenhydramine HCl & pseudoephedrine-diphenhydramine/pseudoephedrine	no	no	no	no	no	no	no	no	no
triprolidine HCl & pseudoephedrine HCl-codeine/triprolidine/pseudoephedrine	no	no	no	no	no	no	no	no	no
cetirizine HCl	no	no	no	no	no	no	no	no	no
mizolastine	no	C/I KE++	no	no	no	no	no	no	no
promethazine HCl	no	C/I KE++/ pr++	no	C/I it++/ pr++	C/I fl++/ pr++	vo++/pr++	po++/pr++	no	no
montelukast	mo-	mo+	no	mo+	mo+	mo+	mo+	no	no
fexofenadine HCl	no	fe-	no	fe-	no	no	no	no	no
Expectatorants; cough suppresants									
cod. Phos.-Codeine	no	no	no	no	no	no	no	no	no
oxomemazine & potassium guaicol sulph. & sod. Benzoate & excip qs- sodium benzoate	no	no	no	no	no	no	no	no	no
acetylcysteine	no	no	no	no	no	no	no	no	no
Inhalations									
terbutaline sulph	no	no	no	no	no	no	no	no	no
reactions (local) on the nasopharynx									
xylometazoline HCl & ipratropium bromide	no	no	no	no	no	no	no	no	no
oxymetazoline	no	no	no	no	no	no	no	no	no

Cardiovascular	griseofulvin	ketoconazole	terbinafine	itraconazole	fluconazole	voriconazole	posaconazole	amphothericin B-Fungizone	caspofungin
Amiodarone	Am--	Am+++C/I QT++	no	Am+++Itra++C/I QT++	Am+++C/I QT++	Am+++V+C/I QT++	Am+++P+C/I QT++	no	no
Carvedilol	no	Car++	no	Car++	Car++	Car++	no	no	no
Dobutamine	no	no	no	no	no	no	no	no	no
Digoxin	no	Dig++	no	Dig++	no	no	Dig++	Dig+++C/I hypokalemia	no
Milrinone	no	no	no	no	no	no	no	no	no
Quinidine	Quin--	Quin+++C/I QT++	no	Quin+++C/I QT++	Quin+++C/I QT++	Quin+++C/I QT++	Quin++P++C/I QT++	no	no
Flecainide	no	C/I QT++	no	C/I QT++	C/I QT++	C/I QT++	C/I QT++	no	no
Amlodipine	Amlo-	Amlo++	no	Amlo++	Amlo++	Amlo++	Amlo+	no	no
Bisoprolol	no	no	no	no	no	no	no	no	no
Ivabradine	Iva---C/I	Keto+Iva+++C/I QT++	no	Keto+Iva+++C/I QT++	Iva+++C/I QT++	V++Iva+++C/I QT++	Iva++C/I	no	no
Propranolol	no	no	no	no	no	no	no	no	no
Diltiazem	Dil--	Keto+Dil+++C/I	no	Itra++Dil+++C/I	Dil++	Dil+++C/I risk of AV block	D++P++	no	no
Isosorbide mononitrate	no	no	no	no	no	no	no	no	no
Isosorbide dinitrate	no	no	no	no	no	no	no	no	no
Nifedipine	Nif-	Keto+Nif++	no	itra--Nif++	Nif++	Nif++	Nif+++	no	no
ASPIRIN (acetylsalicylic acid)	As--	no	no	no	no	no	no	no	no
Enoxaparin	no	no	no	no	no	no	no	no	no
Clopidogrel	Clop++	Clop---C/I	no	Clop---C/I	Clop---C/I	Clop---C/I	Clop---C/I	no	no
Heparin	no	no	no	no	no	no	no	no	no
Rivaroxaban	no	Riv+++C/I bleeding risk	no	Riv+++C/I bleeding risk	Riv+++C/I bleeding risk	no	no	no	no
Tranexamic	no	no	no	no	no	no	no	no	no
Clonidine	no	no	no	no	no	no	no	no	no
MIGRALEVE	no	no	no	no	no	no	no	no	no
Spironolactone	no	no	no	Itra++Dil+++C/I	no	no	Posa++	no	no
Acetazolamide	no	no	no	no	no	no	no	no	no
Amlodipine	Amlo-	Amlo++	no	Amlo++	Amlo++	Amlo++	Amlo+	no	no
Doxazosin	no	no	no	no	no	no	no	no	no
Valsartan	no	Val++	no	no	no	no	no	no	Val ++
Hydrochlorothiazide	no	no	no	no	no	no	no	no	no
Enalapril	no	Enal++	no	Enal++	no	no	no	no	no
Ramipril	no	no	no	no	no	no	no	no	no
Pentoxifylline	no	no	no	no	no	no	no	no	no
Atorvastatin	Ator--	Ator+++C/I	no	Ator+++Itra++C/I limit 20 mg	Ator+++	Ator+++	Ator+++	no	no
Rosuvastatin	no	no	no	no	no	no	no	no	no
Ezetimibe	no	no	no	no	no	no	no	no	no
Fluvastatin	no	Fluv+	no	no	Fluv+	Fluv+	no	no	no
Ciprofibrate	no	no	no	no	no	no	no	no	no
Pravastatin	no	no	no	no	no	no	no	no	no
Simvastatin	Sim--- C/I	Sim+++C/I rhabdomyolysis	no	Sim+++Itra++ C/I rhabdomyolysis	Sim+++C/I rhabdomyolysis	Sim+++C/I rhabdomyolysis	Sim+++P++C/I rhabdomyolysis	no	no

References

[1] St-Germain, Guy, and Richard Summerbell.Identifying filamentous fungi: A clinical laboratory handbook. Star Publishing Company, 1996.

[2] Schwartz, Robert A. "Superficial fungal infections." *The Lancet,* 364.9440 (2004): 1173-1182.

[3] Guarro, Josep, Josepa Gené, and Alberto M. Stchigel. "Developments in fungal taxonomy." *Clinical microbiology reviews,* 12.3 (1999): 454-500.

[4] Richardson, Malcolm, and Boni E. Elewski. *Superficial fungal infections*. Health press, 2000.

[5] Blanco, Jose L., and Marta E. Garcia. "Immune response to fungal infections." *Veterinary Immunology and Immunopathology,* 125.1 (2008): 47-70.

[6] Romani, L. "Immune resistance and tolerance to fungi." *G. Ital. Dermatol. Venereol,* 148 (2013): 551-561.

[7] Casadevall, Arturo. "Antibody immunity and invasive fungal infections." *Infection and immunity,* 63.11 (1995): 4211.

[8] Glocker, Erik-Oliver, et al. "A homozygous CARD9 mutation in a family with susceptibility to fungal infections." *New England Journal of Medicine,* 361.18 (2009): 1727-1735.

[9] Ferwerda, Bart, et al. "Human dectin-1 deficiency and mucocutaneous fungal infections." *New England Journal of Medicine,* 361.18 (2009): 1760-1767.

[10] Bellocchio, Silvia, et al. "The contribution of the Toll-like/IL-1 receptor superfamily to innate and adaptive immunity to fungal pathogens in vivo." *The Journal of Immunology,*172.5 (2004): 3059-3069.

[11] Baran, R., N. McLoone, and R. J. Hay. "Could proximal white subungual onychomycosis be a complication of systemic spread? The lessons to be learned from Maladie Dermatophytique and other deep infections." *British Journal of Dermatology,* 153.5 (2005): 1023-1025.

[12] Zaias, Nardo.*The nail in health and disease*. McGraw-Hill/Appleton & Lange, 1990.

[13] Croxatto, Antony, Guy Prod'hom, and Gilbert Greub. "Applications of MALDI-TOF mass spectrometry in clinical diagnostic microbiology." *FEMS microbiology reviews,* 36.2 (2012): 380-407.

[14] Zhang, Xinyi, et al. "Evaluation of a novel, integrated approach using functionalized magnetic beads, bench-top MALDI-TOF-MS with prestructured sample supports, and

pattern recognition software for profiling potential biomarkers in human plasma." *Journal of biomolecular techniques: JBT*15.3 (2004): 167.

[15] Erhard, Marcel, et al. "Identification of dermatophyte species causing onychomycosis and tinea pedis by MALDI-TOF mass spectrometry." *Experimental dermatology,* 17.4 (2008): 356-361.

[16] Seng, Piseth, et al. "MALDI-TOF-mass spectrometry applications in clinical microbiology." *Future microbiology,* 5.11 (2010): 1733-1754.

[17] Marinach-Patrice, C., et al. "Use of mass spectrometry to identify clinical Fusarium isolates." *Clinical Microbiology and Infection,* 15.7 (2009): 634-642.

[18] Lynch, Tom, and Price Amy. "The effect of cytochrome P450 metabolism on drug response, interactions, and adverse effects." *American family physician,* 76.3 (2007): 391.

[19] De Montellano, Paul R. Ortiz, ed.*Cytochrome P450: structure, mechanism, and biochemistry*. Springer Science & Business Media, 2005.

[20] Dixon, Dennis M. and Walsh, Thomas J "Antifungal Agents" *Medical Microbiology. 4th edition*. Ed. Samuel Baron, Galveston (TX): University of Texas Medical Branch at Galveston, 1996, chapter 76. Print.

[21] Casadevall, Arturo, and Matthew D. Scharff. "Return to the past: the case for antibody-based therapies in infectious diseases." *Clinical infectious diseases,* 21.1 (1995): 150-161.

[22] Como, Jackson A., and William E. Dismukes. "Oral azole drugs as systemic antifungal therapy." *New England Journal of Medicine,* 330.4 (1994): 263-272.

[23] Bossche, Hugo Vanden, Patrick Marichal, and Frank C. Odds. "Molecular mechanisms of drug resistance in fungi." *Trends in microbiology,* 2.10 (1994): 393-400.

[24] Roberts, D. T., W. D. Taylor, and J. Boyle. "Guidelines for treatment of onychomycosis." *British Journal of Dermatology,* 148.3 (2003): 402-410.

[25] Sheehan, Daniel J., Christopher A. Hitchcock, and Carol M. Sibley. "Current and emerging azole antifungal agents." *Clinical microbiology reviews,* 12.1 (1999): 40-79.

[26] Moudgal, Varsha V., and Jack D. Sobel. "Antifungal drugs in pregnancy: a review." *Expert opinion on drug safety,* 2.5 (2003): 475-483.

[27] Ginter-Hanselmayer, Gabriele, et al. "Epidemiology of tinea capitis in Europe: current state and changing patterns." *Mycoses,* 50.s2 (2007): 6-13.

[28] Shemer, Avner, et al. "Treatment of tinea capitis–griseofulvin versus fluconazole–a comparative study." *JDDG: Journal der Deutschen Dermatologischen Gesellschaft,* 11.8 (2013): 737-741.

[29] Rippon, John Willard. "The changing epidemiology and emerging patterns of dermatophyte species."*Current topics in medical mycology*. Springer New York, 1985. 208-234.

[30] Grunwald, M. H., B. Amichai, and A. Shemer. "Fingertip contamination after a brief touch of tinea capitis lesions caused by Microsporum canis." *British Journal of Dermatology,* 172.1 (2015): 291-292.

[31] Hay, R. J., et al. "Tinea capitis in south-east London—a new pattern of infection with public health implications." *British Journal of Dermatology,* 135.6 (1996): 955-958.

[32] Neil, Gail, et al. "Control of the carrier state of scalp dermatophytes." *The Pediatric infectious disease journal,* 9.1 (1990): 57.

[33] Elewski, Boni Elizabeth. "Tinea capitis: a current perspective." *Journal of the American Academy of Dermatology,* 42.1 (2000): 1-20.

[34] Abdel-Rahman, S. M., M. C. Nahata, and D. A. Powell. "Response to initial griseofulvin therapy in pediatric patients with tinea capitis." *The Annals of pharmacotherapy,* 31.4 (1997): 406-410.

[35] Quero, Roberto. "Allergic reaction to griseofulvin." *J. est. Derm.*34.5 (1960): 283-284.

[36] Hamm, H., et al. "Short duration treatment with terbinafine for tinea capitis caused by Trichophyton or Microsporum species. The Study Group." *The British journal of dermatology,* 140.3 (1999): 480-482.

[37] López-Gómez, S., et al. "Itraconazole versus griseofulvin in the treatment of tinea capitis: a double-blind randomized study in children." *International journal of dermatology,* 33.10 (1994): 743-747.

[38] Gupta, Aditya K., et al. "Therapeutic options for the treatment of tinea capitis caused by Trichophyton species: griseofulvin versus the new oral antifungal agents, terbinafine, itraconazole, and fluconazole." *Pediatric dermatology,* 18.5 (2001): 433-438.

[39] Elewski, Boni E., et al. "Terbinafine hydrochloride oral granules versus oral griseofulvin suspension in children with tinea capitis: Results of two randomized, investigator-blinded, multicenter, international, controlled trials< sup>*</sup>." *Journal of the American Academy of Dermatology,* 59.1 (2008): 41-54.

[40] Coutinho, Agnes E., and Karen E. Chapman. "The anti-inflammatory and immunosuppressive effects of glucocorticoids, recent developments and mechanistic insights." *Molecular and cellular endocrinology,* 335.1 (2011): 2-13.

[41] Lin, Richie L., Jacek C. Szepietowski, and Robert A. Schwartz. "Tinea faciei, an often deceptive facial eruption." *International journal of dermatology,* 43.6 (2004): 437-440.

[42] del Boz, Javier, Vicente Crespo, and Magdalena de Troya. "Pediatric Tinea Faciei in Southern Spain: A 30-Year Survey." *Pediatric dermatology,* 29.3 (2012): 249-253.

[43] Nicola, Aste, et al. "A 20-year survey of tinea faciei." *Mycoses,* 53.6 (2010): 504-508.

[44] Bardazzi, Federico, et al. "Tinea faciei in a newborn: a new case." *Pediatric dermatology,* 17.6 (2000): 494-495.

[45] Wilmer, Axel, and Uwe Wollina. "Oral terbinafine in the treatment of griseofulvin-resistant Tinea capitis et faciei et corporis in a 10-month-old girl." *Acta dermato-venereologica,* 78.4 (1998): 314-314.

[46] Hiruma, M., and A. Kukita. "Tinea faciei caused by Microsporum canis in a newborn." *Dermatology,* 176.3 (1988): 130-132.

[47] Virgili, A., M. Corazza, and M. R. Zampino. "Atypical features of tinea in newborns." *Pediatric dermatology,* 10.1 (1993): 92-92.

[48] Atzori, Laura, et al. "Tinea faciei due to Microsporum canis in children: a survey of 46 cases in the District of Cagliari (Italy)." *Pediatric dermatology,* 29.4 (2012): 409-413.

[49] Jorquera, E., J. C. Moreno, and F. Camacho. "[Tinea faciei: epidemiology]." *Annales de dermatologie et de vénéréologie.* Vol. 119. No. 2. 1991.

[50] Gorani, Alberto, Alfio Oriani, and Stefano Cambiaghi. "Seborrheic Dermatitis-like Tinea Faciei." *Pediatric dermatology,* 22.3 (2005): 243-244.

[51] Surpam, R. B., et al. "Trichophyton violaceum: A rare isolate in 18-day-old neonate." *Indian journal of medical microbiology,* 24.4 (2006): 292.

[52] Shrum, Joseph P., Larry E. Millikan, and Omar Bataineh. "Superficial fungal infections in the tropics." *Dermatologic clinics,* 12.4 (1994): 687-693.

[53] Adams, Brian B. "Tinea corporis gladiatorum." *Journal of the American Academy of Dermatology,* 47.2 (2002): 286-290.

[54] Szepietowski, Jacek C., and R. A. Schwartz. "Tinea faciei." *Emedicine Dermatology. St. Petersburg: eMedicine Corp* (2001).

[55] Kang, Daoxian, et al. "Impetigo-Like Tinea Faciei Around the Nostrils Caused by Arthroderma vanbreuseghemii Identified Using Polymerase Chain Reaction–Based Sequencing of Crusts." *Pediatric dermatology,* 30.6 (2013): e136-e137.

[56] Alteras, I., et al. "15-Year Survey of Tinea f aciei in the Adult." *Dermatology,* 177.2 (1988): 65-69.

[57] Basak, S. Alison Finger, et al. "Common features of periocular tinea." *Archives of ophthalmology,* 129.3 (2011): 306-309.

[58] Arenas RToussaint SIsa-Isa RKerion and dermatophytic granuloma: mycological and histopathological findings in 19 children with inflammatory tinea capitis of the scalp.*Int J Dermatol,* 2006;45 (3) 215-219

[59] Koçak MDeveci MSEkşioğlu MGünhan OYağli SImmunohistochemical analysis of the infiltrated cells in tinea capitis patients.*J Dermatol,* 2002;29 (3) 131-135.

[60] Rasmussen JEAhmed ARTrichophytin reactions in children with tinea capitis.*Arch Dermatol*1978;114 (3) 371-372

[61] Khaled, Aida, et al. "Tinea faciei: a report on four cases." *ACTA DERMATOVENEROLOGICA ALPINA PANONICA ET ADRIATICA*16.4 (2007): 170.

[62] Meymandi, Simin, Marni C. Wiseman, and Richard I. Crawford. "Tinea faciei mimicking cutaneous lupus erythematosus: a histopathologic case report." *Journal of the American Academy of Dermatology,* 48.2 (2003): S7-S8.

[63] Baker, Roger Denio. "The pathologic anatomy of mycoses. Human infection with fungi, actinomycetes and algae." *The pathologic anatomy of mycoses. Human infection with fungi, actinomycetes and algae.* (1971).

[64] Scully C: The oral cavity. In*In Rook/ Wilkinson/Ebling Textbook of dermatology*. 6th edition. Edited by Champion RH, Burton JL, Burns DA, Breathnach SM. Oxford: Blackwell Science Ltd; 1998:3047-3123.

[65] Kligman, A. M., H. Mescon, and E. D. DeLamater. "The Hotchkiss-McManus stain for the histopathologic diagnosis of fungus diseases." *American journal of clinical pathology,* 21.1 (1951): 86-91.

[66] Weedon D.*Skin Pathology*. 2nd ed.Philadelphia, PA: Churchill Livingstone, Elsevier Ltd;2002.

[67] Elder, David E.*Lever's histopathology of the skin*. Lippincott Williams & Wilkins, 2014.

[68] Nakayama, Juichiro. "Four cases of sebopsoriasis or seborrheic dermatitis of the face and scalp successfully treated with 1a-24 (R)-dihydroxycholecalciferol (tacalcitol) cream." *European Journal of Dermatology,* 10.7 (2000): 528-32.

[69] Patel, G. K., and C. M. Mills. "Tinea faciei due to Microsporum canis abscess formation." *Clinical and experimental dermatology,* 25.8 (2000): 608-610.

[70] Coleman Iii, William P. "Skin Infections: Diagnosis and Treatment Edited By: John C. Hall And Brian J. Hall." *Dermatologic Surgery,* 37.12 (2011): 1776-1776.

[71] Piérard, Géerald E., Jorge E. Arrese, and Claudine Piérard-Franchimont. "Treatment and prophylaxis of tinea infections." *Drugs,* 52.2 (1996): 209-224.

[72] Szepietowski, J. C. "Terbinafine exacerbates psoriasis: case report with a literature review." *Acta dermatovenerologica Croatica: ADC*11.1 (2002): 17-21.

[73] Calcaterra, Roberta, et al. "Rosacea-Like Tinea Incognito due to Trichophyton mentagrophytes vr. mentagrophytes." *Acta Dermatovenerologica Croatica,* 21.4 (2014).

[74] Szepietowski J. The contemporary therapy of superficial fungal infections. Terapia Leki 2000; 28: 18–23.

[75] Metkar, Amol, et al. "Extensive neonatal dermatophytoses." *Pediatric dermatology,* 27.2 (2010): 189-191.

[76] Ohno, Sayoko, et al. "Tinea corporis with acute inflammation caused by Trichophyton tonsurans." *The Journal of dermatology,* 35.9 (2008): 590-593.

[77] Silveira-Gomes, Fabíola, et al. "Dermatophytosis diagnosed at the Evandro Chagas Institute, Pará, Brazil." *Brazilian Journal of Microbiology,* 44.2 (2013): 443-446.

[78] Sellami, A., et al. "Childhood dermatomycoses study in Sfax hospital, Tunisia." *Mycoses,* 51.5 (2008): 451-454.

[79] Gupta RK: Opportunistic infections in renal allograft recipients. Transplant Proc, 2007; 39: 731

[80] Budihardja, Debby, Viviane Freund, and Peter Mayser. "Widespread erosive tinea corporis by Arthroderma benhamiae in a renal transplant recipient: case report." *Mycoses,* 53.6 (2010): 530-532.

[81] Güleç, A. Tülin, et al. "Superficial fungal infections in 102 renal transplant recipients: a case-control study." *Journal of the American Academy of Dermatology,* 49.2 (2003): 187-192.

[82] Virgili, Annarosa, Maria Rosaria Zampino, and Lucia Mantovani. "Fungal skin infections in organ transplant recipients." *American journal of clinical dermatology,* 3.1 (2002): 19-35.

[83] Romano, Clara, et al. "Tinea corporis purpurica and onychomycosis caused by Trichophyton violaceum." *Mycoses,* 54.2 (2011): 175-178.

[84] Kawachi, Yasuhiro, et al. "Chronically Recurrent and Disseminated Tinea Faciei/Corporis—Autoinoculation from Asymptomatic Tinea Capitis Carriage." *Pediatric dermatology,* 27.5 (2010): 527-528.

[85] Burkhart, Craig N., Howard Chang, and Lorie Gottwald. "Tinea corporis in human immunodeficiency virus-positive patients: case report and assessment of oral therapy." *International journal of dermatology,* 42.10 (2003): 839-843.

[86] Rajpara, Vidya, et al. "Trichophyton tonsurans associated tinea corporis infection with the development of Majocchi's granuloma in a renal transplant patient." *Journal of drugs in dermatology,* 4.6 (2005): 767.

[87] Brocq, L. "Les parapsoriasis." *Ann Dermatol Syphiligr (Paris)*3 (1902): 433-468.

[88] Morishita N, Ninomiya J, Sei Y, Takiuchi I. Experimental studies on the penetration of dermatophytes into thehuman stratum corneum and the effect of washing. *Jpn J Med Mycol* 2004; 45: 247–252.

[89] Kasai, T. "[Epidemiological survey of Trichophyton tonsurans infection in Tohoku district and its clinical problems]." *Nihon Ishinkin Gakkai zasshi= Japanese journal of medical mycology,* 46.2 (2004): 87-91.

[90] Parent, Dominique, Jacques Decroix, and Michel Heenen. "Clinical experience with short schedules of itraconazole in the treatment of tinea corporis and/or tinea cruris." *Dermatology,* 189.4 (1994): 378-381.

[91] Imwidthaya, S., and M. Thianprasit. "A study of dermatophytoses in Bangkok (Thailand)." *Mycopathologia,* 102.1 (1988): 13-16.

[92] Al-Sogair, S. M., M. K. Moawad, and Y. M. Al-Humaidan. "Fungal infection as a cause of skin disease in the eastern province of Saudi Arabia: tinea corporis and tinea cruris." *Mycoses,* 34.9-10 (1991): 423-427.

[93] Ajello, Libero, and Morton E. Getz. "Recovery of Dermatophytes from Shoes and Shower Stalls1." *Journal of Investigative Dermatology,* 22.1 (1954): 17-24.

[94] Knudsen, Erik A. "Isolation of dermatophytes from footwear with adhesive tape strips." *Medical Mycology,* 25.1 (1987): 59-61.

[95] Khosravi, Ali Reza, et al. "Unusual presentation of tinea cruris due to Trichophyton mentagrophytes var. mentagrophytes." *The Journal of dermatology,* 35.8 (2008): 541-545.

[96] Devroey, Ch. "Epidemiology of Ringworm (Dermatophytosis)." *Seminars In Dermatology*. Vol. 4. No. 3. 1600 John F Kennedy Boulevard, Ste 1800, Philadelphia, Pa 19103-2899 USA: Wb Saunders Co-Elsevier Inc, 1985.

[97] Otero, L., V. Palacio, and F. Vazquez. "Tinea cruris in female prostitutes." *Mycopathologia,* 153.1 (2002): 29-31.

[98] Chakrabarti, A., S. C. Sharma, and P. Talwar. "Isolation of dermatophytes from clinically normal sites in patients with tinea cruris." *Mycopathologia,* 120.3 (1992): 139-141.

[99] Odom, Richard. "Pathophysiology of dermatophyte infections." *Journal of the American Academy of Dermatology,* 28.5 (1993): S2-S7.

[100] Venkatesan, G., et al. "Trichophyton rubrum-the predominant etiological agent in human dermatophytoses in Chennai, India." (2007).

[101] Das, Shukla, Renu Goyal, and S. N. Bhattacharya. "Laboratory-based epidemiological study of superficial fungal infections." *The Journal of dermatology,* 34.4 (2007): 248-253.

[102] Ameen, Mahreen. "Epidemiology of superficial fungal infections." *Clinics in dermatology,* 28.2 (2010): 197-201.

[103] Kemna, Maggi E., and Boni E. Elewski. "A US epidemiologic survey of superficial fungal diseases." *Journal of the American Academy of Dermatology,* 35.4 (1996): 539-542.

[104] Silva-Tavares, H., M. M. A. Alchorne, and O. Fischman. "Tinea cruris epidemiology (Sao Paulo, Brazil)." *Mycopathologia,* 149.3 (2001): 147-149.

[105] Nadalo, Dana, and Cathy C. Montoya. "What is the best way to treat tinea cruris?." *Clinical Inquiries, 2006 (MU)*(2006).

[106] Hainer, Barry L. "Dermatophyte infections." *American family physician,* 67.1 (2003): 101-110.

[107] Shobhana, A., Subhasish Kamal Guha, and D. K. Neogi. "Mucocutaneous manifestations of HIV infection." *Indian Journal of Dermatology, Venereology, and Leprology,* 70.2 (2004): 82.

[108] Kaviarasan, P. K., et al. “Clinical variations in dermatophytosis in HIV infected patients.” *Indian Journal of Dermatology, Venereology, and Leprology,* 68.4 (2002): 213.

[109] Aly, Raza, and Timothy Berger. “Common superficial fungal infections in patients with AIDS.” *Clinical infectious diseases,* 22.Supplement 2 (1996): S128-S132.

[110] Sentamil Selvi, G., et al. “Clinical and mycological features of dermatophytosis in renal transplant recipients.” *Mycoses,* 42.1-2 (1999): 75-78.

[111] Danesh-Pazhooh, Maryam. “The frequency of tinea pedis in patients with tinea cruris in Tehran, Iran.” *Mycoses,* 43.1-2 (2000): 41-44.

[112] Drake, Lynn A., et al. “Guidelines of care for superficial mycotic infectionsof the skin: Tinea corporis, tinea cruris, tinea faciei, tinea manuum, and tinea pedis.” *Journal of the American Academy of Dermatology,* 34.2 (1996): 282-286.

[113] Fulton, James E. “Miconazole therapy for endemic fungal disease.” *Archives of dermatology,* 111.5 (1975): 596-598.

[114] Bogaert, Huberto, et al. “Multicentre double-blind clinical trials of ciclopirox olamine cream 1% in the treatment of tinea corporis and tinea cruris.” *Journal of international medical research,* 14.4 (1986): 210-216.

[115] Sakurai, K., et al. “Mode of Action of 6-Cyclohexyl-l-hydroxy-4-methyl-2 (1H)-pyridone Ethanolamine Salt (Hoe 296).” *Chemotherapy,* 24.2 (1978): 68-76.

[116] Bogaert, Huberto, et al. “Multicentre double-blind clinical trials of ciclopirox olamine cream 1% in the treatment of tinea corporis and tinea cruris.” *Journal of international medical research,* 14.4 (1986): 210-216.

[117] Lesher, Jack L., et al. “Butenafine 1% cream in the treatment of tinea cruris: a multicenter, vehicle-controlled, double-blind trial.” *Journal of the American Academy of Dermatology,* 36.2 (1997): S20-S24.

[118] Lesher, Jack L. “Oral therapy of common superficial fungal infections of the skin.” *Journal of the American Academy of Dermatology,* 40.6 (1999): S31-S34.

[119] Montero-Gei, F., and A. Perera. “Therapy with fluconazole for tinea corporis, tinea cruris, and tinea pedis.” *Clinical infectious diseases,* 14.Supplement 1 (1992): S77-S81.

[120] Djeridane, Assya, Yasmina Djeridane, and Aomar Ammar-Khodja. “Epidemiological and aetiological study on tinea pedis and onychomycosis in Algeria.” *Mycoses,* 49.3 (2006): 190-196.

[121] Ilkit, Macit, et al. “Epidemiology of tinea pedis and toenail tinea unguium in worshippers in the mosques in Adana, Turkey.” *The Journal of dermatology,* 32.9 (2005): 698-704.

[122] Aste, N., M. Pau, and P. Biggio. “Tinea pedis observed in Cagliari, Italy, between 1996 and 2000.” *Mycoses,* 46.1-2 (2003): 38-41.

[123] Cheng, Sauyi, and Laiyin Chong. “A prospective epidemiological study on tinea pedis and onychomycosis in Hong Kong.” *Chinese medical journal,* 115.6 (2002): 860-865.

[124] Kamihama, T., et al. “Tinea pedis outbreak in swimming pools in Japan.” *Public Health,* 111.4 (1997): 249-253.

[125] Al Hasan, Muhannad, et al. “Dermatology for the practicing allergist: Tinea pedis and its complications.” *Clinical and Molecular Allergy,* 2.1 (2004): 5.

[126] Ledezma, Eliades, et al. “Efficacy of ajoene in the treatment of tinea pedis: a double-blind and comparative study with terbinafine.” *Journal of the American Academy of Dermatology,* 43.5 (2000): 829-832.

[127] Weinstein, Andrew. And Brian Berman "Topical treatment of common superficial tinea infections." *American family physician,* 65.10 (2002): 2095-2102.

[128] Semel, Jeffery D., and Harry Goldin. "Association of athlete's foot with cellulitis of the lower extremities: diagnostic value of bacterial cultures of ipsilateral interdigital space samples." *Clinical infectious diseases,* 23.5 (1996): 1162-1164.

[129] Shemer, A., et al. "New criteria for the laboratory diagnosis of nondermatophyte moulds in onychomycosis." *British Journal of Dermatology,* 160.1 (2009): 37-39.

[130] Haneke, Eckart, and Diane Roseeuw. "The scope of onychomycosis: epidemiology and clinical features." *International journal of dermatology,* 38.S2 (1999): 7-12.

[131] Kilkenny, M., et al. "The prevalence of common skin conditions in Australian school students: 1. Common, plane and plantar viral warts." *British Journal of Dermatology,* 138.5 (1998): 840-845.

[132] Shemer, A., et al. "A novel two-step kit for topical treatment of tinea pedis–an open study." *Journal of the European Academy of Dermatology and Venereology,* 24.9 (2010): 1099-1101.

[133] Leibovici, Vera, et al. "Population-based epidemiologic study of tinea pedis in Israeli children." *The Pediatric infectious disease journal,* 21.9 (2002): 851-853.

[134] Noguchi, H., et al. "Tinea pedis survey in members of the Japanese Self-Defense Forces undergoing ranger training." *Mycoses,* 37.11-12 (1994): 461-467.

[135] Leyden, James L. "Tinea pedis pathophysiology and treatment." *Journal of the American Academy of Dermatology,* 31.3 (1994): S31-S33.

[136] Clayton, Y. M. "Clinical and mycological diagnostic aspects of onychomycoses and dermatomycoses." *Clinical and experimental dermatology,* 17.s1 (1992): 37-40.

[137] Vella Zahra, Loranne, et al. "Characteristics of superficial mycoses in Malta." *International journal of dermatology,* 42.4 (2003): 265-271.

[138] Hay, R. J., et al. "A comparative study of dermatophytosis in coal miners and dermatological outpatients." *British journal of industrial medicine,* 40.3 (1983): 353-355.

[139] Shemer, A., et al. "A novel two-step kit for topical treatment of tinea pedis–an open study." *Journal of the European Academy of Dermatology and Venereology,* 24.9 (2010): 1099-1101.

[140] Bergstresser, Paul R., et al. "Topical terbinafine and clotrimazole in interdigital tinea pedis: a multicenter comparison of cure and relapse rates with 1-and 4-week treatment regimens." *Journal of the American Academy of Dermatology,* 28.4 (1993): 648-651.

[141] Gupta, Aditya K., et al. "Itraconazole for the treatment of tinea pedis: a dosage of 400 mg/day given for 1 week is similar in efficacy to 100 or 200 mg/day given for 2 to 4 weeks." *Journal of the American Academy of Dermatology,* 36.5 (1997): 789-792.

[142] Weinberg, Jeffrey M., and Evelyn K. Koestenblatt. "Efficacy of once-daily treatment of interdigital tinea pedis with sertaconazole 2% cream." *Journal of the American Academy Of Dermatology*. Vol. 62. No. 3. 360 Park Avenue South, New York, NY 10010-1710 USA: Mosby-Elsevier, 2010.

[143] Elewski, Boni E.*Cutaneous fungal infections*. No. Ed. 2. Blackwell Science Inc., 1998.

[144] Macura, Anna B. "Dermatophyte infections." *International journal of dermatology,* 32.5 (1993): 313-323.

[145] Ilkit, Macit, Murat Durdu, and Mehmet Karakas. "Cutaneous id reactions: a comprehensive review of clinical manifestations, epidemiology, etiology, and management." *Critical reviews in microbiology,* 38.3 (2012): 191-202.

[146] Brenner, Sarah, Ronni Wolf, and Marina Landau. "Scabid: An Unusual Id Reaction To Scabies." *International Journal of Dermatology,* 32.2 (1993): 128-129.

[147] Kaaman, T., and J. Torssander. "Dermatophytid--a misdiagnosed entity?."*Acta dermato-venereologica*63.5 (1982): 404-408.

[148] Veien, N. K., T. Hattel, and G. Laurberg. "Plantar Trichophyton rubrum infections may cause dermatophytids on the hands." *Acta dermato-venereologica,* 74.5 (1994): 403-404.

[149] Iglesias, M. E., et al. "Generalized skin reaction following tinea pedis (dermatophytids)." *The Journal of dermatology,* 21.1 (1994): 31-34.

[150] Szepietowski, Jacek C., et al. "Factors influencing coexistence of toenail onychomycosis with tinea pedis and other dermatomycoses: a survey of 2761 patients." *Archives of dermatology,* 142.10 (2006): 1279-1284.

[151] Daniel, C. Ralph, et al. "Two feet–one hand syndrome: a retrospective multicenter survey." *International journal of dermatology,* 36.9 (1997): 658-660.

[152] Aste, N., and M. Pau. "Tinea manuum bullosa." *Mycoses,* 48.1 (2005): 80-81.

[153] Summerbell, R. C., J. Kane, and S. Krajden. "Onychomycosis, Tinea Pedis and Tinea Manuum Caused by Non-Dermatophytic Filamentous Fungi Nicht-Dermatophyten-Fadenpilze als Erreger von Onychomykosen, Tinea pedis und Tinea manuum." *Mycoses,* 32.12 (1989): 609-619.

[154] Mochizuki, Takashi, et al. "The first isolation in Japan of Trichophyton mentagrophytes var. erinacei causing tinea manuum." *International journal of dermatology,* 44.9 (2005): 765-768.

[155] Djeridane, Assya, Yasmina Djeridane, and Aomar Ammar-Khodja. "Epidemiological and aetiological study on tinea pedis and onychomycosis in Algeria." *Mycoses,* 49.3 (2006): 190-196.

[156] Welsh, Oliverio, Lucio Vera-Cabrera, and Esperanza Welsh. "Onychomycosis." *Clinics in dermatology,* 28.2 (2010): 151-159.

[157] Effendy, I., et al. "Epidemiology and clinical classification of onychomycosis." *Journal of the European Academy of Dermatology and Venereology,* 19.s1 (2005): 8-12.

[158] Young, Lindsay S., Harvey A. Arbuckle, and Joseph G. Morelli. "Onychomycosis in the denver pediatrics population, a retrospective study." *Pediatric dermatology,* 31.1 (2014): 106-108.

[159] Larsen, Gitte Kiellberg, Merete Haedersdal, and ELSE L. Svejgaard. "The prevalence of onychomycosis in patients with psoriasis and other skin diseases." *Acta dermato-venereologica,* 83.3 (2003): 206-209.

[160] Gupta, A. K., et al. "A higher prevalence of onychomycosis in psoriatics compared with non-psoriatics: a multicentre study." *British Journal of Dermatology,* 136.5 (1997): 786-789.

[161] Hamnerius, N., Johan Berglund, and J. Faergemann. "Pedal dermatophyte infection in psoriasis." *British Journal of Dermatology,* 150.6 (2004): 1125-1128.

[162] Leibovici, Vera, et al. "Increased prevalence of onychomycosis among psoriatic patients in Israel." *Acta dermato-venereologica,* 88.1 (2008): 31-33.

[163] Kaçar, N., et al. "The prevalence, aetiological agents and therapy of onychomycosis in patients with psoriasis: a prospective controlled trial." *Clinical and experimental dermatology,* 32.1 (2007): 1-5.

[164] Pawlaczyk, M., et al. "Does onychomycosis more frequently affect patients suffering from psoriasis?.",*Mikologia Lekarska,* 14.1 (2007): 52.

[165] Staberg, B., M. Gammeltoft, and P. Onsberg. "Onychomycosis in patients with psoriasis." *Acta dermato-venereologica,* 63.5 (1982): 436-438.

[166] Zawirska, A., Z. Adamski, and L. Kurek. "Dermatophyte infections in psoriatic patients." *Mikologia Lekarska,* 13.4 (2006): 287.

[167] Klaassen, K. M. G., et al. "The prevalence of onychomycosis in psoriatic patients: a systematic review." *Journal of the European Academy of Dermatology and Venereology,* 28.5 (2014): 533-541.

[168] Shemer, Avner, et al. "Onychomycosis in psoriatic patients–rationalization of systemic treatment." *Mycoses,* 53.4 (2010): 340-343.

[169] Hay, R. J., et al. "Candida onychomycosis—an evaluation of the role of Candida species in nail disease." *British Journal of Dermatology,* 118.1 (1988): 47-58.

[170] Tosti, A., R. Hay, and R. Arenas-Guzmán. "Patients at risk of onychomycosis–risk factor identification and active prevention." *Journal of the European Academy of Dermatology and Venereology,* 19.s1 (2005): 13-16.

[171] Elewski, Boni E. "Onychomycosis: pathogenesis, diagnosis, and management." *Clinical microbiology reviews,* 11.3 (1998): 415-429.

[172] Martínez, Erick, et al. "Microsporum spp. onychomycosis: disease presentation, risk factors and treatment responses in an urban population." *Brazilian Journal of Infectious Diseases,* 18.2 (2014): 181-186.

[173] Shemer, Avner. "Update: medical treatment of onychomycosis." *Dermatologic therapy,* 25.6 (2012): 582-593.

[174] Shemer, Avner, et al. "Onychomycosis: A simpler in-office technique for sampling specimens." *Journal of Family Practice,* 61.9 (2012): 552.

[175] Eenglish, Mary P. "Nails and fungi." *British Journal of Dermatology,* 94.6 (1976): 697-701.

[176] Summerbell, R. C., J. Kane, and S. Krajden. "Onychomycosis, Tinea Pedis and Tinea Manuum Caused by Non-Dermatophytic Filamentous Fungi Nicht-Dermatophyten-Fadenpilze als Erreger von Onychomykosen, Tinea pedis und Tinea manuum." *Mycoses,*32.12 (1989): 609-619.

[177] Campbell, C. K., and J. L. Mulder. "Skin and nail infection by Scytalidium hyalinum sp. nov." *Sabouraudia,* 15.2 (1977): 161-166.

[178] Crespo-Erchiga, Vicente, Silvestre Martínez-García, and Leandro Martínez-Pilar. "Dermatomicosis por Scytalidium." *Piel,* 20.10 (2005): 498-503.

[179] Kotrajaras, Renoo, et al. "Hendersonula toruloidea infection in Thailand." *International journal of dermatology,* 27.6 (1988): 391-395.

[180] Jones, S. K., et al. "Hendersonula toruloidea infection of the nails in Caucasians." *Clinical and experimental dermatology,* 10.5 (1985): 444-447.

[181] Hennequin, C., et al. "Invasive Fusarium infections: a retrospective survey of 31 cases." *Medical Mycology,* 35.2 (1997): 107-114.

[182] Elewski, Boni E., and Maria A. Charif. "Prevalence of onychomycosis in patients attending a dermatology clinic in northeastern Ohio for other conditions." *Archives of dermatology,* 133.9 (1997): 1172-1173.

[183] Faergemann, Jan, et al. "Genetic predisposition–understanding underlying mechanisms of onychomycosis." *Journal of the European Academy of Dermatology and Venereology,* 19.s1 (2005): 17-19.

[184] Haneke, E. "Fungal infections of the nail." *Seminars in dermatology*. Vol. 10. No. 1. 1991.

[185] Kemna, Maggi E., and Boni E. Elewski. "A US epidemiologic survey of superficial fungal diseases." *Journal of the American Academy of Dermatology,* 35.4 (1996): 539-542.

[186] Zaias, Nardo. "Onychomycosis." *Archives of dermatology,* 105.2 (1972): 263-274.

[187] Baran, R., et al. "A new classification of onychomycosis." *British Journal of dermatology,* 139 (1998): 567-571.

[188] Hay, Roderick J., and Robert Baran. "Onychomycosis: a proposed revision of the clinical classification." *Journal of the American Academy of Dermatology,* 65.6 (2011): 1219-1227.

[189] Hay, Roderick J., Robert Baran, and E. Haneke. "Fungal (onychomycosis) and other infections involving the nail apparatus." *Baran and Dawber's diseases of the nails and their management*. Blackwell Science Oxford, 2001. 129-171.

[190] Baran, R., R. Hay, and Ch Perrin. "Superficial white onychomycosis revisited." *Journal of the European Academy of Dermatology and Venereology,* 18.5 (2004): 569-571.

[191] Baran, Robert, Jan Faergemann, and Roderick J. Hay. "Superficial white onychomycosis—A syndrome with different fungal causes and paths of infection." *Journal of the American Academy of Dermatology,* 57.5 (2007): 879-882.

[192] Shemer, Avner, and C. Ralph Daniel. "Common nail disorders." *Clinics in dermatology,* 31.5 (2013): 578-586.

[193] Avner, S., N. Nir, and T. Henri. "Fifth toenail clinical response to systemic antifungal therapy is not a marker of successful therapy for other toenails with onychomycosis." *Journal of the European Academy of Dermatology and Venereology,* 20.10 (2006): 1194-1196.

[194] Arca E, Saracli MA, Akar A, et al. "Polymerase chain reaction in the diagnosis of onychomycosis." *European Journal of Dermatology,* 14.1 (2004): 52-55.

[195] Escobar, Martha Lucía, and Jaime Carmona-Fonseca. "Onicomicosis por hongos ambientales no dermatofíticos." *Rev Iberoam Micol,* 20 (2003): 6-10.

[196] Moreno, Gabriela, and Roberto Arenas. "Other fungi causing onychomycosis." *Clinics in dermatology,* 28.2 (2010): 160-163.

[197] Piraccini, Bianca Maria, Giulia Rech, and Antonella Tosti. "Photodynamic therapy of onychomycosis caused by Trichophyton rubrum." *Journal of the American Academy of Dermatology,* 59.5 (2008): S75-S76.

[198] Sotiriou, Eleni, et al. "Photodynamic therapy for distal and lateral subungual toenail onychomycosis caused by Trichophyton rubrum: Preliminary results of a single-centre open trial." *Acta dermato-venereologica,* 90.2 (2010): 216-217.

[199] Kalokasidis, Kostas, et al. "The effect of Q-switched Nd: YAG 1064 nm/532 nm laser in the treatment of onychomycosis in vivo." *Dermatology research and practice,* 2013 (2013).

[200] Hochman, Lisa G. "Laser treatment of onychomycosis using a novel 0.65-millisecond pulsed Nd: YAG 1064-nm laser." *Journal of Cosmetic and Laser Therapy,* 13.1 (2011): 2-5.

[201] Carney, Caitlin, et al. "Treatment of onychomycosis using a submillisecond 1064-nm neodymium: yttrium-aluminum-garnet laser." *Journal of the American Academy of Dermatology,* 69.4 (2013): 578-582.

[202] Utako Kimura, M. D., et al. "Treating onychomycoses of the toenail: clinical efficacy of the sub-millisecond 1,064 nm Nd: YAG laser using a 5 mm spot diameter." *Journal of Drugs in Dermatology,* 11.4 (2012): 496-504.

[203] Moon, Seong Hun, et al. "Treatment of onychomycosis with a 1,064-nm long-pulsed Nd: YAG laser." *Journal of Cosmetic and Laser Therapy,* 16.4 (2014): 165-170.

[204] Noguchi, Hiromitsu, et al. "Treatment of onychomycosis using a 1064nm Nd: YAG laser." *Medical mycology journal,* 54.4 (2013): 333-339.

[205] Landsman, Adam S., et al. "Treatment of mild, moderate, and severe onychomycosis using 870-and 930-nm light exposure." *Journal of the American Podiatric Medical Association,* 100.3 (2010): 166-177.

[206] Nenoff, Pietro, Sonja Grunewald, and Uwe Paasch. "Laser therapy of onychomycosis." *JDDG: Journal der Deutschen Dermatologischen Gesellschaft,* 12.1 (2014): 33-38.

[207] Anderson, R. Rox, and John A. Parrish. "Selective photothermolysis: precise microsurgery by selective absorption of pulsed radiation." *Science,* 220.4596 (1983): 524-527.

[208] Paasch, Uwe, et al. "Antifungal efficacy of lasers against dermatophytes and yeasts in vitro." *International Journal of Hyperthermia,* 29.6 (2013): 544-550.

[209] Dupuy, Alain, et al. "Risk factors for erysipelas of the leg (cellulitis): case-control study." *Bmj,* 318.7198 (1999): 1591-1594.

[210] Sunenshine, Peter J., Robert A. Schwartz, and Camila K. Janniger. "Tinea versicolor." *International journal of dermatology,* 37.9 (1998): 648-655.

[211] Terragni, L., et al. "Pityriasis versicolor in the pediatric age." *Pediatric dermatology,* 8.1 (1991): 9-12.

[212] Congly, H. "Pityriasis versicolor in a 3-month-old boy." *Canadian Medical Association Journal,* 130.7 (1984): 844.

[213] Wyre, H. W., and W. Taylor Johnson. "Neonatal pityriasis versicolor." *Archives of dermatology,* 117.11 (1981): 752-753.

[214] Vuran, Emre, et al. "Identification of malassezia species from pityriasis versicolor lesions with a new multiplex PCR method." *Mycopathologia,* 177.1-2 (2014): 41-49.

[215] Romano, C., et al. "Perineal and genital pityriasis versicolor due to Malassezia globosa." *Journal of the European Academy of Dermatology and Venereology,* (2014).

[216] Hellgren, L., and J. Vincent. "The incidence of tinea versicolor in central Sweden." *Journal of medical microbiology,* 16.4 (1983): 501-502.

[217] Hu, Stephanie W., and Michael Bigby. "Pityriasis versicolor: a systematic review of interventions." *Archives of dermatology,* 146.10 (2010): 1132-1140.

[218] Crespo-Erchiga V, G_omez-Moyano E, Crespo M. Pityriasis versicolor and the yeasts of genus Malassezia. Actas Dermosifiliogr 2008; 99:764–71.

[219] Gaitanis, Georgios, et al. "The Malassezia genus in skin and systemic diseases." *Clinical microbiology reviews,* 25.1 (2012): 106-141.

[220] Cafarchia, Claudia, et al. "Advances in the identification of Malassezia." *Molecular and cellular probes,* 25.1 (2011): 1-7.

[221] Crespo-Erchiga, Vicente, and Vicente Delgado Florencio. "Malassezia yeasts and pityriasis versicolor." *Current opinión in infectious diseases,* 19.2 (2006): 139-147.

[222] Gupta, Aditya K., et al. "Skin diseases associated with Malassezia species." *Journal of the American Academy of Dermatology,* 51.5 (2004): 785-798.

[223] maeda, manubu, and hideyo yamaguchi. "Pityriasis versicolor rubra."*European Journal of Dermatology*12.2 (2002): 160-4.

[224] Mendez-Tovar, Luis J. "Pathogenesis of dermatophytosis and tinea versicolor." *Clinics in dermatology,* 28.2 (2010): 185-189.

[225] Park, Hyun Jung, et al. "Skin characteristics in patients with pityriasis versicolor using non-invasive method, MPA5." *Annals of dermatology,* 24.4 (2012): 444-452.

[226] Chetty, G. N., A. Kamalam, and A. S. Thambiah. "Pityriasis versicolor-A Study of 200 Cases in a Tropical Skin Clinic: Pityriasis versicolor—Eine Untersuchung an 200 Fällen in einer tropischen Hautklinik." *Mycoses,* 22.7 (1979): 234-246.

[227] Sodre, Celso Tavares, T. L. Assis, and Rubem David Azulay. "Pitiriase vesicolor. Atualizacao." *An. bras. dermatol,* 59.6 (1984): 275-80.

[228] Saadatzadeh, M. R., et al. "Cell-mediated immunity to the mycelial phase of Malassezia spp. in patients with pityriasis versicolor and controls." *British Journal of Dermatology,* 144.1 (2001): 77-84.

[229] Hafez, M., and S. El-Shamy. "Genetic susceptibility in pityriasis versicolor." *Dermatology,* 171.2 (1985): 86-88.

[230] Olerud, J. E. "Ellenburg & Rifkin's Diabetes Mellitus." (2003): 895-908.

[231] Rivard, Shayna C. "Pityriasis Versicolor: Avoiding Pitfalls in Disease Diagnosis and Therapy." *Military medicine,* 178.8 (2013): 904-906.

[232] Faergemann J. The role of Malassezia yeasts in skin diseases. Mikol Lek 2004; 11: 129–133.

[233] Pedrosa, Ana Filipa, Carmen Lisboa, and Acácio Gonçalves Rodrigues. "Malassezia infections: A medical conundrum." *Journal of the American Academy of Dermatology,* 71.1 (2014): 170-176.

[234] Sampaio SAP, Rivitti EA. Micoses superficiais. In: Sampaio SAP, Rivitti EA (eds), Dermatologia, 3rd edn. S~ao Paulo: Artes M_edicas Ltda, 2007; 703–22.

[235] Gupta, A. K., et al. "In vitro susceptibility of the seven Malassezia species to ketoconazole, voriconazole, itraconazole and terbinafine." *British Journal of Dermatology,* 142.4 (2000): 758-765.

[236] Faergemann, Jan, et al. "Efficacy of itraconazole in the prophylactic treatment of pityriasis (tinea) versicolor." *Archives of dermatology,* 138.1 (2002): 69-73.

[237] Horta, Paulo. "Sobre uma nova forma de piedra." *Memórias do Instituto Oswaldo Cruz,* 3.1 (1911): 86-107.

[238] Axéll, Tony, et al. "A proposal for reclassification of oral candidosis." *Oral Surgery, Oral Medicine, Oral Pathology, Oral Radiology, and Endodontology,* 84.2 (1997): 111-112.

Authors' Contact Information

Professor Avner Shemer, MD
Department of Dermatology,
Chaim Sheba Medical Center,
Affiliated to the Tel-Aviv University,
Sackler School of Medicine,
Tel Hashomer, Israel
Email: ashemer1@gmail.com

Dr. Nicole Sakka, MD
PgD, Department of Dermatology,
Chaim Sheba Medical Center,
Affiliated to the Tel-Aviv University,
Sackler School of Medicine,
Tel Hashomer, Israel

Dr. Sharon Baum, MD
Department of Dermatology,
Chaim Sheba Medical Center,
Affiliated to the Tel-Aviv University,
Sackler School of Medicine,
Tel Hashomer, Israel

Index

A

access, viii
accounting, 22
acid, 22, 106, 107, 176, 184, 190, 191, 199, 208, 213
acidity, 193
acne, 41, 68, 78, 80, 103, 183, 191, 205
acne vulgaris, 68, 78, 205
adaptation, 193
adaptive immune response, 11
adaptive immunity, 11, 12, 231
adhesion, 193
adolescents, 63, 99, 100, 113, 141, 179
adrenal gland, 194
adults, viii, 37, 38, 41, 42, 43, 44, 48, 49, 51, 52, 61, 63, 64, 80, 83, 88, 99, 107, 113, 120, 132, 136, 180, 186, 200
adverse effects, 23, 25, 58, 173, 175, 232
adverse event, 109
Africa, 5, 38, 40, 124, 193
agar, 16, 57, 114, 126, 171, 190, 193, 197, 203
age, 3, 15, 22, 48, 61, 83, 93, 113, 115, 127, 141, 142, 160, 177, 178, 180, 201, 211, 242
agranulocytosis, 200, 205
AIDS, 7, 103, 115, 195, 200, 237
alcoholism, 200
algae, 234
Algeria, 237, 239
algorithm, 173
allergens, 17, 136
allergic reaction, 11, 107
allergist, 237
allergy, 17
allylamine, 58
alopecia, 38, 39, 41, 44, 45, 51, 52, 54, 57, 59, 162
alopecia areata, 44, 45, 57, 162
amino, 22
amino acid, 22
anaerobic bacteria, 123
analgesic, 25
anatomy, 61, 234
anemia, 167
annealing, 18
annular rings, 2
anorexia, 58
antibiotic, 79, 81, 124, 132, 164, 201
antibody, 232
antidepressants, 21, 200
antiepileptic drugs, 21
antifungal drugs, viii, 7, 12, 27, 28, 31, 33, 34, 35, 66, 74, 174, 208
antigen, 16, 85, 131, 203, 207
antihistamines, 29
antimycotic treatment, viii, 43, 161
apex, 2, 180
aplastic anemia, 200
areolae, 183
arrest, 169
arthralgia, 105, 136
arthritis, 105, 123, 136
Asia, 5, 38, 40, 115, 193
aspergillosis, 3, 6, 7, 16, 29
assessment, 235
assimilation, 207
asthma, 136
asymptomatic, 7, 44, 63, 64, 89, 90, 110, 117, 125, 132, 137, 183, 186, 192, 193, 195, 196, 202, 203, 206, 212
athletes, 83, 84, 87, 115, 142
atmosphere, 101
atopic dermatitis, 40, 48, 49, 50, 70, 84, 87, 90, 93, 94, 107, 108, 136, 162, 180, 186
atopy, 136
at-risk populations, 6
atrophy, 127, 201

attachment, 67
Austria, 38
authorities, 27
autoantibodies, 67
autoimmune disease, 206
autosomal dominant, 95, 138, 152
autosomal recessive, 85, 138
awareness, 28
axilla, 105, 106, 138, 211

B

bacillus, 211
bacteremia, 211
bacteria, 18, 19, 27, 42, 52, 55, 57, 79, 116, 120, 123, 124, 128, 132, 171, 188, 196, 200
bacterial cells, 27
bacterial infection, 54, 59, 65, 74, 78, 81, 121, 122, 124, 128, 130, 132, 196, 212
bacterium, 52, 73, 78, 79
balanitis, 207
barriers, 9, 11, 199
base, 2, 44, 57, 107, 177, 204
beams, 176
benign, 68, 72, 163, 165, 168
benzoyl peroxide, 213
beta blocker, 21
bilateral, 90, 137
bioavailability, 29
biochemistry, 232
biomarkers, 18, 232
biopsy, 16, 66, 69, 73, 81, 91, 93, 94, 96, 104, 105, 118, 136, 138, 164, 165, 166, 169, 171, 172, 183, 189, 195, 205, 207, 208, 213
biosynthesis, 27, 29
biotechnology, 12
black and white piedra, vii, 195, 196
blastomycosis, 7, 16, 29
bleeding, vii, 25, 46, 158, 165
blepharitis, 74
blood, viii, 13, 19, 22, 23, 51, 52, 80, 139, 158, 168, 169, 188, 194, 208
blood cultures, 208
blood flow, 22
blood pressure, 194
blood stream, 13
blood supply, 169
blood vessels, 80, 158
bloodstream, 208
blue-collar workers, 115
bone(s), 7, 89, 97, 159, 194
bone growth, 159
bowel, 206
Brazil, 101, 195, 235, 236
brevis, 74
brittleness, 167
bronchiectasis, 163, 168
bronchoscopy, 208
buccal mucosa, 201
budding, 1, 2

C

cancer, 31
candida, 106, 202
candidiases, vii
candidiasis, 6, 29, 32, 35, 99, 102, 150, 172, 200, 201, 202, 203, 204, 205, 206, 207, 208
capsule, 11
carbon, 1, 21, 22, 207
carbon monoxide, 21, 22
carbuncle, 41
cardiovascular disease(s), 160, 168
caregivers, 168
Caribbean, 38, 124, 125
cascades, 12
catheter, 211
cattle, 63, 78, 88
caucasians, 22, 240
CBC, 139
cell death, 176
cell division, 27, 28
cell membranes, 1, 12, 29
cell surface, 12
cellulitis, 41, 122, 128, 173, 178, 211, 238, 242
central nervous system, 89, 97
cervix, 207
challenges, 16
changing environment, 1
cheilitis, 203, 206
chemical(s), 19, 21, 27, 79, 106, 162, 175, 197, 208
chemokines, 11
chemotherapy, 115, 199, 206
childhood, 48, 61, 80, 92, 150
children, 37, 38, 41, 42, 43, 44, 49, 51, 52, 54, 56, 58, 59, 61, 63, 64, 67, 70, 83, 84, 93, 100, 101, 113, 115, 120, 127, 138, 141, 142, 143, 169, 175, 179, 186, 200, 233, 234, 238
chitin, 1, 12, 28
chlamydia, 189
chloasma, 186
cholesterol, 12, 21, 28
cilia, 10
cimetidine, 24
circulation, 113, 143, 199
cirrhosis, 168

classes, 28, 29, 74, 99, 108
classification, 1, 2, 18, 33, 96, 144, 201, 239, 241
climate(s), 7, 48, 61, 63, 84, 101, 103, 115, 143, 179, 180, 184, 195, 212
clinical diagnosis, 49, 50, 105, 106, 118
clinical presentation, vii, viii, 6, 17, 39, 49, 51, 53, 65, 67, 69, 73, 74, 81, 87, 90, 92, 96, 102, 106, 114, 117, 118, 125, 130, 131, 138, 144, 146, 154, 157, 158, 159, 162, 163, 166, 169, 188, 189, 195, 206, 215
clinical problems, 235
clinical symptoms, 43, 127, 194
clinical trials, 12, 23, 34, 178, 237
closure, 207
clothing, 7, 84, 101
clozapine, 24
clubbing, 168
clustering, 1
CMC, 150
CO2, 115
coal, 238
cobalt, 136
coccidioidomycosis, 5, 7, 16, 29
coding, 23
cold compress, 136
collaboration, 59, 75
collateral, 177
collateral damage, 177
colonization, 9, 56, 84, 199, 205
color, vii, 3, 17, 48, 56, 73, 88, 95, 105, 117, 120, 123, 136, 144, 148, 149, 150, 152, 160, 163, 165, 167, 168, 179, 182, 183, 185, 187, 188, 189, 207, 212
coma, 194
commercial, 16
community, 113, 115, 179
competition, 6, 10, 48
complement, 11, 12, 16, 199
complementary DNA, 208
compliance, 57, 108, 127
complications, 85, 111, 237
composition, 184
compost, 193
compounds, 1, 12, 21, 22, 175, 189, 190, 191
conditioning, 199
configuration, 70, 188
conidiophore, 2
consolidation, 29
consumption, 101
contact dermatitis, 65, 69, 106, 107, 108, 135
contaminant, 10, 16, 57, 171
contamination, 57, 73, 78, 84, 87, 114, 142, 194, 199, 200, 232
contraceptives, 25, 180, 184
control group, 141, 176
controlled studies, 33, 177
controlled trials, 174, 233
cooling, 18
cornea, 207
correlation, 21, 177, 187, 202
corticosteroid cream, 127
corticosteroids, 65, 85, 87, 101, 184, 200
cosmetic(s), 63, 65, 97, 127, 183, 192
cost, 18, 19, 23, 57, 59, 74, 108, 177, 190, 213
cotton, 56
covering, 194
cracks, 206
Croatia, 63
crops, 195
crust, 95
cryptococcosis, 3, 6, 7, 16, 29
CT scan, 208
culture, 1, 3, 15, 16, 17, 19, 43, 44, 56, 57, 60, 66, 73, 79, 81, 90, 100, 104, 114, 120, 125, 128, 130, 131, 132, 136, 138, 145, 164, 170, 171, 172, 176, 177, 189, 190, 193, 197, 203, 206, 213
culture media, 114, 190, 213
culture medium, 1, 3, 17
cure(s), viii, 15, 30, 58, 79, 81, 97, 109, 110, 124, 127, 128, 152, 154, 155, 156, 157, 161, 173, 174, 175, 176, 177, 178, 191, 238
cuticle, 13, 157, 172
cyanotic, 168
cycles, 18
cyclosporine, 24, 103
cytochrome, viii, 22, 23, 24, 25, 29, 58, 232
cytokines, 11, 12
cytosine, 30

D

damages, 197
dandruff, 107
danger, 22
DASP, 95
database, 19, 20
deaths, 5
deep systemic mycoses, vii
defects, 200
defence, 11
defense mechanisms, 10, 11, 199
deficiencies, 162
deficiency, 22, 109, 115, 167, 183, 202, 231
deformation, 152, 153, 154, 157, 159, 160, 161, 168, 169, 178, 197
degradation, 22

dehiscence, 2
dendritic cell, 10, 11, 12
dentures, 200, 203, 206
deposition, 84
depression, 87, 200
depth, 64, 172, 187
derivatives, 174
dermatitis, 39, 40, 47, 48, 49, 50, 66, 69, 70, 73, 74, 90, 93, 94, 106, 107, 108, 117, 130, 135, 136, 159, 164, 213
dermatology, 13, 232, 233, 234, 235, 236, 237, 238, 239, 240, 241, 242, 243
dermatophytid, 59, 121, 122, 132
dermatoses, 61, 64
dermatosis, 72
dermis, 7, 55, 67, 191
desorption, 18
destruction, 142, 147
detachment, 2
detection, 16, 18, 23, 66, 104, 203, 207
detergents, 162
deviation, 10
diabetes, 9, 84, 102, 106, 115, 141, 143, 173, 180, 183, 184, 200, 204, 205, 206, 207, 211, 212, 243
diabetic patients, 143
dialysis, 143
diarrhea, 57, 175
differential diagnosis, vii, 44, 52, 54, 66, 71, 80, 104, 105, 138, 159, 162, 167, 168, 184, 189, 205, 215
diffusion, 110
dimethylsulfoxide, 170
diphenhydramine, 24
discomfort, 97, 127, 174, 178, 200
diseases, vii, 3, 5, 6, 7, 9, 10, 12, 15, 31, 34, 65, 87, 94, 95, 96, 97, 115, 118, 125, 130, 141, 143, 162, 180, 183, 188, 199, 200, 201, 215, 232, 234, 236, 237, 238, 241, 243
disorder, 6, 9, 27, 41, 46, 47, 48, 50, 52, 66, 67, 80, 97, 102, 137, 138, 143, 152, 161, 163, 169, 183, 192, 194
distress, 57
distribution, 5, 7, 27, 69, 83, 99, 100, 116, 142, 183, 191
dizziness, 25
DNA, 2, 16, 18, 23, 30, 173, 180, 190, 208
DNA polymerase, 18
DNA sequencing, 2
dogs, 38, 84, 142, 195
domestication, 142
dosage, 238
dosing, 58, 175, 191
double bonds, 28
double-blind trial, 237
drainage, 208
drug abuse, 205
drug interaction, viii, 21, 29, 109, 127, 173, 175, 177, 178
drug metabolism, 24
drug reactions, 21
drug resistance, 30, 31, 127, 232
drug safety, 232
drug therapy, 12, 84, 142
drug treatment, 200
drugs, viii, 7, 12, 21, 22, 23, 27, 28, 29, 30, 31, 33, 34, 35, 66, 74, 91, 102, 173, 174, 177, 178, 200, 208, 213, 215, 232, 235
drying, 197
dyes, 107
dyspareunia, 207
dysphagia, 206
dysplasia, 206
dysuria, 207

E

eczema, 93, 94, 99, 102, 119, 121, 124, 130, 131, 135, 159, 160, 164
edema, 46, 48, 80, 90, 200, 203, 206
education, 101, 111
educational programs, 75
elbows, 46, 105, 136
electron, 122
electron microscopy, 122
electrophoresis, 190
ELISA, 203
emotional distress, 190
endocrine, 9, 168, 194, 200
endocrine disorders, 168
endocrine system, 194
endocrinology, 233
endoscopy, 208
energy, 176
environment(s), 5, 6, 9, 43, 63, 80, 84, 101, 182, 184, 193, 195, 199, 204, 211
environmental conditions, 5
environmental factors, 7, 100, 180, 197
environmental influences, 100
enzyme(s), viii, 1, 21, 22, 23, 25, 29, 30, 58, 192
epidemic, 87
epidemiologic, 143, 236, 238, 241
epidemiology, 37, 61, 232, 233, 236, 238, 239
epidermis, 10, 54, 67, 87, 100, 138, 158, 164, 172, 191, 204
epidermolysis bullosa, 122
epithelial cells, 10
epithelium, 149, 172

Epstein-Barr virus, 91
erosion, 125, 200
erysipelas, 122, 128, 131, 173, 242
erythema multiforme, 91
erythema nodosum, 131
erythrasma, 125, 183, 188, 206, 211, 212, 213, 214
esophagus, 200, 206, 208
ethanol, 175
ethnicity, 189
etiology, 239
eukaryotic, 1, 12, 22, 27
eukaryotic cell, 27
Europe, 5, 38, 115, 125, 232
evidence, 23, 33, 58, 141, 172, 177, 180, 184, 189, 192, 195, 213
evolution, 38
examinations, 15, 60
exclusion, 178
exercise, 106
expertise, 15
exposure, 9, 11, 22, 31, 62, 63, 65, 80, 88, 92, 106, 136, 143, 180, 183, 192, 206, 242
extensor, 56, 105, 136
extraction, 190, 204
exudate, 207

F

factories, 125
FAD, 22
false negative, 17, 45, 172
false positive, 17, 18
families, 22
family history, 143
family members, 12, 57, 62, 184
family physician, 232, 236, 238
farmers, 63
farms, 125
fatty acids, 10
fauna, 9
FDA, 23, 27, 29, 33
fetus, 33, 35, 188
fever, 39, 206
fibers, 107
Fiji, 124
filament, 1
filiform, 202
filtration, 28
first-generation cephalosporin, 213
fishing, 179
fixation, 16, 171
flame, 170
flight, 18
flora, 9, 10, 11, 84, 180, 183, 190, 195, 199, 211
fluid, 10, 78, 79, 121, 124, 126, 164
fluorescence, 39, 40, 42, 56, 176, 189, 211, 213
fluoxetine, 24
fluvoxamine, 24
folate, 202
follicle(s), 74, 79, 80, 111, 191, 205
folliculitis, 39, 41, 52, 65, 74, 79, 85, 103, 180, 183, 204, 205, 208
food, 18, 58, 80
food intake, 58
footwear, 113, 114, 115, 141, 143, 236
formaldehyde, 107
formation, 30, 39, 59, 75, 79, 169, 180, 207, 234
fragility, 161
fragments, 150, 173
France, 143
friction, 105, 106, 122, 194, 204
functional changes, 100
fungal disease, vii, 3, 5, 6, 9, 34, 96, 181, 236, 237, 241
fungal infection, 3, 5, 6, 7, 9, 10, 11, 15, 16, 18, 19, 30, 31, 33, 35, 37, 42, 49, 60, 63, 65, 67, 72, 73, 77, 84, 85, 93, 96, 97, 99, 100, 102, 109, 110, 111, 114, 123, 124, 126, 127, 130, 131, 132, 133, 136, 141, 142, 152, 158, 160, 161, 162, 195, 199, 206, 208, 231, 234, 235, 236, 237, 238
fungi, vii, viii, 1, 2, 3, 5, 6, 7, 9, 10, 11, 12, 13, 15, 16, 17, 18, 19, 27, 28, 30, 38, 39, 40, 42, 48, 57, 63, 65, 74, 79, 83, 84, 87, 114, 115, 123, 124, 134, 142, 143, 145, 147, 149, 151, 152, 153, 155, 170, 171, 172, 176, 178, 190, 193, 195, 199, 207, 208, 231, 232, 234, 240, 241
fungus, vii, 1, 3, 5, 6, 9, 10, 11, 12, 13, 15, 16, 17, 18, 37, 42, 66, 79, 85, 86, 87, 102, 110, 115, 117, 120, 124, 125, 126, 127, 130, 132, 142, 146, 152, 153, 157, 161, 165, 166, 168, 170, 171, 172, 173, 176, 179, 190, 193, 196, 197, 200, 234
furuncle, 41

G

gastric ulcer, 206
gastrointestinal tract, 9
gel, 109, 110, 126, 190, 191
genetic disorders, 152
genetic factors, 142, 180, 184
genetic mutations, 9
genetic predisposition, 92, 143, 184
genotype, 21, 23
genotyping, 23
genus, 3, 7, 19, 78, 142, 179, 180, 199, 200, 242, 243
genus Candida, 199

geographical mobility, 5
geography, 15
Germany, 38
gingivitis, 102
gland, 179, 184, 191, 196
glucocorticoids, 58, 233
glucose, 126
glycol, 190
glycoproteins, 1
gonorrhea, 189
granules, 233
growth, 2, 3, 42, 43, 101, 163, 169, 171, 180, 184, 190, 193, 196, 205
growth rate, 3
gyms, 63

H

HAART, 201, 209
habitat(s), 2, 37, 180
hair, 6, 11, 13, 15, 37, 38, 39, 40, 42, 43, 44, 45, 46, 50, 52, 56, 57, 59, 60, 65, 74, 77, 78, 79, 80, 81, 82, 84, 85, 86, 97, 99, 103, 104, 183, 195, 196, 197, 198, 204, 206
hair follicle, 52, 57, 65, 74, 79, 80, 82, 84, 85, 99, 103, 104, 183, 204
hair loss, 39, 46, 197
half-life, 22, 23
handedness, 143
hay fever, 136
headache, 57, 58
healing, vii, 52, 70, 73, 74, 87, 88, 90, 92, 94, 96, 97, 105, 106, 108, 120, 130, 136, 194
health, 115, 231
heme, 21, 22, 23
hemodialysis, 143
hepatocytes, 21
herpes, 91, 103, 207
herpes simplex, 91
high fat, 7
hirsutism, 127
histological examination, 125
histology, 173
histoplasmosis, 5, 7, 16, 29
history, 9, 16, 54, 87, 98, 143, 159, 184, 205, 206, 207
HIV/AIDS, 147
Hong Kong, 124, 128, 237
hormones, 194
horses, 78, 88, 195
host, vii, 5, 6, 7, 9, 10, 11, 12, 13, 27, 28, 30, 31, 37, 38, 39, 43, 79, 84, 86, 101, 117, 180, 184, 199, 200
HPV, 163
human, 6, 9, 11, 12, 18, 19, 27, 38, 62, 74, 81, 84, 97, 109, 114, 142, 158, 163, 180, 193, 199, 205, 211, 232, 235, 236
human body, 9, 205
human immunodeficiency virus (HIV), 5, 7, 9, 12, 23, 31, 87, 101, 102, 103, 109, 136, 142, 143, 147, 149, 189, 193, 200, 201, 206, 208, 235, 236, 237
human skin, 81, 193, 211
humidity, 84, 101, 143, 174, 180, 183, 184, 211
Hungary, 38
hybridization, 16
hydrogen, 18
hydrogen bonds, 18
hydroxide, 15, 56, 65, 66, 104, 170, 171, 189, 197
hydroxyl, 190
hygiene, 70, 84, 101, 111, 200, 211
hyperhidrosis, 114, 115, 133, 143, 180, 184, 211
hypersensitivity, 91, 203
hyperthyroidism, 200
hypoparathyroidism, 206
hypothesis, 180
hypothyroidism, 160, 205, 206
hypotrichosis, 196

I

ibuprofen, 24
ideal, 106
identification, 2, 3, 6, 15, 18, 19, 53, 172, 190, 192, 197, 203, 207, 240, 243
identity, 143
idiopathic, 161
images, viii
immersion, 120, 205
immigrants, 125
immigration, 5, 86, 102
immune defense, 12
immune disorders, 200
immune function, 31, 141
immune response, 10, 11, 12, 39, 73, 87, 127
immune system, 9, 10, 11, 42, 48, 52, 81, 87, 109, 117, 180, 192, 203
immunity, 10, 12, 13, 31, 85, 100, 102, 199, 201, 202, 231, 243
immunocompromised, 5, 6, 7, 29, 31, 84, 149, 195, 199, 208, 211, 214
immunodeficiency, 50, 102, 142, 150, 201, 205
immunoglobulin(s), 136, 199
immunohistochemistry, 16
immunosuppression, 84, 85, 101, 103, 143, 147, 150, 184, 200, 207

immunosuppressive drugs, 103, 141
impetigo, 41, 54, 71
improvements, 48
in utero, 188
in vitro, 27, 30, 176, 177, 191, 242
in vivo, 27, 30, 171, 191, 231, 242
incidence, 5, 6, 7, 37, 38, 61, 83, 113, 115, 125, 141, 142, 211, 242
incubation period, 86
India, 100, 236
individuals, 5, 6, 7, 16, 43, 44, 63, 100, 114, 141, 183, 199, 205, 211
inducer, 22, 25
induction, 22, 23
ineffectiveness, 29
inefficiency, 190
infancy, 48, 138, 150, 201, 206
infants, 22, 49, 52, 54, 63, 65, 75, 106, 107, 179, 200, 201
infection, 5, 6, 7, 9, 10, 11, 12, 13, 15, 16, 35, 37, 38, 39, 43, 44, 45, 48, 54, 57, 59, 61, 62, 63, 64, 65, 66, 73, 75, 77, 81, 83, 84, 86, 87, 89, 97, 98, 99, 100, 101, 102, 103, 104, 106, 110, 111, 114, 115, 118, 120, 122, 123, 124, 125, 126, 127, 128, 130, 132, 134, 136, 141, 142, 143, 144, 145, 146, 147, 149, 150, 151, 152, 153, 158, 169, 170, 171, 172, 173, 178, 179, 180, 183, 189, 190, 192, 193, 195, 196, 200, 201, 203, 204, 205, 206, 207, 208, 211, 212, 232, 234, 235, 236, 239, 240, 241
infectious agents, 195
inflammation, 39, 40, 42, 45, 46, 50, 56, 58, 64, 86, 102, 103, 117, 121, 149, 159, 164, 172, 205, 235
inflammatory cells, 189
inflammatory disease, 46, 105, 136
ingestion, 5, 11
ingredients, 107
inguinal, 104
inheritance, 196
inhibition, 23, 27, 28, 197
inhibitor, 23, 25, 184, 192
initiation, 15, 132, 170
injure, 153
injury, 10, 12, 55, 153
inmates, 109
inoculation, 100, 193
inoculum, 3, 43
insertion, 7
integument, 10, 13
interdependence, 11
interference, 10
interferon, 11
interstitial lung disease, 168
intertrigo, 106
intervention, 12
intra-abdominal abscess, 208
intravenously, 28, 29
iodine, 59
ionization, 18
ipsilateral, 238
Iran, 237
iris, 91
iron, 22, 167, 202
isolation, 126, 171, 203, 239
isoniazid, 24
Israel, 38, 115, 239, 245
Italy, 63, 233, 237

J

Japan, 5, 128, 237, 239
jock itch, vii, 101
joints, 105, 136, 194

K

keratin, 11, 48, 126, 142, 172, 174, 189, 191, 196, 200, 211
keratinocytes, 66
keratosis, 137, 171
kidney(s), 21, 54
kill, 11, 154, 177, 191
knees, 46, 105, 136
KOH, 56, 65, 66, 104, 110, 126, 170, 171, 203, 205

L

labeling, 172
laboratory tests, 104
Langerhans cells, 85
lasers, 176, 177, 242
leakage, 28
legs, 54, 85, 88, 89, 93, 95
leishmaniasis, 80, 81
leisure, 62
lentigo, 165
leprosy, 73
lesions, 15, 39, 40, 45, 46, 47, 48, 49, 50, 54, 57, 60, 64, 65, 67, 69, 72, 73, 74, 78, 79, 80, 81, 84, 85, 86, 87, 88, 89, 90, 91, 92, 93, 95, 97, 99, 102, 103, 104, 106, 109, 111, 116, 117, 118, 120, 124, 127, 132, 134, 136, 137, 138, 143, 149, 154, 164, 180, 181, 182, 183, 186, 187, 188, 189, 190, 194, 195, 201, 202, 203, 204, 206, 207, 208, 211, 213, 214, 232, 242
leukemia, 102

leukocytes, 172
leukopenia, 57
leukoplakia, 202
lichen, 17, 46, 73, 156, 157, 162, 203
lichen planus, 17, 73, 156, 157, 162, 203
lifetime, 207
light, vii, 19, 22, 56, 61, 65, 66, 67, 176, 189, 213, 242
lipids, 161, 180, 190, 193
liver, 21, 22, 29, 58, 139, 175, 208
liver enzymes, 58, 175
liver function tests, 139
livestock, 62, 63
living environment, 115
loci, 2
lung cancer, 168
lupus, 56, 57, 61, 65, 67, 69, 94, 203, 234
lupus erythematosus, 56, 61, 67, 69, 234
Luvox, 24
lying, 172
lymph, 39, 89, 97
lymph node, 39, 89, 97
lymphadenopathy, 39
lymphangitis, 136
lymphedema, 163
lymphocytes, 131
lymphoid, 11
lymphoid organs, 11
lymphoma, 102
lysis, 2, 12

M

macrophages, 10, 11
magnetic resonance, 208
majority, 2, 6, 7, 12, 22, 44, 65, 92, 126, 170, 177, 181
MALDI, 18, 19, 231, 232
malignancy, 195, 206
malignant melanoma, 165
malignant tumors, 205
malnutrition, 180, 184
management, 6, 29, 173, 192, 239, 240, 241
manipulation, 12
manual workers, 115
masking, 79
mass, 1, 2, 18, 19, 22, 196, 197, 207, 231, 232
mass spectrometry, 18, 231, 232
matrix, 18, 119, 128, 153, 154, 157, 159, 160, 161, 163, 164, 166, 168, 169, 172, 175
matter, 58, 195
media, 114, 190, 207
median, 158
medical, viii, 9, 16, 18, 38, 100, 177, 199, 206, 215, 232, 233, 235, 237, 240, 242, 243
medical history, 9, 206
medication, 17, 33, 34, 35, 74, 101, 122, 152, 161, 176, 191
medicine, 3, 31, 238, 243
Mediterranean, 38
melanin, 3, 184, 193, 206
melanoma, 164, 165
mellitus, 9, 84, 115, 143, 173, 180, 183, 200, 205, 206, 207, 211
membranes, 22
meningitis, 5, 30, 211
metabolic disorder, 160
metabolism, 10, 21, 22, 23, 29, 232
metabolites, 10, 18, 21, 23
metabolized, 21, 22, 23
metabolizing, 21, 22
methylene blue, 208
microorganism(s), 10, 11, 18, 19
microscope, 66, 126, 189, 197
microscopy, 15, 56, 66, 81, 100, 104, 125, 126, 132, 138, 145, 170, 171, 173, 176, 177, 189, 203
microsomes, 21
Middle East, 38, 124
migration, 5
military, 191
mitosis, 30
modifications, 84
moisture, 105, 106
mold(s), viii, 6, 11, 15, 28, 57, 100, 114, 120, 124, 126, 141, 142, 143, 147, 148, 149, 152, 158, 162, 169, 171, 172, 173, 174, 175
molecular biology, 104
molecules, 11, 12, 21, 28, 29, 30, 199
Moon, 242
morbidity, 19, 111
morphology, 1, 2, 15, 48, 49, 90, 162, 171, 196
mortality, 5, 19, 111, 208
mother cell, 2
mucoid, 2, 193
mucormycosis, 7
mucosa, 78, 194, 200, 201, 203, 206
mucous membrane(s), 6, 9, 10, 203, 206
mucus, 73
mutation(s), 9, 122, 196, 231
mycelium, 1
mycology, viii, 128, 168, 175, 176, 232, 235, 242
mycosis fungoides, 96
mycotic disease, vii, 215

N

NADH, 22
nail biting, 46
nanoparticles, 208
nausea, 29, 57, 175, 206
necrosis, 200
neodymium, 242
neonates, 62, 63, 65, 200
nephrotic syndrome, 167
nervous system, 73
nested PCR, 190
neutropenia, 57, 200
neutrophils, 66
nevus, 165
New England, 231, 232
New Zealand, 38
nickel, 136
nitrogen, 29
nodules, 52, 78, 97, 195, 196
non-dermatophyte molds, viii, 6, 15, 57, 114, 120
non-mycotic lesion, vii
North America, 124
nuclear membrane, 12
nucleic acid, 190, 204
nucleotides, 18
nucleus, 12
nummular eczema, 48, 88, 93, 94
nutrients, 1
nutrition, 1, 115
nutritional state, 84

O

obesity, 111, 115, 205, 211
occlusion, 111, 176, 204
odynophagia, 206
oil, 47, 154, 175, 191
olive oil, 110
omeprazole, 22
onycholysis, 143, 145, 146, 147, 152, 153, 154, 157, 172
onychomycosis, vii, 9, 13, 17, 19, 33, 64, 83, 85, 97, 103, 113, 114, 115, 118, 119, 128, 132, 139, 141, 142, 143, 144, 145, 146, 147, 148, 149, 150, 152, 153, 154, 155, 156, 157, 158, 159, 160, 161, 162, 163, 164, 165, 167, 168, 169, 170, 171, 172, 173, 174, 175, 176,177, 178, 195, 205, 208, 231, 232, 235, 237, 238, 239, 240, 241, 242
opacification, 144
opacity, 147
oral antibiotic, 213
oral cavity, 200, 203, 234
oral lesion, 201
organ(s), 1, 5, 7, 10, 13, 22, 102, 115, 172, 199, 206, 235
organic matter, 7
organism, 9, 10, 11, 38, 57, 58, 63, 81, 111, 124, 131, 143, 148, 171, 175, 195, 200, 203, 205
outpatients, 238
oxidative stress, 184

P

pain, 39, 45, 58, 116, 136, 174, 194, 206
PAL, 203
palate, 201, 206
palpation, 39
paracoccidioidomycosis, 7
parallel, 109, 127, 130, 157, 172
parasite(s), 9, 11, 66, 81, 142
parasitic infection, 10
parents, 65, 84
paronychia, 143, 144, 146, 147, 148, 158, 164, 178, 205, 208
paroxetine, 24, 25
pathogenesis, 10, 11, 63, 168, 180, 200, 205, 240
pathogens, 1, 5, 6, 7, 12, 27, 28, 30, 37, 38, 39, 57, 63, 84, 100, 104, 114, 126, 142, 149, 199, 231
pathology, 28, 151, 152, 153, 154, 234
pathophysiology, 238
pathway, 11, 22, 30, 114
pattern recognition, 10, 232
Paxil, 24, 25
PDT, 176, 213
penicillin, 57, 171
penis, 46, 103, 207
peptides, 11
perineum, 104, 183, 200
peripheral vascular disease, 128
peritonitis, 208
personal hygiene, 38, 125, 132
person-to-person contact, 63, 142
petroleum, 197
pH, 27, 115
phalanx, 150
pharmacotherapy, 233
phenotype, 211
phenytoin, 22, 24, 25
Philadelphia, 234, 236
phlebitis, 28
photosensitivity, 57, 66, 67
phylum, 193
physical activity, 61
physical exercise, 101

physicians, viii, 43, 132, 215
physiology, 61
pigmentation, 165, 182, 183, 192, 193, 194
pilot study, 110
pityriasis versicolor, vii, 7, 29, 125, 179, 180, 182, 183, 184, 185, 186, 187, 188, 189, 190, 191, 192, 242, 243
placebo, 109, 110, 177, 190, 191, 192
placental barrier, 35
plants, 1, 5, 7, 184
plaque, 39, 67, 78, 80, 87, 88, 96, 102, 103, 105, 106, 123, 136, 201
plasma membrane, 12, 28
pleural effusion, 163
Poland, 38
polar, 21
pollution, 63
polymerase, 16, 18, 104, 173
polymerase chain reaction (PCR), 16, 18, 19, 66, 104, 126, 138, 173, 190, 203, 208, 242
polymorphism(s), 21, 23, 190
polysaccharides, 1
pools, 63, 83, 115, 125, 237
population, 5, 9, 12, 73, 83, 84, 92, 99, 102, 113, 115, 125, 141, 143, 179, 193, 200, 206, 239
porphyrins, 213
port of entry, 13, 128, 171
post-streptococcal glomerulonephritis, 54
potassium, 15, 35, 56, 65, 66, 104, 170, 171, 189, 197
potential benefits, 33
prednisone, 74, 103
pregnancy, 25, 33, 34, 35, 180, 183, 200, 232
preparation, 18, 19, 66, 125, 197, 205
preservation, 170
prevalence rate, 115
prevention, 75, 111, 240
prevention of infection, 75
probability, 17, 171
prognosis, 75, 214
proliferation, 86, 158
propagation, 13
prophylactic, 111, 189, 191, 192, 243
prophylaxis, 192, 235
propylene, 190
prostacyclins, 21
protection, 7, 11, 12
protein synthesis, 12, 28
proteins, 1, 12, 18, 21
Prozac, 24, 25
pruritus, 117, 136, 183, 207, 212
pruritus ani, 212
psoriasis, 17, 40, 41, 46, 47, 49, 50, 53, 54, 61, 74, 88, 91, 92, 96, 105, 106, 118, 123, 136, 137, 141, 143, 151, 152, 153, 154, 155, 156, 160, 162, 172, 180, 235, 239, 240
pterygium, 157
puberty, 37
public health, 111, 125, 132, 232
pus, 39, 42, 52, 55, 121, 123, 132
pyelonephritis, 208, 211
pyogenic, 164

Q

QT interval, 25
quality control, 18
quality of life, 97
quantification, 27

R

race, 179, 191
radiation, 242
radiotherapy, 200
rash, 46, 67, 68, 70, 74, 90, 91, 92, 94, 121, 130, 131, 186, 189, 203, 204, 207
reactions, 21, 57, 59, 65, 131, 207, 234, 239
reactive oxygen, 11, 176
real time, 104
receptor(s), 10, 12, 231
recognition, 193, 203, 232
recreational, 136
recurrence, 104, 109, 111, 141, 192, 194
red wine, 165
regrowth, 60
regulations, 3
relapses, 64, 74, 111
relevance, 17
remission, 80, 87, 123, 197
renal failure, 200
replication, 10
reproduction, 1, 2, 6, 10, 19
requirements, 190
residuals, 186
resistance, 7, 11, 12, 31, 38, 111, 191, 192, 231
resolution, 13, 57, 74, 87, 88, 91
resorcinol, 127
response, vii, 11, 12, 13, 16, 31, 38, 57, 60, 66, 85, 86, 87, 100, 102, 109, 111, 126, 127, 145, 148, 164, 172, 231, 232, 241
restriction fragment length polymorphis, 104, 190
reticulum, 21
rhabdomyolysis, 25

ribosomes, 12
rings, 29, 87, 88, 189
ringworm, 37, 83
risk(s), 6, 9, 12, 25, 29, 31, 33, 34, 35, 43, 101, 102, 111, 113, 115, 125, 132, 143, 173, 175, 183, 193, 199, 200, 207, 208, 240
risk factors, 115, 143, 183, 207, 208, 240
risperidone, 24
RNA, 16, 30, 173
RNA processing, 30
rods, 213
roots, 97
rosacea, 68, 69, 74, 80, 94, 103
rules, 34
rural population, 7

S

safety, 12, 57, 176
salinity, 193
salmon, 154
sampling error, 66, 170
SAP, 243
saprophyte, vii, 16, 17, 18, 74, 114, 142, 157
saprophyte fungus, vii
sarcoidosis, 69, 94
Saudi Arabia, 236
scabies, 50, 138
scaling, 39, 40, 46, 47, 48, 50, 56, 64, 65, 72, 88, 93, 97, 103, 116, 118, 121, 124, 132, 135, 181, 182, 189, 212
scatter, 2
school, 43, 59, 61, 63, 100, 115, 238
science, 3
scrotum, 101, 103, 207
seborrheic dermatitis, 41, 47, 48, 50, 61, 65, 66, 107, 180, 234
sebum, 37, 110, 191
secrete, 1, 11
secretion, 207
seizure, 29
selenium, 162, 190, 197
self-image, 178
sensation, 64, 68, 73, 90, 94, 96, 101, 107, 127, 130, 137, 138, 186, 188, 194, 206
sensations, 117
sensitivity, vii, 136, 190, 203, 207
sensitization, 131
sepsis, 206
septum, 2
sequencing, 19
serotonin, 25
serotonin syndrome, 25
serum, 13, 16, 23, 25, 123
services, 59, 75
sex, 15, 113, 142, 179, 180
sex hormones, 180
sexual contact, 207
sexual reproduction, 1, 6
sexually transmitted diseases, 189
shade, vii, 160
shape, 2, 70, 73, 81, 88, 92, 95, 105, 136, 157, 165, 167, 186, 208
showing, viii, 31
side effects, 28, 29, 58, 74, 110, 127
signals, 11, 12
signs, 39, 46, 47, 68, 94, 165, 189, 206
silver, vii, 46, 190, 208
sinusitis, 136, 163
skeleton, 126
skin, vii, viii, 6, 7, 9, 10, 11, 13, 16, 17, 39, 42, 45, 47, 48, 49, 50, 51, 52, 53, 54, 55, 57, 58, 60, 61, 63, 64, 65, 66, 67, 68, 69, 72, 73, 74, 77, 78, 79, 80, 81, 83, 84, 86, 87, 88, 89, 90, 91, 93, 94, 95, 96, 97, 100, 101, 102, 103, 104, 105, 106, 107, 108, 110, 113, 114, 117, 118, 119, 120, 122, 123, 124, 125, 126, 127, 128, 131, 132, 136, 137, 138, 141, 143, 144, 152, 154, 156, 157, 160, 163, 179, 180, 182, 183, 184, 185, 186, 189, 190, 191, 193, 194, 195, 196, 203, 204, 205, 206, 211, 212, 213, 215, 234, 235, 236, 237, 238, 239, 243
skin diseases, vii, 65, 66, 100, 163, 191, 215, 239, 243
SLE, 56
small intestine, 21, 22
smoking, 200, 202
soccer, 115
social class, 115
socioeconomic status, 38
sodium, 28
software, 232
solution, 56, 66, 108, 110, 126, 127, 170, 174, 175, 189, 197, 213
South America, 7, 38, 193, 195
South Pacific, 83, 84
Southeast Asia, 6, 195
Spain, 63, 128, 233
specialization, viii
species, 1, 2, 3, 5, 6, 7, 10, 11, 15, 18, 19, 28, 31, 37, 38, 44, 57, 58, 63, 66, 78, 81, 114, 115, 128, 133, 134, 142, 143, 146, 176, 180, 189, 190, 191, 192, 193, 195, 199, 200, 203, 205, 207, 208, 232, 233, 240, 242, 243
spleen, 208
spore, 2, 19, 39, 211
sporotrichosis, 7, 29, 30, 32

sputum, 195
St. Petersburg, 234
stable complex, 23
stable complexes, 23
standardization, 16
staphylococci, 116
stasis, 130
state(s), 1, 23, 44, 150, 211, 232
sterile, 126, 131
steroid cream, 70
steroids, 15, 21, 65, 66, 75, 84, 87, 90, 93, 97, 102, 103, 115, 127, 136, 141, 201, 205, 206
sterols, 28, 29
stimulation, 130
stomach, 22, 206, 208
stomatitis, 203, 206
stress, 16, 57, 80, 136, 152, 161, 165, 169
stretching, 182
striae, 148
structural changes, 100
structure, 1, 10, 28, 29, 64, 161, 232
subacute, 53, 159, 164
subcutaneous mycoses, vii, 7
subcutaneous tissue, 7, 11, 78
substrate(s), 22, 24, 207
success rate, 175
succession, 100
sulfate, 35
sulfur, 22, 161, 190, 197
superficial mycoses, vii, 84, 99, 100, 238
superparamagnetic, 208
survival, 6, 43
survival rate, 6
susceptibility, 9, 12, 31, 180, 191, 208, 231, 243
sweat, 183, 191, 193, 196
Sweden, 179, 242
swelling, 158, 168, 194
symptoms, 64, 65, 127, 189, 194, 206
syndrome, 134, 146, 162, 163, 167, 168, 239, 241
synthesis, 11, 22, 23, 27, 28, 29, 30, 184, 213
syphilis, 51, 94, 118, 188, 189

T

T cell(s), 11, 12
tar, 190
target, 12, 18, 91, 178, 208
taxonomy, 231
technician, 17
techniques, 15, 17, 19, 104, 138, 190, 232
technological advances, 199
technologies, 104
technology, 18
teeth, 200
telangiectasia, 68, 80, 94, 127
temperature, 3, 18, 73, 101, 184
tension, 115, 182
tertiary syphilis, 189
testing, 21, 30, 31, 170, 173, 182, 208
texture, 3, 80, 88, 97
Thailand, 124, 236, 240
therapeutic effect, 21
therapy, 22, 33, 57, 58, 66, 74, 75, 87, 97, 109, 111, 127, 132, 136, 146, 148, 150, 173, 175, 176, 177, 180, 192, 193, 201, 208, 213, 232, 233, 235, 237, 240, 241, 242
thinning, 162
thorax, 204
thrush, 200, 206
thyroid, 206
tin, 64, 90, 186
tinea barbae, vii, 62, 67, 79, 80, 81, 82
tinea capitis, vii, 30, 37, 38, 39, 40, 41, 42, 43, 44, 45, 46, 47, 48, 50, 51, 52, 54, 56, 57, 58, 59, 63, 64, 65, 67, 69, 81, 88, 125, 131, 142, 175, 232, 233, 234
tinea corporis, vii, 9, 17, 51, 61, 63, 64, 69, 73, 83, 84, 85, 86, 87, 88, 89, 90, 91, 92, 93, 95, 96, 97, 98, 100, 103, 105, 109, 110, 120, 136, 142, 205, 235, 236, 237
tinea cruris, vii, 88, 89, 99, 100, 101, 102, 103, 104, 105, 108, 109, 110, 111, 236, 237
tinea faciale, vii, 51, 61, 62, 63, 64, 65, 66, 67, 68, 69, 70, 71, 73, 74, 75, 93, 94
tinea manuum, vii, 33, 100, 133, 134, 136, 137, 138, 139, 237, 239
tinea nigra palmaris, vii, 194
tinea pedis, vii, 9, 33, 83, 88, 100, 103, 113, 114, 115, 116, 117, 118, 120, 121, 122, 123, 124, 125, 127, 128, 130, 131, 132, 134, 136, 141, 143, 144, 173, 232, 237, 238, 239
tinea versicolor, 179, 183, 191, 242, 243
tissue, 11, 16, 30, 78, 168, 171, 172, 176, 178, 200, 203, 208, 213
TLR, 12
TLR2, 10, 12
TLR4, 12
TLR9, 12
tobacco, 24
topical antibiotics, 164
tourism, 5
toxic effect, 27
toxicity, 23, 25, 27, 28, 29, 109
training, 238
traits, 19
transcription, 12

transferrin, 13
transformation, 2, 180, 183, 184
transfusion, 12, 188
translation, 12
transmission, 37, 43, 59, 84, 114, 125, 200
transparency, 160
transplant, 102, 103, 200, 235, 237
transplant recipients, 235, 237
transplantation, 199
transport, 15, 104
trauma, 63, 84, 115, 128, 133, 142, 143, 153, 154, 160, 161, 167, 169, 193
treatment, vii, viii, 3, 6, 7, 12, 15, 17, 28, 29, 30, 33, 34, 35, 43, 54, 57, 58, 59, 60, 75, 81, 82, 90, 92, 97, 101, 108, 109, 110, 111, 117, 119, 124, 125, 126, 127, 128, 130, 131, 132, 136, 139, 148, 150, 152, 154, 155, 157, 158, 160, 161, 168, 170, 171, 173, 174, 175, 176, 177, 178, 183, 186, 187, 188, 189, 190, 191, 192, 197, 198, 200, 203, 208, 213, 214, 215, 232, 233, 236, 237, 238, 240, 242, 243
treatment methods, vii
trial, 109, 191, 240, 241
triglycerides, 37
tuberculosis, 6, 168
tumor, 11, 164, 168
tumor necrosis factor, 11
Turkey, 237
turnover, 10, 125

U

ulcer, 16, 194
ulcerative colitis, 168
underlying mechanisms, 241
United States (USA), 63, 179, 236, 238
upholstery, 100
urban, 38, 240
urban areas, 38
urban population, 240
urea, 175, 176
urticaria, 131
UV light, 189

V

vagina, 207
vaginitis, 207
valvular heart disease, 214
vancomycin, 213
variations, 178, 237
vasoconstriction, 187
VDRL, 51
vegetation, 7
venereal disease, 188
Venezuela, 179
ventilation, 106
vesicle, 65, 126
Viagra, 24
violence, 87, 117
viral infection, 92, 184
viruses, 18, 91
visualization, 66
vitiligo, 162, 184, 206
vomiting, 29, 57, 206
vulnerability, 11
vulva, 212

W

war, 43, 83
warts, 158, 238
water, 115, 161, 195, 205
wavelengths, 176
weakness, 161, 194
wear, 7, 106, 113, 123, 160, 206
web, 113, 114, 117, 121, 123, 124, 130, 204, 211, 212
weight reduction, 111
West Africa, 125
Western Europe, 37, 100
work environment, 113
workers, 77
worldwide, 1, 5, 6, 27, 38, 61, 83, 84, 99, 142, 148, 176, 179, 215
wound infection, 214
wrestling, 84
wrists, 85

Y

yeast(s), 1, 5, 9, 10, 11, 15, 41, 57, 106, 114, 120, 143, 170, 180, 183, 184, 189, 190, 192, 193, 199, 200, 207, 208
yield, 170, 209
young adults, 41, 44, 120, 179, 186, 199
yttrium, 242

Z

zinc, 59, 162, 190, 197